RHEUMATOID ARTHRITIS:

Natural Treatments for Pain-Free Living

Dr George J Georgiou, Ph.D.,N.D.,D.Sc (AM)

Dedication

First, I would like to deeply bow to the thousands of patients who have helped me understand the complexities of Candida and who need to take credit for the time spent with them in refining this protocol over many years.

All these patients over the years have been my "laboratory" for developing many treatment protocols through trial and error, backed by research.

I would also like to thank all the researcher scientists, lecturers and teachers who dedicate their life to helping others, and all the courageous health professionals who go against the grain of the establishment, while thinking outside the box.
A loving hug of gratitude to my wife and 4 children for their support and understanding during my professional endeavours throughout these years – they are all blessed.

Finally, I deeply embrace the Divine faith that I have been blessed with, that has helped me believe in the innate healing abilities of the body, through the power of Natural healing, without chemical intervention.

A profound blessing to you all and may your healing journey be fruitful and fulfilling!

Disclaimer

The information contained within this book is offered for you to make educated health decisions so that you can optimize your health. If there are serious health conditions, then you should always consult your primary care physician before beginning any other treatment regime.

The health information in this book is not advice and should not be treated as such – it is provided without any representations or warranties, express or implied. We do not warrant or represent that the medical information in this book is true, accurate, complete, current or non-misleading.

You must not rely on the information in this book as an alternative to medical advice from your doctor or other professional healthcare provider. If you have any specific questions about any medical matter, you should consult your doctor or other professional healthcare provider. If you think you may be suffering from any medical condition, you should seek immediate medical attention. You should never delay seeking medical advice, disregard medical advice or discontinue medical treatment because of information in this book.

While every attempt has been made to provide information that is both accurate and cutting-edge, the author cannot be held responsible for any decision that the reader may take while reading the guide, nor can a guarantee be provided that this guide and the remedies that it recommends will help everyone.

Published by:

Da Vinci Health Publishing
Panayia Aimatousa 300
Aradippou 7101
Larnaca
Cyprus
admin@davincipublishing.com

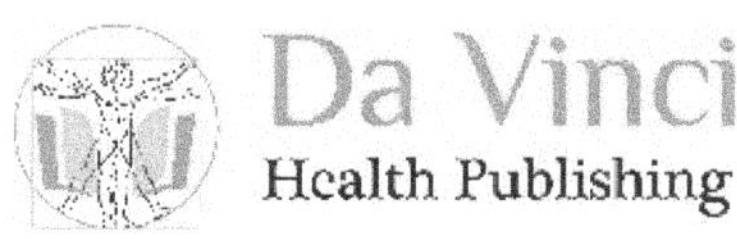

ISBN: 978-9925-569-36-6

Table of Contents

Chapter 1

The Da Vinci Natural Rheumatoid Arthritis Protocol

Natural Treatments without Drugs!

Rheumatoid arthritis (RA) is an autoimmune disease in which the body's immune system – which normally protects its health by attacking foreign substances like bacteria and viruses – mistakenly attacks the joints. This creates inflammation that causes the tissue that lines the inside of joints (the synovium) to thicken, resulting in swelling and pain in and around the joints. The synovium makes a fluid that lubricates joints and helps them move smoothly.

The result is very similar to inflammation that you may have seen if you've had an infected cut or wound – it goes red, swells, produces extra fluid and hurts. The redness is caused by the flow of blood increasing. As a result, the inflamed joint may feel warmer than usual. The inflammation is caused by a build-up of fluid and cells in the synovium. Your joint hurts for two reasons:

- Your nerve endings are irritated by the chemicals produced by the inflammation.
- The capsule is stretched by the swelling in your joint.

If inflammation goes unchecked, it can damage cartilage, the elastic tissue that covers the ends of bones in a joint, as well as the bones themselves. Over time, there is loss of cartilage, and the joint spacing between bones can become smaller. Joints can become loose, unstable, painful and lose their mobility. Joint deformity also can occur. Joint damage cannot be reversed, and because it can occur early, doctors recommend early diagnosis and aggressive treatment to control RA.

Rheumatoid arthritis most commonly affects the joints of the hands, feet, wrists, elbows, knees and ankles. The joint effect is usually symmetrical. That means if one knee or hand is affected, usually the other one is, too. Because RA also can affect body systems, such as the cardiovascular or respiratory systems, it is called a systemic disease. Systemic means "entire body."

Rheumatoid arthritis is a condition that affects the joints. However, it is a progressive condition, which means that a lot of people find that it starts to affect other parts of the body as well. The eyes are commonly affected.

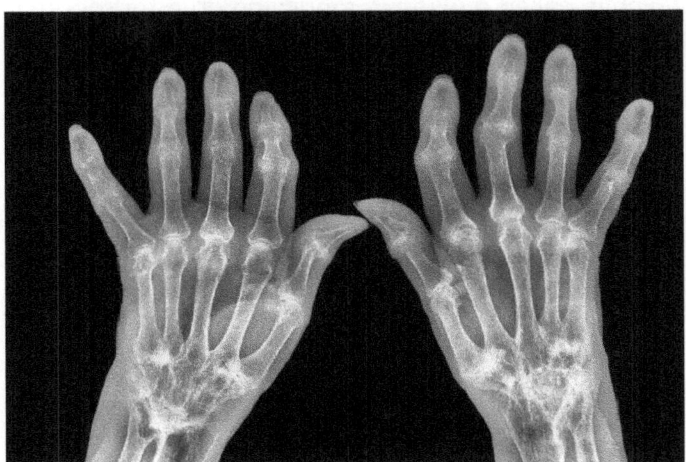

Usually, the symptoms of rheumatoid arthritis start to appear quite quickly, only taking a few weeks for them to fully appear. Some people experience the full range of symptoms within just a few days. It should be noted, however, that every person is unique, and this means that each one will experience the condition in different ways. Many people find that their symptoms change over time, and that they have periods without any symptoms at all.

However, as a progressive condition, most people ultimately find that the symptoms become more frequent and more severe over time.

Changes in joints in rheumatoid arthritis

Although the exact trigger of RA likely varies from patient to patient, the following events occur in rheumatoid arthritis joints. A stress causes an insult to your joints and your joints send a help signal to your immune cells.

When the first immune cells arrive, they request more immune cells and nutrients to help repair the damage by sending chemical messengers (cytokines such as TNF-alpha, VEGF, IL-1 or IL-6) into the bloodstream.

These cytokines spur the growth of more blood vessels (angiogenesis) usually in the synovium. They make the blood vessels more porous (leaky) to easily allow immune cells and fluid to reach the joint. Your synovial cells (synoviocytes) begin to proliferate, making the synovial membrane thicker. The synovial cells change in shape, becoming more fibroblast- like.

Some scientists directly describe synoviocytes' increased growth as cancer-like. Methotrexate, which is called a disease modifying drug for rheumatoid arthritis is often used for cancer therapy.

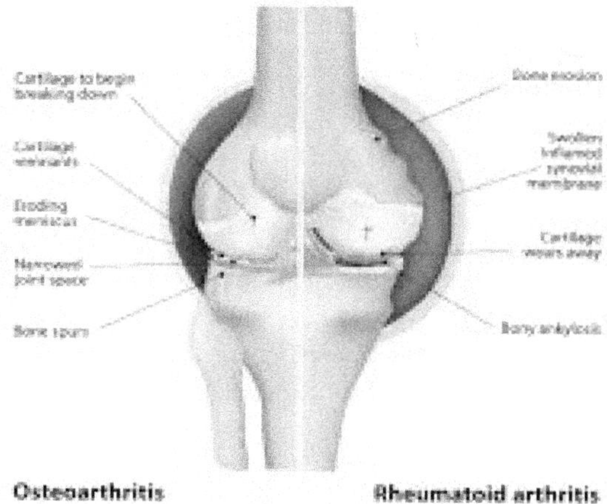

The synovium produces excess synovial fluid and enlarges the joint space. The cytokines also signal the immune cells to divide. The joint becomes swollen by fluid accumulation and warm. This response is called an inflammatory response and plays a major role in developing the degenerative disease of the joint.

Thus, the synovium in rheumatoid arthritis joints becomes very thick and contains blood vessels, immune cells, and many layers of synovial cells that act more like fibroblasts. This structure is called pannus. The pannus fills the joint space and grows so aggressively that it erodes the cartilage and underlying bone. The cartilaginous surface becomes rough and pitted. The large, warm mass in the joint is mainly the pannus and inflammation. The pannus causes much of the pain.

The immune cells begin reacting against these abnormal synovial cells as well as cartilage and bone cells. The cartilage and bone cells divide and grow, attempting to repair the damage.

In about one third of RA patients, their disease resolves within the first 2-3 years. In other RA patients, the new joint tissue may not form correctly. Degenerative disease of the joints often continues in these patients.

Some patients with rheumatoid arthritis in their hands develop deformities as part of the degenerative disease of the joint. Others with RA in their feet may develop a limp.

12 Early Signs and Symptoms of Rheumatoid Arthritis

Most people start to experience 12 specific symptoms when the condition is just starting.

These are:

1. Joint pain, which can be anything from a sharp, shooting pain, to a constant, nagging, dull ache.
2. Fatigue and feeling lethargic.
3. Joint swelling, which may or may not be visible to the naked eye.
4. Joint tenderness, with some people finding that the softest touch to the affected joint is agony.
5. Joint warmth, which can be noticed if people don't experience too much joint tenderness.
6. Joint redness, generally visible to the naked eye, making the joint look inflamed. This is in part due to the swelling, which causes stress on the skin.
7. Reduction in the range of movements of the joints.
8. Joint stiffness, which often cannot be relieved through simple stretching or movement.
9. Limping, particularly if the joints of the knees are affected.
10. Polyarthritis, meaning multiple joints are affected all over the body.
11. Symmetric arthritis, meaning the joints on both side of the body are affected.
12. Joint deformity.

These 12 signs and symptoms tend to continue to be present in the life of people with rheumatoid arthritis, and they get progressively worse. Overall, the symptoms of rheumatoid arthritis are characterized by pain, stiffness, redness, warmth, and swelling. However, some people also start to experience weight loss, poor appetite, sweating, fevers, and lack of energy. These symptoms are usually interrelated, which means that if you experience one, the others are likely to follow.

A Progressive Condition

Rheumatoid arthritis is progressive and there is no current medical cure for it. However, there are many things that can be done in order to significantly slow down its progression, thereby ensuring those who suffer from it can continue to enjoy a high quality of life.

We will discuss some of the causes of rheumatoid arthritis that are not often known to the medical profession, so it is unlikely that your medical doctor will look for these causes. If they are not dealt with, then it is likely that they will continue causing symptoms and aggravating the condition. We will also discuss specific natural treatment protocols that can be used to offload these.

The symptoms and effects of rheumatoid arthritis may come and go. A period of high disease activity (increases in inflammation and other symptoms) is called a flare. A flare can last for days or months.

Ongoing high levels of inflammation can cause problems throughout the body. Here of some ways rheumatoid arthritis can affect organs and body systems:

- Eyes. Dryness, pain, redness, sensitivity to light and impaired vision
- Mouth. Dryness and gum irritation or infection
- Skin. Rheumatoid nodules – small lumps under the skin over bony areas
- Lungs. Inflammation and scarring that can lead to shortness of breath
- Blood Vessels. Inflammation of blood vessels that can lead to damage in the nerves, skin and other organs
- Blood. Anaemia, a lower than normal number of red blood cells.

A primary care physician may suspect rheumatoid arthritis based in part on a person's signs and symptoms. If so, the patient will be referred to a rheumatologist – a specialist with specific training and skills to diagnose and treat rheumatoid arthritis. In its early stages, rheumatoid arthritis may resemble other forms of inflammatory arthritis. No single test can confirm rheumatoid arthritis. To make a proper diagnosis, the rheumatologist will ask questions about personal and family medical history, perform a physical exam and order diagnostic tests.

Rheumatoid arthritis can make simple tasks like getting out of bed and getting dressed in the morning challenging, let alone holding down a regular job. People with rheumatoid arthritis are more likely to:

- change occupations
- reduce their work hours
- lose their job
- retire early
- be unable to find a job (compared to people without RA).

Rheumatoid arthritis costs over $6,500 per year, for each person who has been diagnosed with the disease. Annual medication costs can reach $15,000 to $20,000 per patient treated with the more expensive biologic agents.

In addition to the financial costs of this disease, the cost of quality of life is high. Compared to those without arthritis, people with rheumatoid arthritis are:

- 40 percent more likely to report fair or poor general health
- 30 percent more likely to need help with personal care
- Twice as likely to have health-related activity limitation

Prevalence of Rheumatoid Arthritis

Rheumatoid arthritis is a common chronic disease that affects about 1% of the world population (Gibofsky, A., 2012). The prevalence of rheumatoid arthritis in the US is currently estimated at approximately 1.5 million people. This is down from an earlier estimate of 2.1 million people. The prevalence and incidence (new cases per year) of RA appears to have declined since the early 1960s (Helmick et al, 2008).

It affects women more than men - nearly three times as many women have the disease as opposed to men. In women, rheumatoid arthritis most commonly begins between ages 30 and 60. In men, it often occurs later in life. Having a family member with rheumatoid arthritis increases the odds of having rheumatoid arthritis; however, the majority of people with rheumatoid arthritis have no family history of the disease.

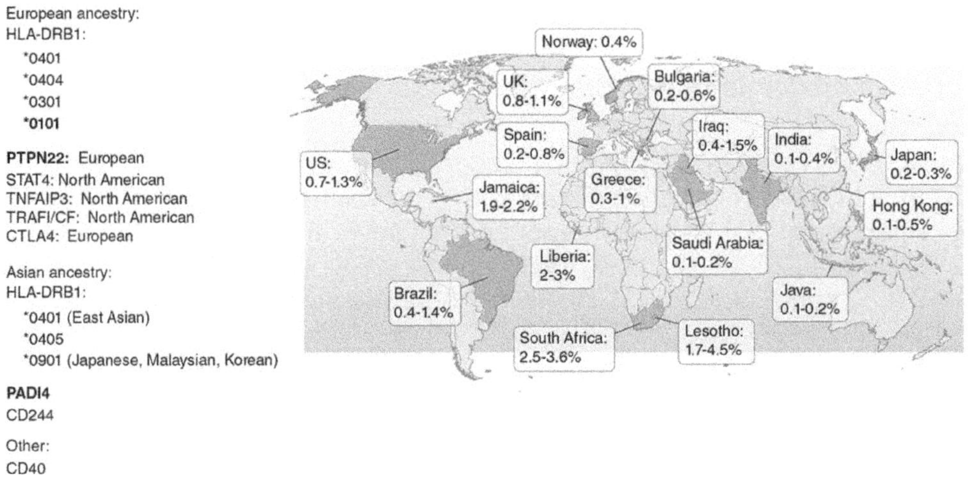

The prevalence of rheumatoid arthritis (RA) is relatively constant in many populations, at 0.5–1.0%. However, a high prevalence of rheumatoid arthritis has been reported in the Pima Indians (5.3%) and in the Chippewa Indians (6.8%). In contrast, low occurrences have been reported in populations from China and

Japan.

These data support a genetic role in disease risk. Studies have so far shown that the familial recurrence risk in rheumatoid arthritis is small compared with other autoimmune diseases. The main genetic risk factor of RA is the HLA DRB1 alleles, and this has consistently been shown in many populations throughout the world.

The strongest susceptibility factor so far has been the HLA DRB1*0404 allele. Tumour necrosis factor alleles have also been linked with RA. However, it is estimated that these genes can explain only 50% of the genetic effect.

Environmental factors have also been studied in relation to RA. Female sex hormones may play a protective role in RA; for example, the use of the oral contraceptive pill and pregnancy are both associated with a decreased risk. However, the postpartum period has been highlighted as a risk period for the development of RA.

Furthermore, breastfeeding after a first pregnancy poses the greatest risk. Exposure to infection may act as a trigger for RA, and a number of agents have been implicated (e.g. Epstein–Barr virus, parvovirus and some bacteria such as *Proteus* and *Mycoplasma*). However, the epidemiological data so far are inconclusive. There has recently been renewed interest in the link between cigarette smoking and RA, and the data presented so far are consistent with and suggestive of an increased risk.

Descriptive epidemiology of RA

The descriptive epidemiology of RA is suggestive of a genetic effect. The occurrence of RA is relatively constant with a prevalence of between 0.5 and 1.0%, a frequency that has been reported from several European (Carmona et al, 2002; Riise et al, 2000; Aho et al, 1998) and North-American populations (Gabriel et al, 1999; Gabriel, SE., 2001). However, there are some interesting exceptions (Fig. 1).

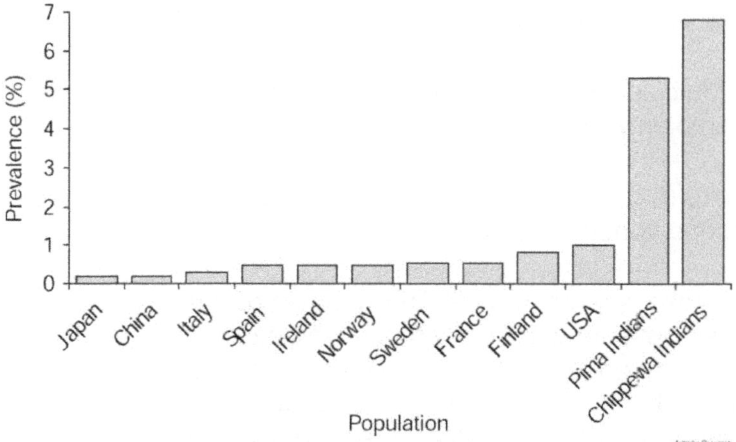

Figure 1 Prevalence of rheumatoid arthritis in various populations

Specifically, native American-Indian populations have the highest recorded occurrence of RA, with a prevalence of 5.3% noted for the Pima Indians (del Puente et al, 1989) and of 6.8% for the Chippewa Indians (Harvey et al, 1981). By contrast, there are several groups with a very low occurrence. Studies in rural African populations, both in South Africa (Brighton et al, 1988) and in Nigeria (Silman et al, 1993), failed to find any RA cases in studies of 500 and 2000 adults, respectively. Studies in populations from Southeast Asia (Dans et al, 1997), including China and Japan (Shichikawa et al, 1999; Zeng et al, 1997), have similarly shown very low occurrences (0.2–0.3%).

What are the risk factors for RA?

Researchers have studied several genetic and environmental factors to determine if they change person's risk of developing RA.

Characteristics that increase risk:

- Age. RA can begin at any age, but the likelihood increases with age. The onset of RA is highest among adults in their sixties.
- Sex. New cases of RA are typically two-to-three times higher in women than men.
- Genetics/inherited traits. People born with specific genes are more likely to develop RA. These genes, called HLA (human leukocyte antigen) class II genotypes, can also make your arthritis worse. The risk of RA may be highest when people with these genes are exposed to environmental factors like

smoking or when a person is obese.

- Smoking. Multiple studies show that cigarette smoking increases a person's risk of developing RA and can make the disease worse.

Cigarette smoke (CS) contains a mixture of approximately 4000 toxic substances including Nicotine concentration in plasma is

Exposure to smoke is a major factor in the onset of rheumatoid arthritis in about 20% of Swedish patients, especially those who carry the HLA-DR4 shared epitope. Smoking releases more than 4000 toxic compounds nicotine, polycyclic aromatic hydrocarbons (carcinogens), unsaturated aldehydes, solvents, free radicals, carbon monoxide, and other gases (Baka et al, 2009), some of which affect bone and joint health.

Smokers have a higher risk for bone fractures, development of osteoporosis, degeneration of intervertebral discs, and slow healing of bone fractures. Smoking lowers bone mineral density increases secretion of proinflammatory cytokines, and augments the risk of citrullination of proteins, which increases the risk for joint erosions. Response rates for smokers are similar between early RA patients and those with chronic RA history.

- History of live births. Women who have never given birth may be at greater risk of developing RA.

- Early Life Exposures. Some early life exposures may increase risk of developing RA in adulthood. For example, one study found that children whose mothers smoked had double the risk of developing RA as adults. Children of lower income parents are at increased risk of developing RA as adults.

- Obesity. Being obese can increase the risk of developing RA. Studies examining the role of obesity also found that the more overweight a person was, the higher his or her risk of developing RA became.

Characteristics that can decrease risk

Unlike the risk factors above which may increase risk of developing RA, at least one characteristic may decrease risk of developing RA.

- Breastfeeding. Women who have breastfed their infants have a *decreased* risk of developing RA.

What are the complications of RA?

For some people, RA causes long-term complications due to increased inflammation throughout the body. This is known as "systematic arthritis" or sometimes "inflammatory arthritis." Studies have found that complications of rheumatoid arthritis can include:

- Higher risk for heart disease and stroke
- Shortness of breath, chest pains, and trouble breathing normally due to lung scarring and damage
- Heart problems and nerve damage, caused by decreased circulation and inflammation of blood vessels (called vasculitis)
- Carpal tunnel syndrome
- Frequent headaches
- Kidney problems and fluid retention
- Bone pain and bone thinning
- Anaemia and fatigue
- Enlarged spleen and low blood cell count
- Small lumps of tissue that develop around swollen joints below the skin - these are called "rheumatoid nodules" and can add to redness or pain. About half of people with RA get rheumatoid nodules, which are most common in bony areas exposed to frequent movement/pressure (like the fingers or elbows)
- Skin rashes, redness, heat, bruising and ulcers near the nail beds
- Impaired vision and eye problems, such as photosensitivity, dryness, redness and pain known as Sjogren's syndrome
- Frequent infections in the mouth and gums
- Appetite changes, weight gain or weight loss
- Employment. RA can make work difficult. Adults with RA are less likely to be employed than those who do not have RA. As the disease gets worse, many people with RA find they cannot do as much as they used to. Work loss among people with RA is highest among people whose jobs are physically demanding. Work loss is lower among those in jobs with few physical demands, or in jobs where they have influence over the job pace and activities.

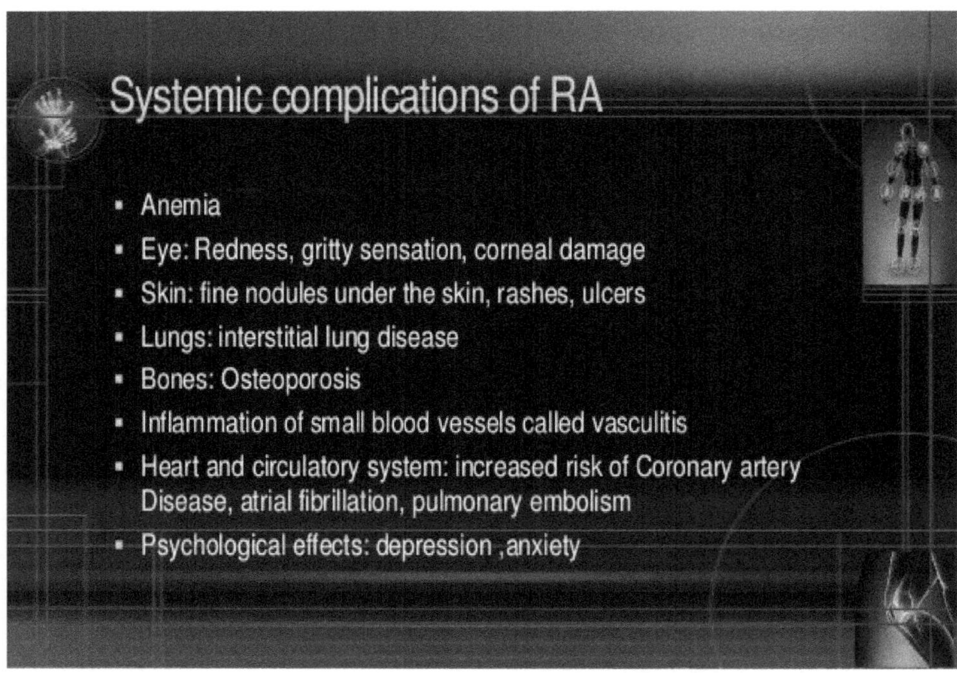

Diagnosis of RA

Blood tests:

There are several blood tests that help a doctor decide whether you're likely to have rheumatoid arthritis (RA). The first set checks to see if you make certain specific antibodies because they're often found in RA patients at high levels. The second set measures the amount of inflammation.

Rheumatoid Factor: Rheumatoid factor_measures how many of one type of your antibodies (IgM, sometimes IgA) binds to a second type of your antibodies (IgG). Initially, only one third of people with RA test positive for the set of antibodies called the rheumatoid factor (Rf).

Most people with rheumatoid arthritis will eventually develop this marker and a positive Rf is considered a sign and symptom of rheumatoid arthritis. However, some people test positive for rheumatoid factor, yet never develop the disease. The level of your Rheumatoid factor in the blood does not predict flares nor your outcome.

When your doctor says you're seronegative (or sero negative), he's indicating that you did not have more Rf than the normal population.

Anti-CCP: These anti-CCP antibodies bind to some self-proteins that are found predominately in the synovial tissue. The citrullinated proteins include filaggrin and its circular form (cyclic citrullinated peptide: CCP). The presence of these antibodies often correlates with some joint destruction. Although this test is relatively recent, a high level of anti-CCP is considered a sign and symptom of rheumatoid arthritis.

Inflammation: Inflammation is your body's response to damage. Your body sends in certain types of white blood cells to pick up debris, fight off infection, promote healing and, if needed, bring in more blood vessels. There is usually a higher state of inflammation in rheumatoid arthritis patients and it is a classic sign and symptom of rheumatoid arthritis. These 2 tests are used to measure it.

Erythrocyte sedimentation rate: This test, often called the ESR, or the sedimentation rate measures the quantity and how quickly the cells are pelleted by spinning in a centrifuge. Indirectly, it measures how many cells are bigger and thus activated.

C-reactive protein. A higher than normal level of C-reactive protein (CRP) in the blood also indicates that your body has chronic inflammation and is a common sign and symptom of rheumatoid arthritis. However, high CRP is also found in chronic heart disease patients.

Improving quality of life

RA affects many aspects of daily living including work, leisure and social activities. Fortunately, there are multiple low-cost strategies in the community that are proven to increase quality of life.

- Get physically active. Experts recommend that ideally adults be moderately physically active for 150 minutes per week, like walking, swimming, or biking 30 minutes a day for five days a week. You can break these 30 minutes into three separate ten-minute sessions during the day. Regular physical activity can also reduce the risk of developing other chronic diseases such as heart disease, diabetes, and depression. We will discuss this in more detail later under natural treatments.

- Go to effective physical activity programs. If you are worried about making the arthritis worse or unsure how to safely exercise, participation in physical activity programs can help reduce pain and disability related to RA and improve mood and the ability to move. Classes take place at local Ys, parks, and community centres. These classes can help people with RA feel better. Learn more about the proven physical activity programs that CDC recommends.

- Join a self-management education class. Participants with arthritis and (including RA) gain confidence in learning how to control their symptoms, how to live well with arthritis, and how arthritis affects their lives. Learn more about the proven self-management education programs that CDC recommends.

- Stop Smoking. Cigarette smoking makes the disease worse and can cause other medical problems. Smoking can also make it more difficult to stay physically active, which is an important part of managing RA.

- Maintain a Healthy Weight. Obesity can cause numerous problems for people with RA and so it's important to maintain a healthy weight.

Causes of Rheumatoid Arthritis

The cause of rheumatoid arthritis is not yet fully understood, although doctors do know that an abnormal response of the immune system plays a leading role in the inflammation and joint damage that occurs. No one knows for sure why the immune system goes awry, but there is scientific evidence that genes, hormones and environmental factors are involved.

Even with these declines, RA occurs at twice the rate in women compared with men, with a prevalence of 1.06% in women (as a percentage of the total population) compared with 0.61% in men (Gibofsky, A., 2012).

The incidence (new cases per year) of RA increases with increasing age in most populations until about the eighth decade of life, when it declines (Silman et al, 2009).

The prevalence of RA varies widely from population to population, with the lowest rates in Asian countries and higher rates among certain Native American populations. This suggests that there is indeed some genetic component underlying susceptibility to the disease.

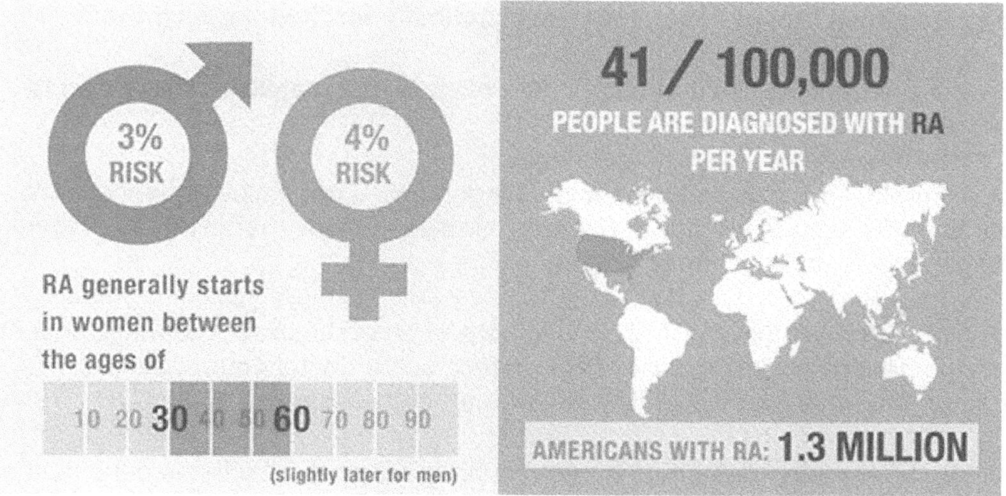

Genetic Factors and Family History

Experts believe that people who develop RA inherit something in the genes involved in the formation and operation of our immune system that increases the likelihood the immune system will attack healthy tissue in the joints.

Results from genetic studies, including twin studies, family studies, and genome-wide linkage studies, have shown that heritability (or the genetic material that we inherit through our parents and family) contributes to the chances of developing RA. One analysis of data from twin studies found that genetics accounted for over 60% of the overall risk for people who develop RA (MacGregor et al, 2000).

Another way of understanding the influence of genes that contribute to RA is to compare the risk of disease development among groups with differing degrees of genetic similarity. The risk of developing RA in the general population is about 1%.

Therefore, about 1 in 100 people in the general population will develop RA. When we look at the chances of developing RA among close family members, such as siblings that share a good deal of genetic material, the risk goes up. The risk of developing RA if your brother or sister (not a twin) has the disease is about 5%. The risk increases further when we consider twins that share the identical genetic material (also called monozygotic twins). If your identical twin has RA, your risk for developing the disease is about 15% (Plenge, RM., 2009).

Selected genes thought to increase susceptibility for rheumatoid arthritis

There are several genes that occur more often in rheumatoid arthritis patients than others.

For example, your human lymphocyte antigen (HLA) gene cluster defines how your immune system will attack bacteria, viruses, moulds, parasites and other foreign objects that get into your body.

The first HLA allele or type that occurs more often in rheumatoid arthritis patients than the general population was DR4. In fact, some doctors currently test whether you have the HLA-DR4 allele as part of their diagnosis.

Another HLA allele, HLA-DR1, is often found in rheumatoid arthritis patients that have anti-CCP antibodies. However, many people with HLA-DR4 or HLA-DR1 do not get rheumatoid arthritis.

Thus, your genes, HLA-DR4 or HLA-DR1 may increase the chances that you get rheumatoid arthritis, but they are not one of the causes of rheumatoid arthritis (Plenge RM., 2009).

Scientists check the prevalence of rheumatoid arthritis in many sets of identical twins to measure the influence of genes on the onset (beginning) and progression of rheumatoid arthritis.

Based on 3 large studies of identical twins, the chance of both twins developing rheumatoid arthritis was only 12.3% to 21%. That is, both twins had rheumatoid arthritis in about 1 out of 5 cases.

These studies mean that only 1 out of 5 genetically identical individuals to you would be expected to get RA.

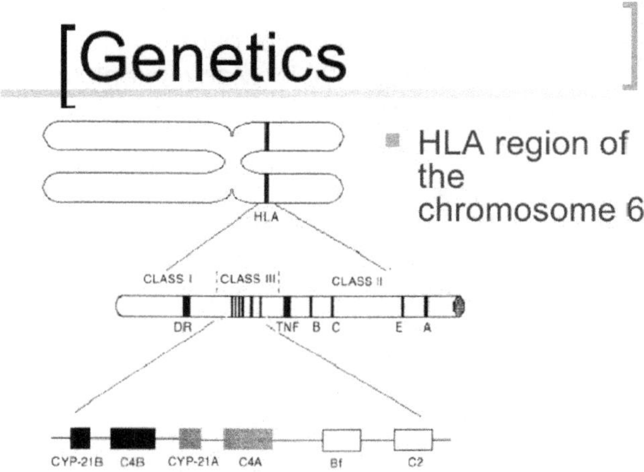

Although your genes may make you more susceptible to getting rheumatoid arthritis, your genes are not one of the causes of rheumatoid arthritis. Thus, environmental factors have a major role in triggering and aggravating your rheumatoid arthritis.

Infections causing Rheumatoid Arthritis

There is much indirect evidence suggesting that exposure to infectious agents may be the trigger for RA. First, epidemiological data come from the observation of a decline in the incidence of RA in several populations. Many studies have indeed shown a halving in incidence over the past 30 years (Jacobsson et al, 1994).

Given the genetically stable population, the most probable explanation is that of a decline in an infectious trigger. This effect of time on occurrence might also be related to the period of birth as well as to the current year of observations. The Pima Indians, for example, showed a decline in occurrence of disease, and an in-depth study based on analysis of birth cohorts has shown a decline in the population occurrence of rheumatoid factor with increasingly recent birth cohorts (Silman et al, 2000; Silman et al, 2001).

Other indirect evidence regarding the role of an infectious agent has arisen from case–control studies suggesting that people who have had a blood transfusion, even some years prior to disease onset, may be at an increased risk of disease (Symmons et al, 1997).

Dr. Leirisalo-Repo concluded that an “infection initiating the process of rheumatoid arthritis is observed in about 20% of patients studied in the early phase of arthritis.” (Leirisalo-Repo et al, 2005). Many scientists have proposed that infection in susceptible people can be one of the initial causes of rheumatoid arthritis.

Many scientists and physicians have searched for that one infectious agent which causes rheumatoid arthritis. Yet, there is no single virus, bacteria, yeast, mould, prion nor mycoplasma that is associated with all cases of rheumatoid arthritis.

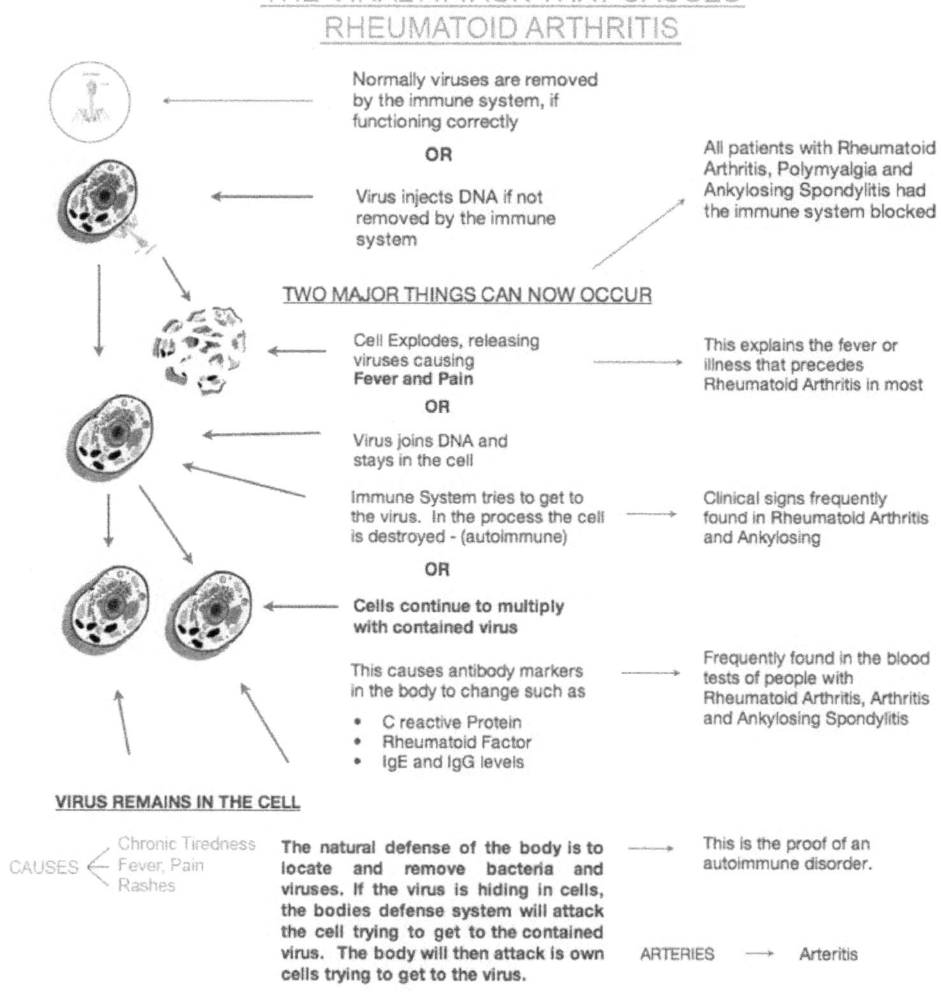

Even when your immune system has cleared or rid your body of the intruder, your immune system may be confused. Your immune system may attack that part of your joints that looks similar or is cross-reactive to the intruder. This is called molecular mimicry because part of the molecules of your joints and the intruder look similar to your immune system.

This cross-reactivity or molecular mimicry between your joint tissue and a part of the intruder probably triggers your initial immune response to your body's tissues or your autoimmune response. Your autoimmune response against your own joint tissues is a major hallmark of rheumatoid arthritis.

Thus, an infection in a susceptible person can be one of the major causes of rheumatoid arthritis. The following infectious agents are being studied for their role in initiating or aggravating arthritis-like symptoms, including rheumatoid arthritis.

The Hepatitis C virus, Epstein Bar Virus, Human Herpes Virus Type 6, Cytomegalovirus, Herpes Simplex Virus, and Parvovirus B-19 are being studied for their role in development of rheumatoid arthritis or other forms of arthritis.

Several bacteria including subclinical Proteus urinary tract infections, the common disease-causing bacteria found in gingivitis, Porphyromonas gingivalis, as well as Mycoplasma arthritidis, Mycoplasma fermentans, Mycoplasma pneumoniae, Ureaplasma urealiticum, and Chlamidia trachomatis are also found to be associated with rheumatoid arthritis in some patients.

At least one researcher found each of these infectious agents (or antibodies reactive with them) in the joint fluid of some rheumatoid arthritis patients at higher levels than in osteoarthritis patients. These studies suggest that infectious agents can be one of the causes of rheumatoid arthritis.

In other cases, joint fluid is infected with Staphylococcus, Streptococcus, or Haemophilus, and the arthritis is then called infectious arthritis.

Interestingly, skeletal evidence suggests that rheumatoid arthritis only became common in the European continent after Christopher Columbus returned from the Americas. This pattern is consistent with Christopher Columbus bringing an infectious agent to Europe from America.

Although infections can be one of the major causes of rheumatoid arthritis, vibrant health thwarts infections from taking hold in individuals. These observations suggest that other factors which affect your overall health also contribute to inducing rheumatoid arthritis.

Smoking and RA

It is perhaps surprising, given how much this exposure has been investigated in other chronic diseases, that very little attention has been given to cigarette smoking until recently. However, findings from a number of recent studies showed that cigarette smoking is associated with an increased risk of RA (Harrison et al, 2001; Hutchinson et al, 2001).

Studies have also suggested that smoking is related to development of rheumatoid factor independent of RA. Indeed, in many of the epidemiological studies showing a relationship between smoking and RA, the positive findings have been restricted to those with rheumatoid factor.

Inflammation and RA

The type of inflammation that causes RA is that which develops in the “synovium,” the tissue that lines the joint. The immune system’s destructive chemicals wear down cartilage that normally cushions the space between joints and bones, causing friction and pain. But the 10-million-dollar question is why would the immune system attack the body and create inflammation in tissues, including the joints?

Inflammation associated with RA can be triggered by a number of factors, and risk factors include:

- Poor gut health or “leaky gut syndrome“
- A poor diet and food allergies (foods that contribute to inflammation include refined carbohydrates, fried foods and too much sugar)
- Obesity (especially if someone was obese before the age of 55)
- Genetic factors (certain genes can affect the immune system may make some people more prone to getting autoimmune disorders)
- Toxicity, due to things like environmental toxin exposure and endocrine disruptors
- Low immune function due to other medical conditions or autoimmune disorders
- Smoking cigarettes

We will examine these in more detail below. However, the development of the rheumatoid arthritis and the onset of flares involves a multistep process (Fig 1).

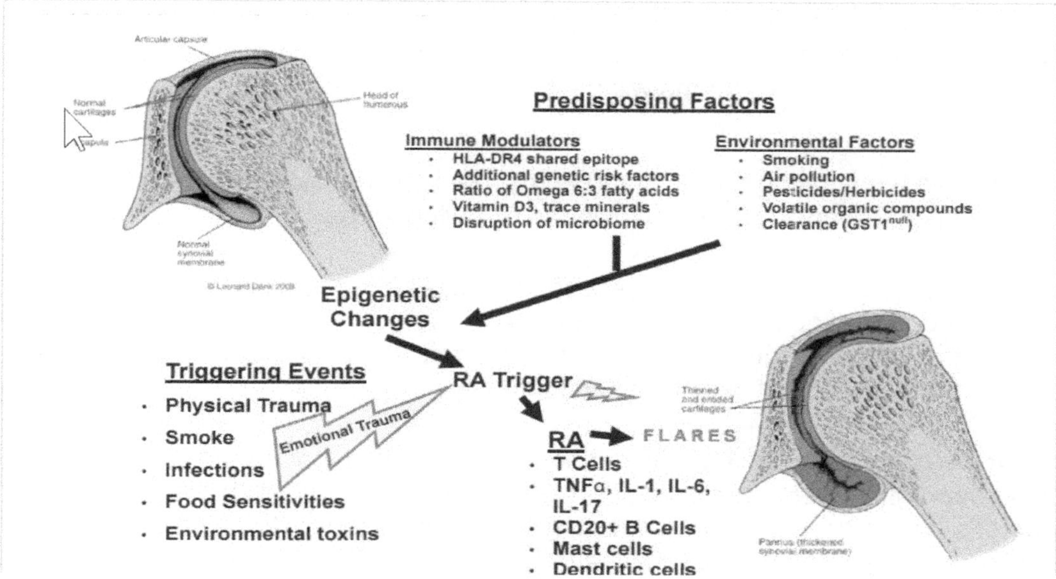

Fig 1. Predisposing Factors for Rheumatoid Arthritis

Predisposing factors were categorized into immune modulators and environmental factors. Genetic risk factors include genes in immune modulation (e.g. HLA-DR4 shared epitope and others) that we have already looked at above.

Diets that are imbalanced in fatty acids - where there is a greater than 5 times amount of omega 6 to omega 3 will increase the risk for prolonged inflammation (Simopoulos, AP., 2008). One of these potential triggering events often coupled with an emotional stress is associated with the onset of RA. Patients exposed to additional triggering events can experience further RA progression and flares, such as food intolerances or sensitivities, infections, environmental toxins, that also include mercury in amalgam fillings and physical trauma.

Food Intolerances and RA

The first thing that I do after taking a history from a RA patient, is to test them for food intolerances. At the Da Vinci Centre where I work, I use Bioresonance testing to test for food intolerances, as after many years of using this method, I find it both accurate and quick.

Whenever I lecture to various practitioners from around the world, food intolerances is something that I place a lot of emphasis on, because it is one of the biggest sources of internal inflammation that we are exposed to. Let's face it, we eat at least three times a day, so if there are any foods that we are intolerant to causing inflammation, then certainly over time this inflammation is going to reach a point where symptoms will develop.

A plausible explanation for the immune mechanisms related to food intolerances which cause or aggravate RA involve the following steps:

- the abnormal entry of large food molecules into the bloodstream
- the formation of immune complexes
- the action of chemical mediators released by activated immune cells
- the activation of cell-mediated immunity

From the many patients that I have seen with RA, I find that the advice that they have been given from medical doctors, is to stop eating certain foods, and every doctor's advice differs. This ad hoc advice does not address the specific food intolerances that each person will have with fibromyalgia, and this certainly differs from person to person.

Generally, the more of the same food that we eat on a regular basis, the higher the probability of developing a food intolerance to that food. Leaky gut, SIBO, dysbiosis, Candida and parasites can also exacerbate and increase food intolerances. One of the golden rules for optimising nutrition, is to avoid eating the same food every day, which in the convenience mode of life that we tend to live, this is very easy to do.

Apart from the specific food intolerances that we find in patients with RA, we also find that many patients react to the nightshade family of vegetables that include potatoes, aubergines or eggplants, all types of peppers as well as tomatoes.

The entire nightshade family contains many of the natural toxins of Belladonna which can create inflammation. In a survey of 5,000 arthritis sufferers, 68% reported complete relief after eliminating nightshades from their diet. Let us look at this in a little more detail as it is important.

As early as 1993, some rheumatologists acknowledged that "There are now sufficient good scientific studies, from the UK and abroad, to suggest that, at least in some patients with RA, dietary therapy may influence at least the symptoms and possibly the progression of the disease."

Recent scientific data shows that 3 of every 4 rheumatoid arthritis patients who eat foods that they are allergic to, experience significantly more stiffness, pain, tender and swollen joint counts, higher Ritchie's articular index, sedimentation rate, C-Reactive Protein levels as well as higher TNF-alpha and IL-1 alpha levels.

Surprisingly, 1 out of 5 rheumatoid patients whose test results did not detect a food allergy still had worse pain when they ate certain foods.

In addition, several physicians of nutritional medicine or integrative medicine write that food allergies are one of the causes of rheumatoid arthritis.

Dietary therapy may reduce rheumatoid arthritis symptoms by eliminating foods that trigger an autoimmune response, according to an article published by Darlington et al in the *British Journal of Rheumatotology* in June 1993. This therapy may even slow the progression of the disease by eliminating all trigger foods from the diet.

Dietary therapy is also useful as a diagnostic tool to discover unique food triggers. The therapy begins with eliminating every possible food trigger for arthritis out of the diet, such as beef, eggs, wheat, oranges, milk, peanuts, malt and soy. Food is then reintroduced one at a time to see if a person reacts to a item.

Nightshades and RA

The nightshades are members of an enormous family of plants called Solanaceae – these include tomatoes, potatoes (not sweet potatoes or yams), eggplant and all types of peppers. Paprika is a sneaky one, showing up in lots of flavouring mixes and often under "spices" on ingredient labels. Other nightshades include goji berries, ashwagandha (an adaptogenic herb), Cape gooseberries (not normal gooseberries), ground cherries and garden huckleberries (not blueberries).

At the Da Vinci Centre in Cyprus where I work, most of my RA patients complain of pain, so I am always trying to find not always to alleviate pain.

What I have found is that by avoiding nightshades, this will lessen your pain, whether the nightshades are the true source of the pain. Other symptoms that nightshades can create include muscle pain and tightness, morning stiffness, poor healing, arthritis, heart burn, reflux insomnia and gall bladder problems.

The nightshades are considered a "calcinogenic" plant; that is, they cause calcinosis, which is a toxic calcification of soft tissues when eaten by animals. This happens because they contain calcitriol (1,25-dihydroxy vitamin D), the most active form of vitamin D. Please note that calcitriol is not vitamin D3 (cholecalciferol), so please do not confuse the two.

In humans, calcitriol is normally the product of vitamin D metabolism – let's see if we can simplify things. Cholecalciferol, or vitamin D3, is produced in the skin by the action of sunlight or can be consumed in food or supplements. In the liver, vitamin D_3 is transformed into calcidiol (25-hydroxycholecalciferol, the compound that we test in the blood as a measure of vitamin D status); then the kidneys transform calcidiol into calcitriol (1,25-dihydroxy vitamin D) (Fig 2).

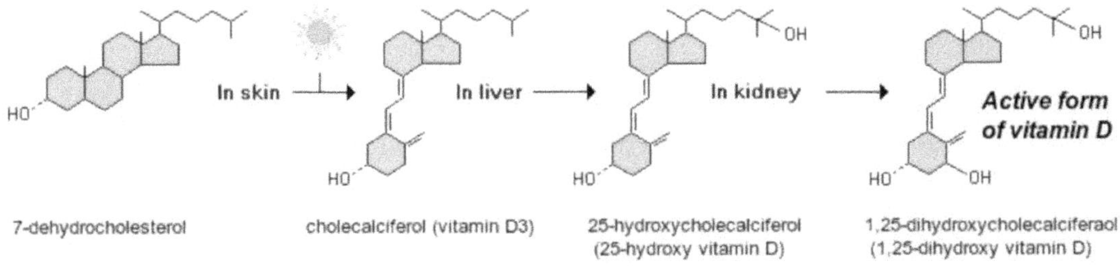

7-dehydrocholesterol — In skin → cholecalciferol (vitamin D3) — In liver → 25-hydroxycholecalciferol (25-hydroxy vitamin D) — In kidney → 1,25-dihydroxycholecalciferaol (1,25-dihydroxy vitamin D) **Active form of vitamin D**

Fig 2. Vitamin D Pathway

Calcitriol is an extremely potent hormone, thousands of times more potent than vitamin D3. It has been said that calcitriol is the most powerful hormone in the human body. Production of calcitriol is very tightly regulated by the kidney.

Calcitriol signals the intestines to absorb calcium from our diet. While we absolutely need calcitriol to maintain proper bone density, too much calcitriol, from any source, leads to hypercalcemia, also known as high blood calcium. The body does not like this situation and wants to get the calcium levels back down to normal as quickly as possible, as an imbalance of minerals in the blood particularly affects the heart. The quickest solution for the body is to deposit the extra calcium into the soft tissues. Each hypercalcemic episode likely lasts for only a short while, however, each episode leaves a small deposit behind. Over time, these deposits lead to the condition known as calcinosis.

Overconsumption of calcitriol from nightshade foods can circumvent the kidney's control and over time lead to calcium deposits in the soft tissues such as the tendons, ligaments, cartilage, cardiovascular tissues, kidneys and skin. Osteoarthritis is basically calcium deposits in the soft tissues of joints. Chronic hypercalcemia can lead to generalized vascular (blood vessel) calcification, which is coronary artery disease. Nephrocalcinosis is calcification of the kidneys.

We are not supposed to bypass the body's control mechanisms for calcitriol. Nightshades do this to our detriment. Many of us do not notice because it happens so slowly and gradually.

There are other chemicals in nightshades that we will not go into detail here, such as Solanine, a glycoalkaloid (Patel et al, 2002), nicotine (Galatz et al, 2006) and capsaicin that can all cause health issues that may indirectly lead to the development of RA and other health problems.

A good experiment that I often recommend to my patients is to try avoiding nightshades for 6 weeks and see the outcome – often they come back reporting far less pain. If they really want to validate the effect, then they can binge on nightshades for a day and then see how they feel.

Nutrients such as vitamin D3 and vitamin K2 (Seyama et al, 1996) can often help, and we will talk about these later in the treatment section.

Gluten Free Diet and RA

The study involved 66 volunteers with rheumatoid arthritis who were randomly assigned to either a diet free of animal products and gluten, found in wheat, rye and barley, or a well-balanced non-vegan diet for 12 months. Thirty-eight were assigned to the vegan diet and 28 to the conventional diet. Average ages for both groups were very close to 50 years and each group's current state of disease activity was very similar.

The results for those eating a vegan diet were significantly better than those on the well-balanced non-vegan diet. After 12 months, patients on the vegan diet reduced their weight from 66.4 to 62.2 kg (9.24 lbs), whereas the other group decreased from 67.8 to only 67.1 kg (1.54 lbs).

After just 3 months, those on a vegan diet had a significant decrease in total cholesterol, LDL, and the LDL/HDL ratio (HDL is often called the "good cholesterol"). The other group did not significantly change.

The rheumatoid arthritis disease activity of the vegan group also substantially decreased after just 3 months. The non-vegan group had a slight decrease. Rheumatoid arthritis disease activity was measured in 28 joints for each patient by considering the number of swollen and tender joints and the patient's overall assessment of their condition.

Leptins, Adipokines and RA

Leptins are hormones often found in fat cells (adipocytes), so the more obese we are, the more leptins the body will be secreting. This overexpression in leptin production can lead to the production of inflammatory factors such as adipokines which can lead to cartilage destruction and osteoarthritis (Terlain et al, 2006; Dumond et al, 2003).

Recently, increased levels of adipokines which are mainly produced by adipocytes have been detected in patients with osteoarthritis. Moreover, studies on different adipokines (proinflammatory), such as leptin, adiponectin, resistin and visfatin have all show a direct link with the initiation and progression of osteoarthritis (Peng-fei et al, 2011).

So, losing weight will play a definitive role in the progression of your rheumatoid arthritis, and this will be discussed later in this chapter.

Obesity and RA

Fat is chemically active, constantly releasing proteins that cause inflammation, which then aggravates RA itself.

Fat cells, or adipocytes, release proteins called cytokines that, in excess, cause constant, low-grade inflammation throughout the body. "Fat, or adipose, tissue is a source of many of the same inflammatory cytokines that are produced by inflamed joint tissue in people with inflammatory arthritis.

The more pounds you add, the more of these proteins circulate in the body, which also seems to lead to more severe RA.

People with rheumatoid arthritis (RA) who are obese are less likely to achieve disease remission than their non-obese counterparts, according to a meta-analysis published in May in *Arthritis Care and Research.* The review also found that obesity was associated with higher levels of disease activity and pain, suggesting excess weight may negatively affect overall outcomes in RA. This meta-analysis supports earlier research, including a study presented at the 2015 annual meeting of the American College of Rheumatology.

There is strong evidence that obesity increases the risk of developing RA, but less is known about its effect on people living with the disease. So, researchers reviewed more than 3,500 studies about the relationship between obesity and four key measures: remission rates, disease activity, patient-reported outcomes at follow-up, and mortality.

Shoenfeld and his co-authors detailed data showing that people with RA who are obese have more active disease, more pain and worse overall health. Inflammation-causing cytokines, which include tumour necrosis factor-*alpha* (TNF-*alpha*), interleukin-1 and interleukin-6, are already overactive in RA.

Every pound of body weight places four to six pounds of pressure on each knee joint.

Recent studies (George et al, 2016) have shown that losing weight will have great benefits for RA and should be part of the holistic treatment of all people with RA.

Candida and RA

From my personal experience, having treated many patients with RA over the years, most of them have Candida. When the Candida is treated, along with the avoidance of food intolerances that are also an important part of the inflammatory cycle, and the balancing of the gut dysbiosis and digestive issues, as well as balancing nutritional deficiencies, then usually the osteoarthritis symptoms will drastically reduce in intensity or disappear altogether, with a little patience and some regenerative work.

Candida can get into joints and cause damage.

A Dutch team of scientists in 2012 injected Candida albicans yeast cells into the knee joints of mice. They found that these mice exhibited not only “joint swelling and inflammation”, but also “enhanced destruction of cartilage and bone”. The study concluded that “minute amounts of fungal components, like C. albicans, are very potent in interfering with the local cytokine environment in an arthritic joint, thereby polarizing arthritis towards a more destructive phenotype." (Marijnissen et al, 2012).

Candida Symptoms

Sinus infections
Intense sweet cravings
Bread, pasta, rice cravings
Vaginal yeast infections
Oral Thrush
White | yellow coated tongue
Gastrointestinal distress
Nausea
Gas
Bloating
Diarrhea

Constipation
Achy joints
Joint soreness, stiffness
Low grade fever
Headache
Flu-like symptoms
Lethargy
Fatigue
Exhaustion
All over body itch
Back itch
Rashes, burning, itchy
Skin breakouts
Muscle ache and pain

Inability to concentrate
Brain fog
Dizzy
Nervousness
Hyperactivity
Irritability
Sadness
Blue feeling
Impending doom
Mood swings
Tired all the time
Fits of rage, anger or tantrums
Food allergies

How does Candida develop?

Inflammation of the gut lining, often involving candida yeast overgrowth, is the primary symptom of leaky gut syndrome and fibromyalgia. The originating cause may be prescription drug use and antibiotics which kill off healthy probiotic flora. Gut inflammation, from candida yeast infection, is usually instigated by one or several of the following factors:

- Prescription hormones (e.g., birth control pills and/or hormone replacement therapy) and prescription corticosteroids (e.g., hydrocortisone).
- Excessive use of antibiotics which kills off health bacteria, causing dysbiosis, candida overgrowth and candida yeast infection.
- Processed foods, as well as foods and beverages contaminated by parasites, fungus, and/or mould which promote the growth of candida yeast infection.
- Increased amounts of refined carbohydrates (e.g., candy bars, cookies, cake, soft drinks, and white bread) which also promote the growth of candida yeast overgrowth and dysbiosis.

- Increased alcohol and caffeine consumption. Remember that alcohol is a natural result of yeast overgrowth and sugar.

It is highly advisable to read the chapter on Candida and get yourself checked out. There is a Candida questionnaire that you can complete at the end of this chapter which will give you a good idea how many symptoms you may have that would lead to a diagnosis of systemic Candidiasis.

Microbiome and RA

Several recent studies have found intriguing links between gut microbes, rheumatoid arthritis, and other diseases in which the body's immune system goes awry and attacks its own tissue.

A study published in 2013 by Jose Scher, a rheumatologist at New York University, found that people with rheumatoid arthritis were much more likely to have a bug called Prevotella copri in their intestines than people that did not have the disease.

Scientists are especially intrigued by how these bacteria influence the immune system. In recent decades, the incidence of many autoimmune diseases has been increasing; many microbiome researchers argue that at least some of this rise is due to changes in our bacterial ecosystem.

Altered diet, the explosion of antibiotic use, and decreasing contact with the microbe-packed natural world of animals and plants have all combined to transform the bacteria that call humans home. “Our microbiome has changed significantly over the past century, and especially over the past 50 years,” says NYU microbiologist Martin Blaser, who puts much of the blame on widespread use of antibiotics. “We're losing microbes with each generation; they are going extinct. These changes have consequences.”

But while many scientists are confident of the link between the microbiome and arthritis, they haven't pinned down what particular role bacteria play in triggering the disease.

Scientists say that *Prevotella copri* may stimulate an immune reaction that then targets joint tissue. Or it may crowd out beneficial microbes that keep immune-system attack cells being too aggressive - a theory supported by the fact that people with high levels of *Prevotella copri* also had reduced amounts of the bacteria *Bacteroides fragilis*, which seems to restrain the immune system.

Other studies have shown that a vegan diet changes the faecal microbial flora in rheumatoid arthritis patients, and changes in the faecal flora are associated with improvement in rheumatoid arthritis activity (Peltonen et al, 1997).

It looks like the microbiome is going to be the centre of attention for a long time to come as new research has suggested that a virus (our own genome is 8% viral in origin) placed into the microbiome can help and repair the gut as well as boosting our immune system.

Reporting on the new study (Kernbauer et al, 2014), in an article well worth reading, the **Science Daily states**:

The new findings are the first strong evidence that viruses in the gastrointestinal tract can help maintain health and heal a damaged gut."

They summarized the study's findings as follows:

The team infected germ-free mice and antibiotic-treated mice with Murine NeoVirus (MNV) and found that the infection triggered the repair of intestinal tissue damaged by inflammation, restored intestinal cell numbers, restored intestinal cell function, and normalized tissue architecture. The results were apparent after just 2 weeks of MNV infection.

Infection with MNV also helped restore the gut's immune system. The investigators do not yet know how the virus supports the immune system. They did find, however, increased signalling by antiviral type 1 interferon proteins, suggesting the virus was playing a key role in driving the immune response.

The investigators also documented a doubling of T-cell levels in the blood and detectable levels of antibodies in the gut and blood of antibiotic-treated mice after MNV infection. These measures were consistent with a normalization of the immune response. The authors conclude that viral infection of the gut may be helpful once antibiotic treatment has wiped out intestinal bacteria.

Treatment with MNV was also able to improve survival in antibiotic-treated mice receiving the damaging chemical dextran sodium sulphate.

As our knowledge of the critical role of microbes increases, a paradigm-shift is occurring in medicine that is only beginning to trickle down to clinical practice. If our very identity depends on 'germs' – e.g. the bacteria within our body account for 10 times more cells and 99% more genetic material that found in the human body itself – the discovery that the viruses in our body – the total number referred to as the virome – also perform indispensable functions in supporting and maintaining our health, turns on its head widely held assumptions about their role in contributing to human disease and various pathologies.

Small intestine bacterial overgrowth (SIBO) and RA

SIBO is a condition characterized by abnormal overgrowth of bacteria in the small intestine. One study reported that up to 84 percent of IBS patients have SIBO and that patients with IBS were 26 times more likely to have SIBO than controls (Pimentel et al, 2000). Eradication of the overgrowth eliminated irritable bowel syndrome in 48% of subjects.

Results from subsequent studies examining the association between SIBO and IBS were mixed. This is in part because there is currently no consistently accepted, gold-standard method of testing for SIBO, and the techniques varied from study to study.

Most bacteria are in your large intestine, but sometimes they can move up into the small intestine. Given that the small intestines should not contain unhealthy bacteria, only the good acidophilus species, then this is not a healthy environment. If the bad bacteria populate the small intestine, they will begin fermenting food that you digest, particularly sugar or starchy foods. So, when you eat starchy foods such as bread, cereals, pasta, rice and sugary foods, the bacteria in your gut ferment the sugars in the food. This fermentation process and its gases expand, and you begin to feel pain and very uncomfortable.

One study shows an increased frequency of bacterial overgrowth in the upper small intestine of patients with RA. Although about one third of our patients had hypochlorhydria or achlorhydria, which is associated with small intestinal overgrowth," (Draser et al, 1969) bacterial overgrowth was also observed in patients with normal acid secretion. This finding indicates that, in addition to hypochlorhydria, other, at present unknown, factors contribute to the development of bacterial overgrowth in patients with RA.

Further, it is of great interest that the patients with RA with bacterial overgrowth had a more pronounced disease activity than the patients with normal microflora. High counts of streptococcal species and Enterobacteriaceae have been recorded in the small intestine of patients with RA, (O'Connor et al, 1989) which in the latter case agrees well with our findings. The bacteriological findings in the upper small intestine largely reflected the oropharyngeal microflora; in addition, Enterobacteriaceae were found in the achlorhydric controls and in the patients with RA irrespective of their gastric acid secretion capacity.

The fact that about one third of our patients with RA had hypochlorhydria or achlorhydria reflects the high incidence of atrophic gastritis in those patients

(Marcolongo et al, 1979). The high frequency of bacterial overgrowth recorded in the achlorhydric controls and in hypochlorhydric or achlorhydric patients with RA indicates indirectly that gastric acid secretion is an important defence factor against exogenous pathogenic micro-organisms.

The bactericidal activity of gastric juices appears to be pH dependent (Gray et al, 1967; Giannella et al, 1972) and even a transient reduction of the gastric pH is effective in clearing gastric bacteria, as previously reported in patients with RA in whom cultivations of gastric juices were obtained before and after stimulation with pentagastrin." (Bennett, JC., 1978). Consequently, we believe that peak acid output is as reliable as other criteria of hypochlorhydria" for predicting small intestinal bacterial overgrowth in patients with RA.

Traditionally, SIBO is being treated by medical doctors using specific antibiotics, sometimes giving these in multiple serial dosages over quite some time. The disadvantage of this is that long-term use of antibiotics is likely to lead to a yeast overgrowth in the gut, or candida, which is another major factor underlying RA.

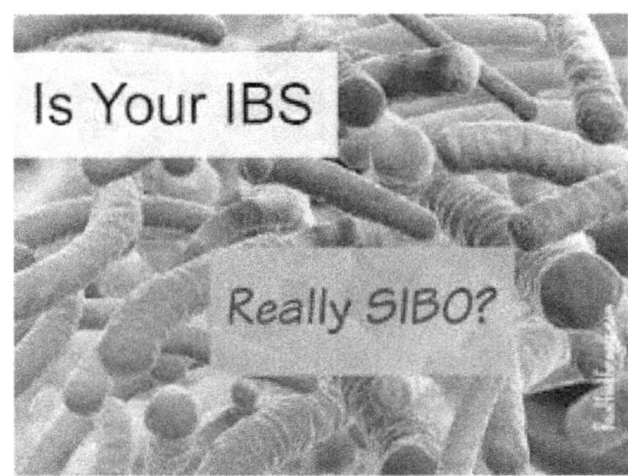

It is probably wiser, if you have or suspect that you have SIBO, to use antibiotic herbs and supplements to help bring back some balance into the gut. Some of these will include grapefruit seed extract, oregano oil, colloidal silver, Echinacea herb, vitamin C, as well as repopulating the gut with friendly bacteria while also eradicating any yeasts. We will talk more about these later in this chapter.

This is more likely to lead to an alleviation of RA symptoms, given that you're working on all of these factors concomitantly. It does not make sense, to work with only one factor at a time, such as SIBO for example, without addressing nutritional deficiencies, candida, parasites, digestive disorders, optimising nutrition and so forth.

This is the premise of the holistic model which I have been using for a number of years in clinical practice with good success. Having said this, all patients are different and there are other factors that also need to be taken into account for the individual patient that I have sitting in front of me.

Nutrient Deficiencies and RA

Among the most important deficiencies that cause inflammation in the body are a low level of omega-3 fatty acids, low vitamin D, and low zinc. These deficiencies are epidemic, even among people who eat a supposedly healthy and balanced diet.

The following studies support that one of the causes of rheumatoid arthritis may be low levels of essential nutrients.

In a study of over 57,000 patients, people who ate more fruits and cruciferous vegetables (broccoli, cabbage, cauliflower, brussel sprouts), certain antioxidant micronutrients, particularly beta-cryptoxanthin, and who took supplemental zinc had lower rates of rheumatoid arthritis.

Vitamin B levels, such as vitamin B6 are often low in rheumatoid arthritis patients and often correlate with higher homocysteine levels, a marker of inflammation.

Vitamin B12 levels were also significantly low in 24% of rheumatoid arthritis patients. Low levels of vitamin D and low vitamin E status are risk factors or increase your chances of getting rheumatoid arthritis. Copper levels are significantly higher in rheumatoid arthritis patients than controls. Selenium levels in both blood and the joints are significantly lower in rheumatoid arthritis patients than those of healthy subjects and osteoarthritis patients.

Thus, low essential nutrients make you more susceptible to RA. Low stomach acid which is associated with poorer protein digestion and mineral uptake is often found in rheumatoid arthritis patients.

Taken together, these data indicate that your diet and nutrient levels influence your risk of getting rheumatoid arthritis. In other words, diet with insufficient vegetables and healthy oils or inadequate digestion of your food is likely one of the causes of rheumatoid arthritis.

There have been remarkably few studies on factors such as diet, although there is a theoretical basis for investigating the role of omega-3 fatty acids. Randomised trials suggest that diets high in eicosapentaenoic acid have a favourable effect on the outcome of RA (Volker et al, 2000; Kremer JM., 2000).

This might be because such fatty acids compete with arachidonic acids, the latter of which are involved in inflammation. Whether such dietary factors have a role in RA onset is much less clear.

Another study, conducted by researchers from *VU Medical University Centre* in Amsterdam and published in the journal *Clinical Rheumatology* in 2008, had eight RA patients consume 20 grams of an antioxidant-rich spread over the course of 10 weeks. All participants were non-smoking women who had been receiving either NSAIDs or "second line" RA drugs for at least three months before the study began.

The antioxidant-rich spread included 400 mg of alpha-tocopherol (vitamin E), 10 mg of lycopene, 10 mg of lutein and five milligrams of palm oil carotenoids, including alpha carotene (vitamin A). The participants were also given a 200 mg daily dose of vitamin C.

The researchers found that at the end of the study, participants had significantly fewer swollen and painful joints than they had at the start of the study, and their overall health had improved. Within four weeks after the end of the intervention; however, their symptoms and health had begun to worsen again - indicating that consistent, on-going antioxidant treatment is needed for long-term symptom relief.

Fish oil and RA

By far, the most well-proven natural RA symptom treatment is fish oil and omega-3 fatty acids. At least 13 separate double-blind, placebo-controlled studies on more than 500 participants have shown that omega-3 supplements significantly reduce RA symptoms and actually enable patients to lower their NSAID usage.

Some research suggests that fish oil becomes even more effective when taken as part of a diet that is low in omega-6s, such as a vegetarian diet, or when olive oil is also taken.

Because severe joint damage occurs early in RA, and because no natural remedies have yet been proven to effectively slow the progression of the disease, it is important that RA patients continue to consult with qualified health professionals even if taking antioxidants, fish oil or other alternative treatments.

A very recent study (Dawczynski et al, 2017) has shown that the use of fish oil in RA patients led to a decline in tender and swollen joints and inflammatory markers such as 5-lipoxygenase product 5-hydroxyeicosatetraenoic acid were significantly reduced.

At the Da Vinci Center we prefer to use KRILLOIL – 1 cap x 2 times daily.

Toxins and RA

Now, for the first time, there's evidence that exposure to chemical toxins could, in fact, trigger the RA.

A new study just published in *Environmental Health Perspectives*, is the first to look at the associations between perfluorooctanoic acid (PFOA), perfluorooctanesulfonic acid (PFOS), and osteoarthritis. This is a potentially huge discovery because these chemicals, (when referred to together, known as PFCs) are widespread in the environment and known to contaminate humans and wildlife. PFCs are used in more than 200 industrial processes and consumer products including grease-proof paper food containers, stain and water-resistant fabrics and personal care products.

"We found that PFOA and PFOS exposures are associated with higher prevalence of osteoarthritis, particularly in women, a group that is disproportionately impacted by this chronic disease," Sarah Uhl, who authored the study along with *Yale* Professor Michelle L. Bell and Tamarra James-Todd, an epidemiologist at the *Harvard Medical School* and Brigham and Women's Hospital, said in a press statement.

The researchers investigated data from six years of the National Health and Nutrition Examination Survey (NHANES, 2003-2008), which allowed them to account for factors such as age, income, and race/ethnicity. When they looked at men and women separately, they found clear, strong associations between the chemical exposure and osteoarthritis for women, but not men. What's more, more exposure meant a higher risk for osteoarthritis. Women in the highest 25 percentile of exposure to PFOAs had about twice the odds of having osteoarthritis compared to those in the lowest 25 percentile of exposure.

Uhl and her team noted that more studies are needed to establish the possible biological mechanisms that could cause PFCs to trigger osteoarthritis. The mechanisms are unclear, but we know that toxins of this nature can cause a tremendous amount of free radical damage in the body, including the joints.

Another study (Parks et al, 2016) that looked at the exposure of women farmers to various pesticides, chemical fertilizers and solvents and found a positive correlation between exposure and the increased risk of developing RA.

Heavy metal toxicity and RA

In the last 50 years, our world has become more laden with many man-made chemicals including pesticides, organic solvents as chloroform and xylene, dioxins, volatile organic compounds such as formaldehyde, and polychlorinated biphenyls.

In addition, we are more exposed to heavy metals including cadmium, and toxic element mercury, than in previous centuries. For example, the toxic element mercury gets into the body from amalgam fillings, fish and vaccinations, as well as from the environment through crematoriums.

Several researchers have also mentioned heavy metals as one of the contributing factors of RA (Naveh et al., 1997; Hannson et al., 1978; Ala et al., 2005; Yazar et al., 2005). Chronic exposure to heavy metals, especially lead (Pb), mercury (Hg) and cadmium (Cd) affects the immune system.

Heavy metals also reduce the number of existing B and T cells (Lehmann et al., 2011). Resultantly, the immune system attacks on its self-molecules, which can lead to RA and other joint diseases (Lehmann et al., 2011).

Scudder et al. (1978) reported significantly higher levels of Cu in RA patients compared to healthy individuals – high levels of copper are known to be toxic to the body. Copper is antagonistic to zinc, so other research has shown that some RA patients were found to be deficient in Zinc levels, but not all (Naveh et al., 1997; Ala et al., 2009).

Toxic mercury causes many of the effects that are found in at least some rheumatoid arthritis patients: adrenal dysfunction, allergy, poor coordination, depression, discouragement, dizziness, fatigue, immune dysfunction, irritability, joint pain, kidney damage, numbness, pain in limbs, tingling, and more.

In addition, formaldehyde, found in many vaccinations, can be used to induce arthritic symptoms in rodents.

Rheumatoid arthritis patients have less ability to rid their bodies of toxins due to low glutathione activity.

Lead (Pb) is known to affect bone, and recent evidence suggests that it has effects on cartilage as well. As osteoarthritis is a highly prevalent disease affecting bone and cartilage, then there is likely a link between lead and osteoarthritis. One study found a correlation between lead levels in the blood and the severity of arthritis (Nelson et al, 2011).

Approximately 95% of the total body Pb burden in adults is stored in bone and has a half-life of decades, which contributes as much as 65% to measured whole blood Pb levels. Pb deposition has been observed in cartilage and bone in human osteoarthritis and is measurable in the synovial fluid of individuals with knee osteoarthritis without a history of excessive metals exposure. Pb stored in bone is released chronically into the blood pool, especially during times of increased bone turnover, such as menopause, and potentially during bone remodelling as seen in osteoarthritis. This makes bone both a target tissue for Pb toxicity and a persistent endogenous source of Pb.

Interestingly, there are studies that have looked at the levels of lead in lipsticks and found these to be quite high in some brands – could this explain why women have a higher prevalence of osteoarthritis? (Stejskal et al, 2013).

Mercury from amalgam fillings or fish mainly is also another culprit as it is a serious neurotoxin that can cause tremendous free-radical damage and the destruction of cartilage and other tissues in the body.

At the Da Vinci Center we often give our patients natural chelators that can mobilize and eliminate these toxic metals from the body such as:

- HMD™ - (Heavy Metal Detox) – pulls toxic metals from inside the cells - 45 drops x 3 times daily for adults
- HMD™ LAVAGE – 25 drops x 3 times daily – an important drainage remedy that help to open-up the detoxification channels to facilitate the elimination of the toxic metals
- HMD™ ORGANIC CHLORELLA (475 mg) – 2 caps x 2 times daily – helps to grab toxic metals in the mesenchyme and the gut, preventing their reabsorption.

These three combined is called the HMD ULTIMATE DETOX PACK

- A-LIPOIC ACID – a water- and fat-soluble antioxidant to help protect the body against free radical damage from circulating toxic metals.

L-GLYCINE – this can help in eliminating other organic toxins such as those we have already discussed, and others such as PFC's, PCB's, Bisphenol A and the like – take 1 cap x 3 times daily.

Causes of your rheumatoid arthritis probably involve multiple factors, including low levels of one or more essential nutrients, possible injury or infection, food or chemical sensitivities, mild dehydration, acid-alkaline imbalance, unreleased stress or past trauma, toxic accumulation, and genetic susceptibility.

High-Fructose Corn Syrup and RA

There is a link between joint and gut inflammation of unknown aetiology in arthritis. Existing research indicates that regular consumption of high-fructose corn syrup sweetened (HFCS) soft drinks, but not diet soft drinks, may be associated with increased risk of seropositive rheumatoid arthritis (RA) in women, independent of other dietary and lifestyle factors.

One unexplored hypothesis for this association is that fructose malabsorption, due to regular consumption of excess free fructose (EFF) and HFCS, contributes to fructose reactivity in the gastrointestinal tract and intestinal in situ formation of enFruAGEs, which once absorbed, travel beyond the intestinal boundaries to other tissues and promote inflammation. In separate studies, the accumulation of advanced glycation end-products has been associated with joint inflammation in RA (DeChristopher et al, 2016).

The researchers concluded: "EFF beverage intake is significantly associated with arthritis in US adults aged 20-30 years, possibly due to the intestinal in situ formation of enFruAGEs."

Vaccinations and RA

There is evidence that has shown that the Hepatitis B vaccination (HBV) significantly increases the odds of developing RA (Geier et al, 2005; Symmons et al, 1993). There are also many toxins in vaccines such as aluminium, formaldehyde and others that may also trigger auto-immune responses.[1]

Statins and RA

There is research (de Jong et al, 2011) to suggest that the use of statin drugs may potentially facilitate autoimmunity, eventually resulting in autoimmune diseases such as RA.

---

[1] https://www.cdc.gov/vaccines/pubs/pinkbook/downloads/appendices/B/excipient-table-2.pdf

Dehydration and RA

Dr. F. Batmanghelidj who studied many chronic and acute signals of dehydration in a stress filled environment in Iran has proposed that dehydration is one of the major causes of rheumatoid arthritis.

However, at present there is no clinical evidence whether or not dehydration is one of the causes of rheumatoid arthritis or affects its progress.

His proposal suggests that even mild dehydration can trigger joint pain in some humans. Furthermore, chronic dehydration would lead to damage to the cartilage, inflammation and angiogenesis, which is consistent with being one of the causes of rheumatoid arthritis.

I include it here as "food for thought". Because of the theory's simplicity, it probably will not receive funding to be adequately tested in a clinical setting.

However, you may want to monitor your water intake in case that his theory of dehydration may be one of your causes of rheumatoid arthritis.

Free Radical Damage – Oxidative Stress

Probably you have all heard of antioxidants that can help us to protect against free radical damage. But what exactly are free radicals and how can these do us harm and cause osteoarthritis.

Our bodies produce free radicals every hour of the day, and there are that there are various reasons for doing so. Free radicals can help eliminate some of the bad microorganisms that may be present in our bodies.

One of the factors that keeps free radicals in check to prevent them from destroying the body are antioxidants that we get from several different foods and nutritional supplements. The problem begins when our antioxidant levels in the body are lower than those of free radicals - when this happens the free radicals begin damaging tissues and organs of the body, including the joints, therefore developing osteoarthritis.

In a recent epidemiological study, Arthritis and Rheumatism reports that antioxidants are correlated to a drop in progression of osteoarthritis in the knees of 640 patients, independent of diet/food allergies (McAlindon et al., 1996).

Vitamin C had the highest correlation (70%), and it was associated with reduced cartilage loss, followed by beta carotene and vitamin E, so these are important supplements to include in your natural treatment protocols.

Our bodies produce free radicals as by-products of cellular respiration, metabolism of foods, breathing, exercising and other vital functions (Cheeseman et al, 1993). The liver produces and uses free radicals for detoxification, while white blood cells send free radicals to destroy bacteria, viruses and damaged cells.

Free radicals ultimately harm and age the body over time because they damage DNA, cellular membranes, lipids (fats) stored within blood vessels and enzymes.

The damage done by free radicals in the body is known as oxidative stress – let us examine what this means:

- When we leave a piece of fruit exposed to the atmosphere, or a metallic nail, they will brown or rust respectively – this is the process of oxidation. This "rusting" process can also take place in the body, and the amount of oxidation in the body is a measure of oxidative stress.
- High levels of oxidative stress affect every organ and system in the body and have been linked with everything from Alzheimer's disease, osteoarthritis, arteriosclerosis, cancer and heart disease to accelerated aging, asthma, diabetes and many other chronic diseases.

Antioxidants counteract free radicals and keep them in balance, preventing them from destroying organs and tissues.

Free radicals have an important role in the pathogenesis of knee osteoarthritis. The excessive production of oxidative stress can damage proteins, lipids, nucleic acids, and matrix components (Sutipornpalangkul et al, 2009).

What Are Antioxidants?

While there are many ways to describe what antioxidants do inside the body, one definition of antioxidants is any substance that inhibits oxidation, especially one used to counteract the deterioration of stored food products or removes potentially damaging oxidizing agents in a living organism.

The major sources of free radicals include:

- Ordinary body functions, such as breathing and digestion
- Exposure to radiation
- Exposure to other environmental pollutants

- Consumption of cigarettes or tobacco, drugs, and alcohol
- Certain medications or high use of antibiotics, which leads to antibiotic resistance
- A poor diet that includes foods like unhealthy fats, too much sugar, pesticides, herbicides or synthetic additives. Many processed and refined foods contain oxidized fats that add free radicals to the body. Excessive amounts of sugar and sweeteners are other sources of free radical growth that contribute to aging, weight gain and inflammation.
- Even too much exercise (overtraining) generates added free radicals
- High amounts of emotional or physical stress. Stress hormones (like too much cortisol) can generate free radicals.

At the Da Vinci Center we recommend the following antioxidants:

<u>ALPHA-LIPOIC ACID</u> - (300 mg) – take 1 cap x 2 times daily

<u>VITAMIN E</u> (200 mg) – take 1 cap x 2 times daily

<u>VITAMIN C BLEND</u> (MIXED ASCORBATES) – take 1 cap x 3 times daily

Combating Free Radical Damage

A recent study (Khojah et al, 2016) has shown that using antioxidants such as one gram of vitamin C daily for 2 months, helped RA patients to significantly reduce free radicals of all kinds, as well as other inflammatory biochemical markers and a drastic reduction in disease activity and morning stiffness. At the Da Vinci Center we would normally give more than double this amount – usually 3 grams daily.

The National Institute on Aging, a part of the National Institutes of Health, has developed a scoring system to measure the amounts of antioxidants in foods. The score given to a particular food is known as its ORAC score. ORAC stands for "Oxygen Radical Absorbance Capacity."

So foods and supplements that have a high ORAC score would be the most powerful antioxidants. Let's look at some of the foods that generally are considered to have a high ORAC score.

Here are just a few foods that have very high ORAC scores:

- Brightly coloured fruits and vegetables – most orange foods like carrots, sweet potatoes, pumpkin and squash, or cantaloupe contain antioxidants called carotenoids. Similarly, to orange veggies, citrus fruits contain a compound called quercetin. Spinach and other leafy greens like kale are high in lutein, and tomatoes and red peppers contain lycopene, all of which have anti-aging effects.

- Berries, grapes and red wine - these dark skin fruits are some of the highest in antioxidants, such as resveratrol.

- Green and white tea - white and green teas are very minimally processed and contain less caffeine than coffee (or even other varieties of tea). They also contain a very high concentration of antioxidants called polyphenols that have been shown to have cancer-fighting properties.

- Cocoa - a study from Seoul National University found that cocoa has a higher antioxidant content that green tea, black tea and even red wine. But you want to make sure the cocoa or dark chocolate you eat is very minimally processed, such as the kinds that are a high percentage of cocoa (more than 65 percent or so) and labelled raw and organic.

- Herbs and spices - these include things like cinnamon, oregano, ginger, turmeric and rosemary. Additionally, essential oils made from the same plants can also be a great source of antioxidant, anti-inflammatory compounds.

High ORAC Foods, Herbs and Supplements

Here are some of the top-10 foods with the highest ORAC scores, based on weight:

1. Goji berries: 25,000 ORAC score
2. Wild blueberries: 14,000 ORAC score
3. Dark chocolate: 21,000 ORAC score
4. Pecans: 17,000 ORAC score
5. Artichoke: 9,400 ORAC score
6. Elderberries: 14,000 ORAC score
7. Kidney beans: 8,400 ORAC score
8. Cranberries: 9,500 ORAC score
9. Blackberries: 5,300 ORAC score
10. Cilantro: 5,100 ORAC score

Top 10 Antioxidant Herbs List

Along with antioxidant foods, certain herbs, spices and essential oils derived from nutrient-dense plants are extremely high in healing antioxidant compounds. Here is another list of the herbs you can try adding to your diet for increased protection against disease. Many of these herbs/spices are also available in concentrated essential oil form. Look for 100 percent pure (therapeutic grade) oils, which are highest in antioxidants.

1. Clove: 314,446 ORAC score
2. Cinnamon: 267,537 ORAC score
3. Oregano: 159,277 ORAC score
4. Turmeric: 102,700 ORAC score
5. Cocoa: 80,933 ORAC score
6. Cumin: 76,800 ORAC score
7. Parsley (dried): 74,349 ORAC score
8. Basil: 67,553 ORAC score
9. Ginger: 28,811 ORAC score
10. Thyme: 27,426 ORAC score

Other antioxidant-rich herbs include garlic, cayenne pepper and green tea. Aim to consume two to three servings of these herbs or herbal teas daily.

Vitamin D Deficiency and RA

A new study led by a Boston University School of Public Health (BUSPH) environmental health expert came up with an unexpected conclusion. The researchers were investigating why women living in the north-eastern United States are more likely to develop rheumatoid arthritis (RA) and they suspected they would find an association with air pollution. Instead, their research has raised the strong possibility that RA results from vitamin D deficiency due to not getting enough exposure to one of nature's most powerful healers - sunlight. The new research, which was just published online in the journal *Environmental Health Perspectives*, found that women in states like Vermont, New Hampshire and southern Maine were more likely to report being diagnosed with RA.

Dr. Veronica Vieira, D.Sc, associate professor of BUSPH environmental health, headed the study using a technique called spatial analysis in 2010. Her research team used data from the Nurses' Health Study, a long-term study of U.S. female nurses. They noted where the women lived, their health status and behavioural risk factors for various diseases during the years from 1988 and 2002; the RA findings were based on 461 women who developed RA, compared to a control group of 9,220.

Bottom line: women living at northern latitudes and receiving less sunlight were at risk of vitamin D deficiency and these were the women who had the greatest incidence of RA. What's more, the risk increased even more if women had been living in the north since the beginning of the study in l988.

The researchers noted that vitamin D deficiency has previously been associated with a variety of other autoimmune diseases. "A geographic association with northern latitudes has also been observed for multiple sclerosis and Crohn's disease, other autoimmune diseases that may be mediated by reduced vitamin D from decreased solar exposure and the immune effects of vitamin D deficiency," the authors wrote.

In a study published in the journal *Nutrients* in June, researchers from the University of Saskatchewan evaluated the vitamin D status in 116 patients at a community clinic, 60 of them suffering from rheumatic diseases. The researchers found that vitamin D levels were significantly worse in patients suffering from autoimmune rheumatic disease (such as rheumatoid arthritis).

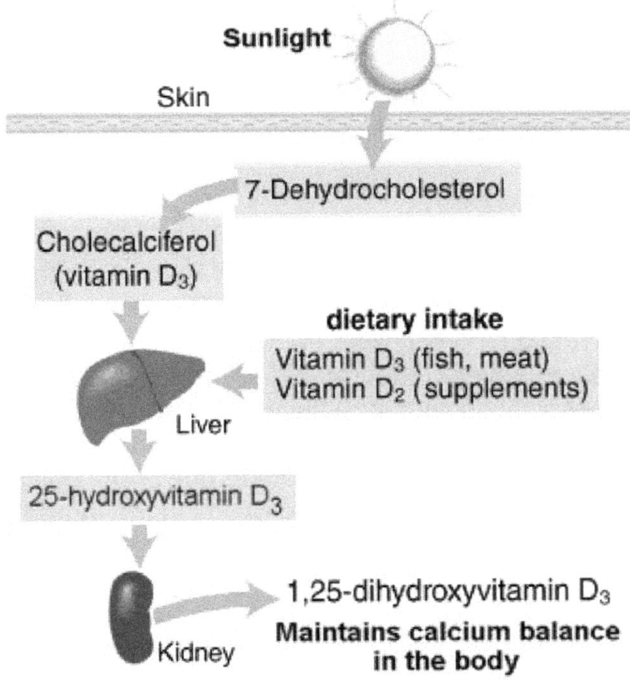

In addition, the researchers found that, among rheumatoid arthritis patients, lower vitamin D levels were directly correlated with more severe symptoms. The effect was so striking that rheumatoid arthritis patients with low blood levels of vitamin D were five times more likely to suffer from active symptoms than patients with higher levels.

A study published in the journal *Arthritis and Rheumatism* in 2004 suggests that high levels of dietary vitamin D may also help prevent the development of rheumatoid arthritis. The researchers analysed data from nearly 30,000 women between the ages of 55 and 69 who had participated in the Iowa Women's Health Study and had been followed for 11 years. Study participants were periodically questioned about their health status, eating habits and use of nutritional supplements. Over the course of the decade-long study, 152 of the participants were diagnosed with rheumatoid arthritis.

The researchers found that women with the highest dietary intake of vitamin D were the least likely to have developed rheumatoid arthritis. In contrast, women whose diet included fewer than 200 International Units of vitamin D per day had a 33 percent higher risk of developing the disease than women whose diets included more. These results remain statistically significant even after adjusting for other potential rheumatoid arthritis risk factors, such as smoking and calcium intake.
Another study (Chandrashekara et al, 2015) found that supplementing with vitamin D for 12 weeks (about 10,000 IU daily) showed a statistically significant improvement in disease activity and a reduction of inflammatory markers such as C-reactive protein (CRP).

A further recent study (Cecchetti et al, 2016) showed that supplementing with vitamin D led to an inverse correlation between vitamin D levels and RA – with a general improvement in most related symptoms.

Get more sunlight

Although certain foods are enriched with vitamin D and the vitamin can also be taken in supplement form, getting more sunlight is still the safest and most effective way to increase your body's levels of this powerful nutrient. Doctors say that your body can produce all the vitamin D it needs from just 15 to 30 minutes per day of skin on the face and hands (without sunscreen) for lighter skinned people, with more time needed for people with darker skin.

And it's not just for reducing your risk of rheumatoid arthritis. Higher levels of vitamin D have been linked to lower rates of various autoimmune diseases, as well as heart disease, diabetes and cancer.

Frequent exposure to sunshine has been linked to the prevention of several serious diseases, from Type II diabetes to between 15-20 types of cancer.

According to a new study published in the *Annals of the Rheumatic Diseases* journal, however, we have yet another reason to love the sun: Older women who enjoy frequent exposure to sunlight throughout their lives are less likely to develop rheumatoid arthritis, an autoimmune condition that affects joints.

The researchers, who are members of the Department of Epidemiology at the *Harvard School of Public Health*, monitored the health of two groups of female nurses. The first group, comprised of over 120,000 women between the ages of 30 to 55, was monitored from 1976 to 2008. The second group, comprised of 115,500 women between the ages of 25 and 32, was monitored from 1989 to 2009.

They found that the older women in the first group with the highest estimated levels of ultraviolet radiation exposure (as determined by factors such as the climate of the state in which they lived) were 21 percent less likely to develop rheumatoid arthritis than the women with the lowest estimated levels.

However, the younger women in the second group demonstrated no correlation between estimated ultraviolet radiation exposure and a decreased risk of rheumatoid arthritis. The study authors believe that this is because younger women are taught from a young age to guard themselves from the sun using sunscreen or avoid it altogether.

"Our study adds to the growing evidence that exposure to UV-B light is associated with decreased risk of rheumatoid arthritis," said Dr. Elizabeth Arkema, co-author of the study. "The mechanisms are not yet understood but could be mediated by the cutaneous production of vitamin D and attenuated by use of sunscreen or sun avoidant behaviour."

Avoiding the sun can pose long-term health problems

This latest study for the *Annals of the Rheumatic Diseases* is one of many to suggest that the sun - the giver of life on Earth - might not be the diabolical purveyor of cancer that several questionable counter-studies (often funded by sunscreen manufacturers) have implied.

Indeed, it has been shown countless times that sunscreen - aside from containing many cancer-causing chemicals, alcohols, parabens, and solvents - blocks vitamin D production. Since vitamin D deficiencies are linked to osteoporosis, depression, and autoimmune disorders like rheumatoid arthritis, it is unsurprising that people (especially young people) who choose to block the sun, rather than embrace it, might suffer from the same in the long-term.

RA and Systemic Inflammation

Inflammation is your body's response to stress from diet, lifestyle and the environment. It causes many diseases like osteoarthritis, cancer, fibromyalgia and general aging.

One of the often-overlooked causes of inflammation in the body and joints is low-grade bacterial, viral or fungal infections in our blood, tissues and cells. Fungus is probably the most common due to the epidemic of systemic Candidiasis we are seeing from an abuse of antibiotics across the Western world.

The Da Vinci Natural Rheumatoid Arthritis Protocol is an all-body approach to healing that provides a road map to wellness for those who suffer from osteoarthritis, by addressing internal health, reducing inflammation by conquering infections (especially Candidaisis), and healing your body from the inside out. There are several factors that can trigger inflammation in the body:

- Chronic low-grade food allergies or food sensitivities that may cause few symptoms.
- An imbalance of bacteria and fungi in your gastrointestinal tract, also known as dysbiosis. This causes your immune system to overreact to bacteria in your gut and can be without notable symptoms.
- Stress! Constant psychological, emotional or physical stress raises the level of cortisol, creating inflammation.
- Environmental toxicity from air, water, food pollutants and toxic metals like mercury and lead all contribute to inflammation and have been linked to many chronic and auto-immune diseases.
- Diet and lifestyle. Too much fat, sugar and protein in your diet, constant dehydration, consumption of too many sodas or caffeine, alcohol, tobacco and other excesses, inactivity, and lack of sleep can all increase inflammation in your body.

The wide-scale adoption of industrial agriculture and food manufacturing has brought us new, high-tech food chemicals that humans have never tried to consume in our entire existence on this planet before now. These create inflammation in the body over time, which leads to chronic disease – we need to avoid as many of these as possible:

- Hexane: Processed, refined, bleached and deodorized high Omega-6 vegetable, Canola, and soybean oils

- Trans-fats and hydrogenated oils
- High fructose corn syrup, refined, granulated sugar and chemical sugar substitutes in huge quantities
- MSG, artificial colours and flavours, preservatives, chemical emulsifiers
- Isolated soy protein; maltodextrin and other industrial by-products
- Bleached, brominated flours and machine-extruded puffs, chips and cereals that are closer to bio-plastics than food
- Fortified foods sprayed with cheap, synthetic vitamins that your body can't properly assimilate
- Toxic pesticide and herbicide residues in almost all food
- BPA, BPS, phthalates, lead, antimony and other toxins from plastic food packaging
- Genetically engineered crops in 80% of the food supply
- Eggs, dairy and meat from grain-fed, filthy, confined animals full of hormones, heavy metals and antibiotics
- Irradiated and ultra-pasteurized foods

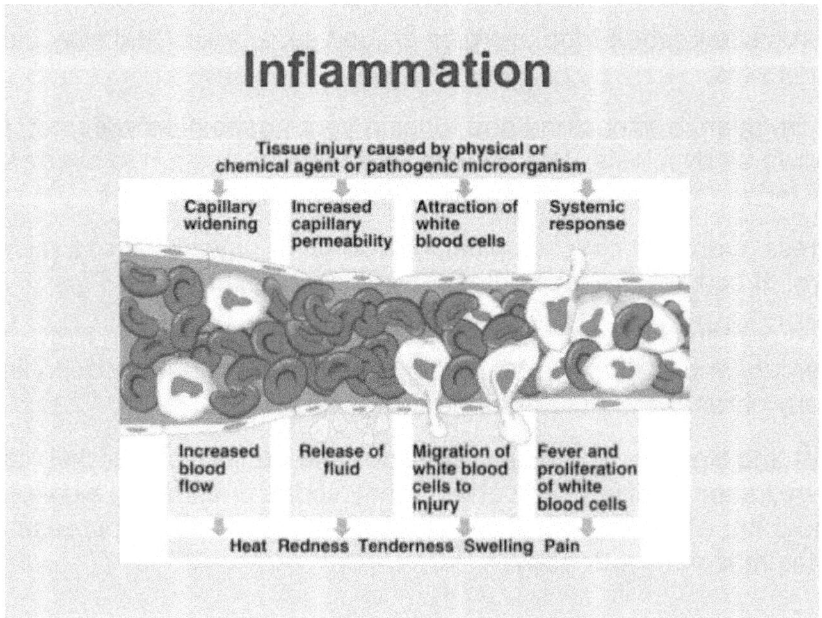

More and more scientific evidence is piling up that it is these modern, industrially-created "foods" that are making us all sick and is one of the main reasons that osteoarthritis is on the increase.

The Anti-inflammatory Diet

Considering the inflammatory nature of osteoarthritis, it is not surprising that anti-inflammatory diets are gaining in popularity among osteoarthritis sufferers looking to find relief from their symptoms through dietary modification rather than drugs. The anti-inflammatory diet that we recommend at the Da Vinci Center looks something like this:

- Eat plenty of fruits and vegetables that are rich in antioxidants
- Reduce the amount of saturated and trans fats in your diet
- Watch your intake of sugar and refined carbohydrates
- Get plenty of omega-3 fatty acids from foods (or supplements)
- Eat lean protein sources, such as fish and organic chicken, and cut back on red meat
- Avoid refined and processed foods.

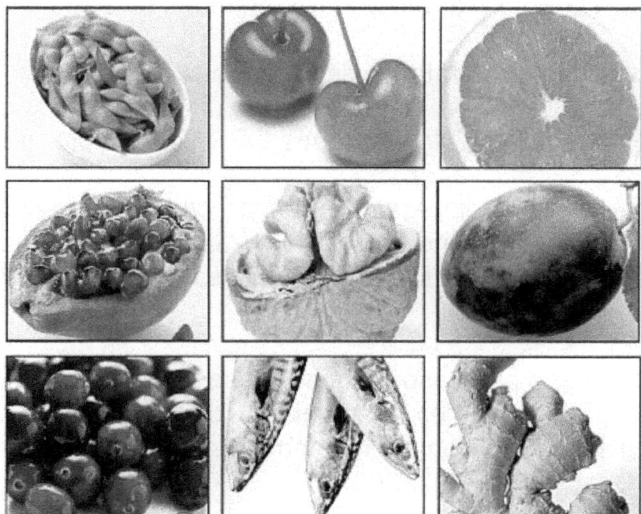

Keeping calories in check is also important as fat cells can release a lot of inflammatory molecules into your bloodstream, so the higher your body fat percentage, the more inflammation you are likely to have.

Vegetarian diets have also been associated with improved eczema symptoms in some studies. Although meat is not typically completely forbidden on anti-inflammatory diets, they do suggest that vegetables and fruits should play a key role in your diet if your goal is to reduce chronic inflammation in your body.

After reading about the potential anti-eczema effects of a high vegetable intake, you might be tempted to embrace a strict vegetarian diet. However, going pescatarian, rather than vegetarian, might make more sense (a pescatarian diet includes fish and other seafood, but not the flesh of land-based animals).

Here are a few more details about the Da Vinci anti-inflammatory diet that we recommend that you follow:

- Eat a wide variety of fruits and vegetables which are rich in antioxidants. A high intake of fruit and vegetables has been inversely associated with plasma concentrations of C-reactive protein (CRP), a key marker of inflammation (Esmaillzadeh et al, 2006).

- Reduce the amount of trans fats in your diet. A high intake of trans fats has been associated with high plasma concentrations of biomarkers of systemic inflammation (Mozaffarian et al, 2004). Foods that contain high amounts of saturated fat are usually restricted on anti-inflammatory diets.

- Get plenty of omega-3 fatty acids from foods (or supplements). These essential fatty acids have been shown to disrupt inflammation cell signalling pathways by binding to the GPR120 receptor (Oh et al, 2012).

- Minimize your intake of sugar and refined carbohydrates, which have high glycaemic loads (GL), and focus on low-GI foods instead. Research suggests that low-GI diets are inversely associated with inflammation (Neuhouser et al, 2012).

- Avoid refined and processed foods. These foods often have high glycaemic loads, plus they often contain food additives, some of which have been shown to promote inflammation in animal studies (Nakanishi et al, 2015; Chassaing et al, 2006).

It is also important to keep your calories in check and your weight in a healthy range. According to a study published in *The American Journal of Clinical Nutrition*, enlarged fat cells in obese individuals promote inflammation, whereas small fat cells in lean individuals promote metabolic homeostasis (Greenberg et al, 2006).

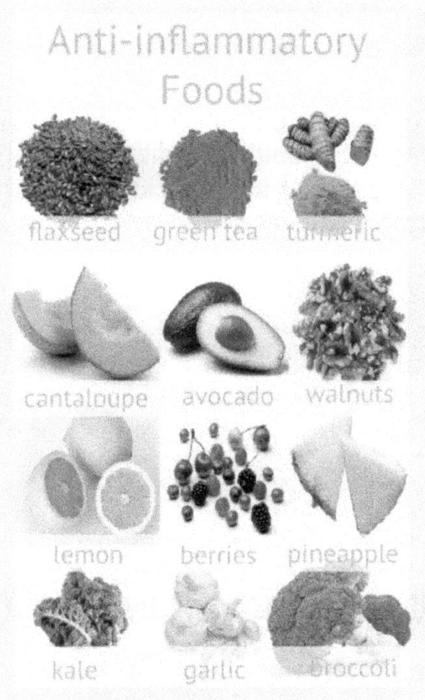

What's more, people with more severe fibromyalgia appear to be more likely to be obese due to inactivity and lack of exercise. The researchers concluded that weight loss may have beneficial effects in obese people with fibromyalgia.

Ginger as a Natural Anti-inflammatory Herb

Ginger (*Zingiber officinale*) has a long history of use as both food and medicine. Among practitioners of herbal medicine, remedies derived from ginger root – such as ginger tea or ginger juice – are well known for their ability to alleviate digestive problems. But, they may also help fight a range of other health problems, especially conditions linked to chronic inflammation.

Ginger has shown promise as a natural remedy for rheumatoid arthritis, a chronic inflammatory condition that causes joint pain which appears to be particularly common among people with fibromyalgia.

A study published in the journal *Medical Hypotheses* found that more than three-quarters of study participants with rheumatoid arthritis or osteoarthritis experienced relief in pain and swelling after treatment with powdered ginger root.

You can use fresh ginger root in so many sweet and savoury recipes, way beyond the typical stir-fries and ginger root tea.

Incorporating ginger into homemade fruit juices or smoothies is also one of the best ways to reap the wonderful health benefits of fresh ginger root. Fruits and vegetables that pair well with ginger in juices include carrots, oranges, mandarins, apples, and grapefruit.

Fruit and Vegetable Smoothies

We have already looked at some of the studies that have shown that eating fruit and vegetables is helpful for your eczema. There is another good way to get the antioxidant nutrients that these fruits and vegetables contain, and that is by drinking smoothies.

Let's look at a few examples that you can add to your daily diet:

Green smoothie with ginger, spinach and flaxseed

This smoothie pairs nutrient-rich baby spinach with mango and banana to create a tasty and nutritious green smoothie. Ground flaxseed and fresh ginger, both of which contain anti-inflammatory compounds, are added to the mix to further boost its health-giving properties.

Ingredients

- About 1 ⅔ cups water and/or non-dairy milk of your choice (rice, almond, coconut)
- 1 small banana
- 1 small mango
- 2 cups baby spinach
- 1 tsp. grated fresh ginger
- 1 Tbsp. ground flaxseed
- 8 ice cubes

Directions

- Peel, rinse, pit and cut the ingredients as needed, and put them in a high-powered blender in the order listed above.
- Secure the lid and process in short bursts until the ice cubes have been thoroughly crushed. Then, slowly increase the speed, and blend at full speed for about 1 minute, or until the smoothie is very smooth and consistent in colour. Add water if needed to adjust the consistency. Makes 2 servings.

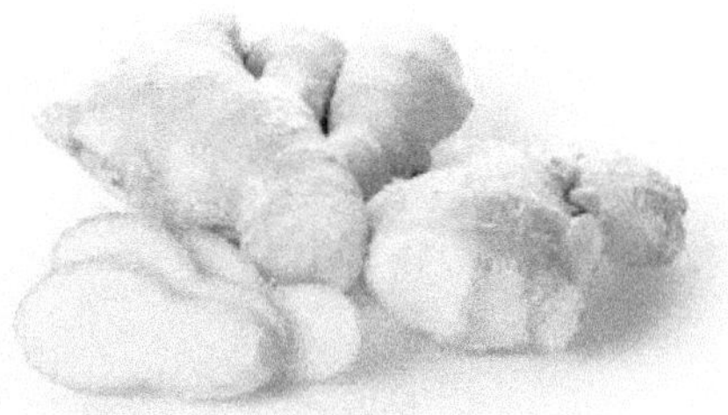

Gingery carrot juice

As you may already know, beta-carotene is a strong antioxidant that helps neutralize free radicals. Free radicals are unstable molecules that can damage DNA and cell membranes, thereby contributing the development of a wide range of health problems, including inflammation in people with fibromyalgia.

The following juicing recipe for eczema sufferers combines fresh carrots with ginger.

Ingredients

- 8 organic carrots
- 1 ½ inch slice fresh ginger

Directions

- Scrub the carrots under cold running water and trim their tops
- Peel the ginger
- Pass the carrots and ginger through a juicer. Clean the juicer right after use
- Serves 1

There is no reason why you cannot drink a couple of these juices daily.

Carrot, mango and turmeric smoothie

This recipe pairs fresh mango with carrot juice to create a luscious, brightly-coloured smoothie. The frozen banana this recipe calls for is added to give this vegan blend a creamy texture, while the turmeric powder ensures your body will get a generous dose of anti-inflammatory compounds.

Ingredients

- 1 ⅔ cups carrot juice

- 1 ripe mango, peeled and pitted
- 1 ½ tsp. pure turmeric powder
- 1 Tbsp. chia seeds
- 1 banana, peeled, sliced and frozen
- Water, as needed

Directions

- Add the carrot juice to a blender, followed by the remaining ingredients.
- Blend until thoroughly combined, stopping to scrape down sides and to check the consistency.
- If the smoothie seems too thick, add some water.
- Pour into tall glasses and serve right away; serves 2.

Pomegranate Juice for RA

Pomegranate juice is rich in polyphenolic compounds that possess antioxidant and anti-inflammatory activities. In a study (Ghavipour et al, 2016), it was shown that pomegranate juice was excellent at reducing inflammatory markers such as C-reactive protein (CRP) and erythrocyte sedimentation rate (ESR), reduced swollen joints as well as increased glutathione peroxidase, an important detoxification nutrient.

Pomegranate extract (POMx) consumption has been shown to reduce the incidence and severity of collagen-induced arthritis in mice (Balbir-Gurman et al, 2011). So drinking pomegranate juice is also good for RA.

Other Useful Juices:

* Carrot, celery, and cabbage juice. Add a little parsley.

* Potato juice (If you are not allergic to this).

* Cherry juice.

* Take juice of half a lemon before every meal and before going to bed.

* Carrot, beet, and cucumber.

* During acute stage, one pint to one quart celery juice daily.

* Radish, garlic

Caution: Certain juices may cause adverse reactions in people with osteoarthritis. Avoid citrus fruits, and be careful with vegetables from the nightshade family, including potatoes, tomatoes, peppers and eggplant. Citrus seems to promote swelling, and nightshades contain psyllium alkaloids, which cause problems for some people.

Homeopathy and RA

In general, homeopathic treatment for chronic conditions such as RA is most effective in consultation with a professional homeopath. However, there are a number of remedies that deserve mention and are most useful for intermittent episodes of pain and other symptoms. If either of these descriptions fits your symptoms, take the remedy in a 30C potency, a few pellets a day when the pain is bad. Limit remedy use to a few times a week.

Rhus Tox – Best Homeopathic medicine for rheumatoid arthritis

Rhus Tox is one of the best Homeopathic medicines for treating rheumatoid arthritis. It proves helpful in rheumatoid arthritis involving any of joint. The guiding symptoms to look out for are pain and stiffness in joints. The stiffness is worse on rising in the morning. It also tends to worsen after a period of inactivity. Movement of joints makes the person feel more comfortable. Warm application over joints also relieves pain. Some may feel better by massaging the affected joint. Also, Rhus Tox is the ideal Homeopathic solution where exposure to cold air or winter makes the joint pain worse.

Actea Spicata – Prominently indicated Homeopathic medicine for rheumatoid arthritis affecting small joints

Actea Spicata is a wonderful Homeopathic medicine for rheumatoid arthritis affecting small joints. The small joints include fingers, toes, wrist and ankles. The affected joints are in severe pain, hot and swollen. The pain is of violent, tearing type. Touch worsens the pain in joints. Movement of affected joints also aggravates pain in cases where Actea Spicata will work best. Where the slightest fatigue worsens pain in small joints, Actea Spicata is the medicine to prescribe.

Pulsatilla and Kalmia Latifolia – Significant Homeopathic medicines for rheumatoid arthritis with shifting/wandering pains

Pulsatilla and Kalmia Latifolia are excellent Homeopathic medicines for rheumatoid arthritis with wandering joint pains. These medicines work wonders where the pain passes from one joint to another in quick succession. Now the pain is experienced in one joint, the next moment in another. The joints are also very swollen and inflamed.

Caulophyllum – Homeopathic medicine for rheumatoid arthritis of small joints where stiffness accompanies pain

Caulophyllum is a most effective Homeopathic medicine for rheumatoid arthritis affecting small joints which are both stiff and in pain. Joints of fingers, wrist, ankles and toes are affected. Caulophyllum is recommended where joint pain is attended with marked stiffness. The joint pain is aching, drawing in nature. Pain wanders from joint to joint every few minutes. The symptoms become majorly worse at night. Finger joints in particular, so that the person has trouble folding his fingers. Nodes may also be observed on finger joints. Significantly, in case of joint pains that start in women especially during pregnancy or childbirth, Caulophyllum is the Homeopathic medicines.

Antimonium Crudum – Top grade Homeopathic medicine for rheumatoid arthritis in finger joints

Antimonium Crudum is the most suitable Homeopathic medicine for rheumatoid arthritis affecting finger joints. In some cases, specific drawing pain is noted in finger joints. Cold application may worsen this pain. Warmth is soothing. Chronic indigestion or gastric complaints may be found in addition to joint pains in persons who need prescribing Antimonium Crudum. A symptom unique to prescription of Antimonium Crudum is that joint pains worsen when taking wine.

Bryonia Alba – Best Homeopathic medicine for rheumatoid arthritis with acute inflammation of joints

Bryonia Alba is a most remarkable Homeopathic medicine for treating rheumatic pains in joints that are acutely inflamed. People who require Bryonia Alba have markedly swollen, red, hot, painful joints. The slightest movement, touch or pressure worsen pain in the affected joint. Warm applications relieve pain.

Causticum – Excellent Homeopathic medicine for hip joint pain in rheumatoid arthritis

Homeopathic medicine Causticum is recommended for hip joint pain in rheumatoid arthritis. The hip joint feels dislocated in persons who will need prescribing Causticum. Standing and walking worsen pain. The gait (walk) is unsteady due to hip pain. Marked stiffness and tension are observed in hip joint. Causticum also works well in cases where the joints are deformed and shortened, contracted tendons are observed.

Ledum Pal – Homeopathic medicine for ankle joint pain in rheumatoid arthritis

Ledum Pal is majorly indicated for ankle joint pain in rheumatoid arthritis. The ankle is swollen. Movement worsens pain. Cold applications may offer some relief in such cases. In addition to this, right-sided hip joint pain also recovers well under Ledum Pal. It is also the Homeopathic remedy for rheumatic pain in joints that start in the feet and then rise upward to the knee or hip.

Sanguinaria Can and Ferrum Met – Homeopathic medicines for shoulder joint pain in rheumatoid arthritis

Sanguinaria Can and Ferrum Met show the most wonderful results in rheumatoid arthritis affecting the shoulder joint. Sanguinaria Can helps right-sided shoulder joint pain. Ferrum Met is most useful for left-sided shoulder joint pain. A person prescribed these medicines will have shoulder pain on raising the arm, which gets worse at night. Marked stiffness is also observed in the shoulder. Homeopathic medicine Ferrum met is best indicated for treating anaemia in rheumatoid arthritis.

Emotional Causes of Osteoarthritis

A report in the Journal of *Chronic Diseases* as long ago as 1964 reviewed the research on personality among those with doctor diagnosed rheumatoid arthritis and found that sufferers tend to be self-sacrificing, **masochistic**, conforming, self-conscious, shy, inhibited, perfectionistic, and interested in sports and games. The *Journal of Psychosomatic Medicine* confirmed these findings more recently, adding that when compared to their non-arthritic siblings, rheumatoid arthritis patients were more nervous, restless, and sensitive to **anger issues**, making them more compliant and solitary.

Those with rheumatoid arthritis are acutely sensitive and aware of their bodies such that their focus is on physical sensations more often than not. “They have a heightened sense of reality that makes them more sensitive to bodily distress”, said one of the lead authors of a study reported in the *Journal of Rheumatology* in 2008. This trait, known as ‘somatic absorption’ was persistent even when other factors such as disease severity, demographics, other illness and psychological distress were considered.

The journal of *Psychotherapy and Psychosomatics* 2009, found that patients who took part in a study where they exchanged feelings and expressed their emotions had lower levels of inflammatory markers in their blood than those who kept their feelings to themselves.

Talking about your feelings has a huge benefit in most chronic diseases including those caused by compromised immune systems. Emotional restriction induces stress, and prolonged stress damages the effectiveness of your immune system. Expressing emotions and sharing feelings releases the body from dealing with the diseases linked to stress, such as auto-immune diseases like rheumatoid arthritis.

Taking Bach Flower Remedies can often help many of these symptoms and help us to relax. Also learning techniques such as the Emotional Freedom Technique is also very helpful, in the same way as meditation, yoga and prayer are all helpful.

Another excellent therapy tool that is easy to self-learn is called Emotional Freedom Technique (EFT). This is defined and described as a clinical procedure for the relief of psychological and physical distress that patients often bring to the attention of nurses. Frequently referred to as "tapping," this technique combines the cognitive reprocessing benefits of exposure and acceptance therapy with the energetic disturbance releases associated with acupuncture and other energy therapies.

More than 60 research articles (Rancour et al, 2015) in peer-reviewed journals report a staggering 98% efficacy rate with the use of this procedure from psychological distress (posttraumatic stress disorder, phobias, anxiety, depression, etc.) to physical conditions (asthma, fibromyalgia, osteoarthritis, pain, seizures).

Summary of Causative Factors

Now that we have looked at the causative factors that holistic medicine examines, let us summarize in brief some of the potential causative factors of RA:

1. *Deficiency of Vital Nutrients.* Joint surfaces are covered with cartilage that must remain smooth, so the bones can move freely. Vitamin C, zinc, copper, manganese, sulphur and other nutrients are needed for maintenance of cartilage. Deficiency of any of these nutrients causes breakdown or slow repair of cartilage surfaces. A deficiency of omega-3 fatty acids found in fish and flaxseed oils can impair joint motion as well.

2. *Calcium Deposits.* Calcium can precipitate or deposit in the joints. This causes pain and stiffness of the joints – taking calcium supplements, or lacking vitamin K would be one of the reasons for calcification of the joints.

3. *Toxic Metals.* Copper, iron, aluminium, mercury and cadmium can deposit in joints, where they can contribute to joint pain and stiffness.

4. *Low Levels of Anti-inflammatory Hormones.* Cortisone and cortisol prevent joint inflammation. Underactivity of the adrenal glands, which produce cortisone, contributes to this type of arthritis. Stiffness and achiness are most noticeable in the morning and the condition improves as the day goes on. Many nutrients such as manganese, boron, vitamins C and E and others are needed by the adrenal glands.

5. *Protein Breakdown or Catabolism.* In this situation, the body consumes its own tissues to burn for energy. Commonly, joint surfaces are affected, and the result is joint pain and inflammation.

6. *An Excess of Pro-inflammatory Hormones, Due to Stress or Nutritional Imbalances.* Pro-inflammatory hormones such as aldosterone tend to increase inflammation in the body that can result in joint pain. Excessive arachadonic acid and other fatty acid imbalances may also contribute to excessive inflammation.

7. *Low Energy.* Normal wear and tear on the joints require constant repair and regeneration. Energy is required to permit repair of joint surfaces. Many people suffer from a low energy level which impairs their ability to properly maintain joint surfaces.

8. *General Toxicity.* High levels of toxins other than heavy metals can also contribute to joint pain and stiffness. These can be organic chemicals, chlorine, solvents and metabolic waste products.

9. *Infections.* Joints can become infected with a wide variety of bacteria, viruses and parasites.

10. *Emotional Causes.* Emotionally charged situations and attitudes of rigidity and anger can contribute to arthritic pain. The mechanism for causing pain and stiffness is usually impairment of the adrenal glands. This in turn causes excessive inflammation.

11. *Structural and Other Causes.* Structural causes include subluxations of bones causing excessive pressure or wear on joints. Other causes may be genetic malformations or other trauma.

Medical Treatment Protocols for RA

The goals of rheumatoid arthritis (RA) treatment are to:

- Stop inflammation (put disease in remission)
- Relieve symptoms
- Prevent joint and organ damage
- Improve physical function and overall well-being
- Reduce long-term complications

One of the most common ways that doctors use to treat RA is by using a variety of different drugs that will most target symptoms but will not alleviate the underlying causative factors. Let us very briefly examine what these drugs are and look at some of their side effects.

- **Nonsteroidal anti-inflammatory drugs (NSAIDs)** are available over-the-counter and by prescription. They are used to help ease arthritis pain and inflammation. NSAIDs include such drugs as ibuprofen, ketoprofen and naproxen sodium, among others. For people who have had or are at risk of stomach ulcers, the doctor may prescribe celecoxib, a type of NSAID called a COX-2 inhibitor, which is designed to be safer for the stomach. These medicines can be taken by mouth or applied to the skin (as a patch or cream) directly to a swollen joint.

- **Corticosteroids**. Corticosteroid medications, including prednisone, prednisolone and methyprednisolone, are potent and quick-acting anti-inflammatory medications. They may be used in RA to get potentially damaging inflammation under control, while waiting for NSAIDs and DMARDs (below) to take effect. Because of the risk of side effects with these drugs, doctors prefer to use them for as short a time as possible and in doses as low as possible.

- **DMARDs**. An acronym for disease-modifying antirheumatic drugs, DMARDs are drugs that work to modify the course of the disease. Traditional DMARDs include methotrexate, hydroxycholorquine, sulfasalazine, leflunomide, cyclophosphamide and azathioprine. These medicines can be taken by mouth, be self-injected or given as an infusion in a doctor's office.

- **Biologics**. These drugs are a subset of DMARDs. Biologics may work more quickly than traditional DMARDs and are injected or given by infusion in a doctor's office. Because they target specific steps in the inflammatory process, they don't wipe out the entire immune response as some other RA treatments do. In many people with RA, a biologic can slow, modify or stop the disease – even when other treatments haven't helped much.

- **JAK inhibitors**. A new subcategory of DMARDs known as "JAK inhibitors" block the Janus kinase, or JAK, pathways, which are involved in the body's immune response. Tofacitinib belongs to this class. Unlike biologics, it can be taken by mouth.

- Surgery – this is usually as a last resort.

Natural Treatments for RA

At the Da Vinci Holistic Health Center in Larnaca, Cyprus, we use a protocol of different treatments for RA. One of the main aims is to identify and eliminate underlying causative factors, and this we do using the IDEL Diagnostic Programme which is a comprehensive diagnostic protocol of functional tests designed to determine a lot of the underlying causative factors discussed in this chapter – see http://www.naturaltherapycenter.com

Let us look at some of the treatments that we use in RA and the reasons behind them.

Glucosamine Sulphate and RA

As important as GS is to healthy cartilage, N-acetyl glucosamine (NAG) is just as important to the extracellular matrix that also helps to comprise our, "cellular cement".

NAG is needed for synthesis of the chondroitin proteoglycans (bigger building blocks) (Biochem J. 1991 Jan; 273(Pt 2): 283-88).

When exogenous GS is given and some is converted to NAG, there are scientists who believe that it is the NAG, "which finally determines the antitoxic and antioxidative properties in this amino sugar" (Eksp Klin Farmakol. 1993. 56(5):53-5).

NAG has the ability to reduce joint pain, swelling, and restricted motion by itself; in fact, the Merck Index puts NAG in an antiarthritic, therapeutic category of its own (p 4353).

A 2007 Japanese study of rheumatoid arthritis patients published in Rheumatology International by Nakamura, H., et al. showed that taking 1500 mg of glucosamine hydrochloride daily for rheumatoid arthritis pain relief significantly improved symptoms according to patient self-evaluation and physician global evaluation. This treatment did not alter measures of inflammation as determined through blood tests. Glucosamine hydrochloride is recommended for rheumatoid arthritis pain relief.

Turmeric and RA

Turmeric (known by its scientific name *Curcuma longa)*, has a long history of use in traditional Indian medicine as a treatment for inflammatory conditions such as RA.

In the study (Chandran et al, 2012) titled, "A randomized, pilot study to assess the efficacy and safety of curcumin patients with active rheumatoid arthritis," forty-five patients diagnosed with RA were randomized into three groups with patients receiving curcumin (500 mg) and diclofenac sodium (50 mg) alone or their combination.

Curcumin is the most thoroughly researched pharmacologically active component of the spice turmeric, and which gives this root its bright, saffron coloured hue. Diclofenac sodium is a non-steroidal anti-inflammatory drug (NSAID) sold under over 100 different trade names throughout the world, e.g. Aclonac, Cataflam, Voltaren.

The primary study endpoints were reduction in Disease Activity Score (DAS) 28. The secondary endpoints included American College of Rheumatology (ACR) criteria for reduction in tenderness and swelling of joint scores.

Remarkably, the researchers found that while patients in all three treatment groups showed statistically significant changes in their DAS scores, the curcumin only group showed the highest percentage of improvement in overall DAS and ACR scores (ACR 20, 50 and 70) and these scores were significantly better than the patients in the diclofenac sodium group. They also noted, "More importantly, curcumin treatment was found to be safe and did not relate with any adverse events." [emphasis added]

They concluded:

Our study provides the first evidence for the safety and superiority of curcumin treatment in patients with active RA and highlights the need for future large-scale trials to validate these findings in patients with RA and other arthritic conditions."

You can also add curcumin to your fruit and vegetable smoothies.

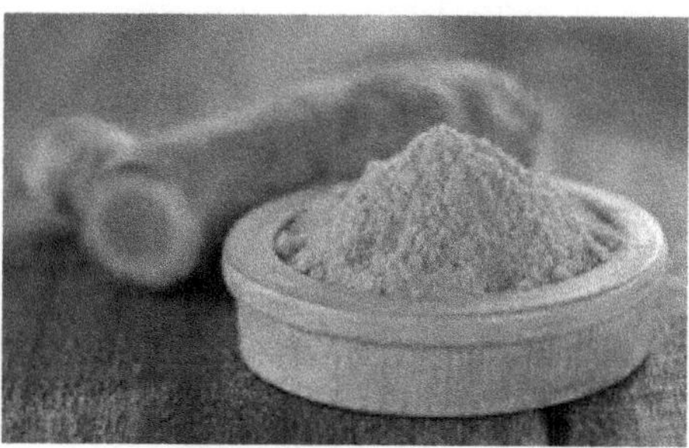

At the Da Vinci Center we recommend taking a high-potency turmeric supplement such as TURMERIC PLUS (10,000 mg) – take one cap x 2 times daily.

Nigella sativa oil (Black cumin oil) and RA
A recent study (Kheirouri et al, 2016) has shown that taking one gram of black cumin seed oil in two divided doses led to improvement in disease activity scores of 28 joints and reduced CD4 (+) CD25 (+) T cell percentage.

Rose Hips and RA
Clinical research has shown that rose hip powder can significantly reduce the severity of symptoms in patients with rheumatoid arthritis.

An estimated 1.5 million adults in the United States suffer from rheumatoid arthritis, a painful and often debilitating autoimmune disorder in which the immune system attacks and even destroys the body's joints, cartilage and bone.

Rheumatoid arthritis is now commonly treated with anti-tumour necrosis factor alpha (anti-TNF) and other drugs that directly target specific molecules in the immune system. But in addition to carrying potential side effects, these drugs are also incredibly expensive. It can cost as much as $16,000 to treat just a single patient for a year with anti-TNF drugs.

In contrast, one year's supply of a rose hip supplement costs just $390.

The most compelling support for rosehips as a rheumatoid arthritis treatment comes from a double-blind study conducted by researchers from the Charite University Medical Centre in Berlin and published in the journal *Phytomedicine* in 2010. The researchers randomly assigned 74 participants (mostly women) to take either 5 grams of encapsulated rose hip powder or a placebo for six months, in addition to their regular rheumatoid arthritis treatments. The participants had suffered from rheumatoid arthritis for an average of more than 18 years.

According to the health assessment questionnaire completed by participants at both the beginning and end of the study, rheumatoid arthritis symptoms significantly improved in the rose hip group but worsened slightly in the placebo group. Likewise, a physicians' assessment found that symptoms improved more in the rose hip group than in the placebo group. No change was observed in the use of pain medication between the two groups.

More specifically, participants in the rose hip group experienced a 20-25 percent improvement in activity and a 40 percent decrease in the number of joints causing discomfort or pain. Placebo participants did not experience any decrease in the number of joints causing discomfort or pain.

These findings suggest that rose hip powder may be a helpful supplemental treatment for rheumatoid arthritis, the researchers concluded. Researcher Kaj Winther suggested that early treatment with rose hip powder may help delay the need for treatment with more expensive drugs.

It remains unclear why rose hips provide relief in rheumatoid arthritis, although it may have something to do with their antioxidant and anti-inflammatory properties. The researchers referred to one of rose hips' active ingredients, the fatty acid GOPO, as a "plant version of fish oil."

"I think we were all surprised to see such meaningful results," researcher Stefan Willich said. "Rheumatoid arthritis is one of the most difficult conditions I'm aware of. It's a tough disease, which makes it all the more remarkable to find such beneficial effects from this remedy."

Cherry juice for arthritis pain

"People with rheumatoid arthritis should include in their daily diets juices high in the anti-inflammatory nutrients," said Cherie Calbom, M.S. Calbom is a certified nutritionist in Kirkland, Washington, and co-author of "Juicing for Life." Calbom adds that parsley, broccoli, and spinach can assist in the treatment of arthritis, since these contain beta-carotene, along with carrots, apples, and ginger, all of which contain copper. She also promotes the drinking of pineapple juice, since it is the only source of the strong anti-inflammatory enzyme bromelain.

Bromelain helps the body breakdown protein. Incomplete protein break down (i.e. poor digestion) is a condition implicated in arthritis. Bromelain also helps break down plaque and fatty tissue deposits that can clog arteries. It also assists in the natural healing of bruises and minor abrasions.

Other juices said to help include bilberry, celery juice, green barley juice, aloe Vera juice, and Boswellia extract.

Not all juices have a positive effect on arthritis symptoms. Spinach juice and spinach itself is bad for arthritis because it contains oxalic acid which can interfere with calcium absorption and exacerbate arthritic symptoms.

Essential Oils for Arthritis

Essential oils are natural plant products that possess anti-oxidant, anti-bacterial, anti-fungal and anti-inflammatory properties (Agarwal and Rangari, 2003; Burt, 2004; Kordali et al., 2005).

Essential oils from ginger, orange and black cumin have been shown to hold promise for the relief of symptoms of arthritis (Osborn et al., 2001; Tekeoglu et al., 2007; Yip and Tam, 2008). Essential oils and their components are rapidly absorbed through the skin and are detectable in plasma after topical application (Jaeger, 1992).

Therefore, topical dermal delivery of essential oils represents an effective method to directly deliver a natural, anti-inflammatory agent to the site of inflammation.

How do essential oils work? Essential oils and their components are rapidly absorbed through the skin and are detectable in plasma after topical application. Therefore, topical dermal delivery of essential oils represents an effective method to directly provide a natural, anti-inflammatory agent to the site of inflammation.

The U.S. National Library of Medicine shares this report and notes a study that used topical application of an ointment containing essential oils that decreased the severity of arthritis. Furthermore, this suppression of arthritis involved changes in the disease-related immunological and biochemical mediators of inflammation (Komeh-Nkrumah et al, 2011).

Here are the five most beneficial essential oils for arthritis:

1. **Ginger**

Ginger essential oil is an amazing healing agent that contains chemicals with analgesic and anti-inflammatory effects on the body. It's been shown to help lessen pain associated with arthritis, making it a great pain reliever. It provides this relief by acting on vanilloid receptors, which are located on sensory nerve endings.

Ginger has that slight burning sensation like the initial intense burning feel you get when you consume spicy pepper. While it typically only lasts a few seconds, researchers discovered that it affects the pain pathways directly and rather rapidly in most cases, relieving the inflammation, which in itself causes pain.

The Arthritis Foundation reports a study from the University of Miami that concluded that ginger extract could be a substitute to non-steroidal anti-inflammatory drugs (NSAIDs).

The study compared the effects of a highly concentrated ginger extract to placebo in 247 patients with osteoarthritis of the knee. The ginger reduced pain and stiffness in knee joints by 40 percent over the placebo., which is a very significant difference.

Researchers at the University of California, Los Angeles showed that ginger affects certain inflammatory processes at a cellular level. Ginger has anti-inflammatory, anti-ulcer and antioxidant activities, as well as a small amount of analgesic properties, making it a great option for arthritis sufferers. (6) It is best to take GINGER capsules – 100 – 200mg daily for about 6 weeks to get the benefits.

2. Turmeric

The most active ingredient in turmeric, curcumin, has become known as a great anti-inflammatory. Turmeric benefits include being highly effective at helping people manage rheumatoid arthritis.

A recent study out of Japan evaluated its relationship with interleukin (IL)-6, the inflammatory cytokine known to be involved in the RA process and discovered that curcumin significantly reduced inflammation. This evidence suggests that regular turmeric use could be a powerful way to combat the development of RA (Wada et al, 2014).

3. Frankincense

Frankincense oil can inhibit the production of key inflammatory molecules associated with conditions like arthritis and can be useful in helping to prevent the breakdown of the cartilage tissue. This has been shown to significantly reduce levels of inflammation, making it a natural treatment option for pain-related conditions that affect the muscles, joints and tendons (Blain et al, 2010).

4. Myrrh

Myrrh oil also had anti-inflammatory properties, and it's often used in tandem to treat arthritis. A study published in *Scientific Reports* showed that frankincense and myrrh are highly effective in treatment of inflammatory diseases, especially when combined.

The study revealed that frankincense and myrrh, especially when used together, help suppress inflammation and the intensity of joint inflammation. Results showed that the individual extract of frankincense or myrrh and combined extracts used to treat groups showed significant differences when compared with the arthritis control group (Shulan Su et al, 2015).

5. Orange

Citrus scents make you feel more awake, and the strong anti-inflammatory properties of orange oil have been researched in regard to their effects for helping fight pain.

A 2009 study published in the *European Journal of Medical Research* investigated the antioxidant potential of various essential oils, reporting that orange was the most highly effective of those studied, which in turn makes it a great essential oil for arthritis treatment (Rantzsch et al, 2009).

Try diluting a few drops of the orange essential oil with 1 teaspoon of avocado or almond oil, and then rub it onto the back of your hand or wherever you have arthritic pain.

How to Use Essential Oils for Arthritis

There are several ways you can use essential oils for arthritis.

To help relieve pain and inflammation while improving your sleep, put a diffuser by your bed and diffuse essential oils while you sleep. You can also rub topically, when blended with a carrier oil (almond oil), directly onto the area where you feel the pain. Be careful to avoid the eyes.

Risks of Essential Oils for Arthritis

Use any essential oils sparingly, whether internally or topically. High levels might cause reactions and sensitivity, so be sure to do a skin patch check before using on a regular basis. You also want to use caution if you take blood pressure medications or have an existing heart condition. Always talk to your doctor before beginning any new treatment.

It's important to make sure that any essential oils you choose are 100 percent pure. If you're pregnant or breastfeeding, check with your doctor first. While most oils are safe for children, please do proper research and review with your physician.

Low Impact Aerobic Exercise

People who have rheumatoid arthritis and exercise regularly will experience less pain, improved sleep, have more energy and better day to day function compared to those who do not exercise. There are several exercises which can be helpful to patients of rheumatoid arthritis. These exercises help in reducing pain that is experienced and making the patients flexible causing a reduction in stiffness. Some of these exercises include:

i. **Low impact aerobic exercises**

These exercises are good for people with rheumatoid arthritis. This is because these kinds of exercises put minimal impact on the affected joints. Some of these exercises include walking, water exercises, low impact aerobic dance and stationery bicycle.

Exercises that have sudden stops, changes in direction such as basketball and soccer are not appropriate. In cases where you have no knee ankle and hip problems jogging can also be helpful.

ii. **Stretching exercises**

You can start by stretching before starting your exercise. This helps in preparing the muscles and joints for the activity. For example, if you are going to jog you can stretch your knees, hips and ankles. You can also do stretching after you are done with the exercise. This helps in preventing stiffness. You can also improvise some form of exercises that can help in reducing stiffness joints that experience limited motion.

iii. **Tai Chi**

Tai Chi is an ancient Chinese practice that usually involve sets of slow flowing movements and this form of practice usually emphasize on mental focus, physical motions and regular breathing. Tai Chi is designed to improve the quality of life, sense of relaxation and mobility. Patients of rheumatoid arthritis can benefit from this exercise because it reduces stiffness and improves strength and balance.

iv. Resistance exercises

Resistance exercises help in strengthening the muscles. Strengthening the muscles can be done using resistance tools such as free weight, elastic bands and machines. In resistance exercises some may be better than others this is usually because of needs of the patients. For example, free weights can be better than machines; this is because they don't force the joints into a specific predetermined movement pattern.

v. Weight-bearing exercises

Patients of rheumatoid arthritis have a high risk of bone thinning. This condition can result to osteoporosis and can also be caused by the medication used to treat rheumatoid arthritis. Weight bearing exercises can be helpful in preserving bones. An example of a good weight bearing exercise is walking.

vi. Swimming

Swimming helps people who have rheumatoid arthritis to reduce the amount of stress on the joints. This is because water supports the body. Walking in a pool can also be helpful. The efforts you put while trying to walk in the water makes your muscles strong. You can do this by walking in water that is up to your waist or chest or you can alternatively put on a flotation belt then walk in deep end water.

Before you start any kind of exercise you should get the right intensity. You can talk with your physical therapist or a trainer who has experience helping people with rheumatoid arthritis so that you can know what is best for you. Generally, people with rheumatoid arthritis should avoid exercising too hard.

You should also choose an exercise that you enjoy. This will help you not to miss exercises on days you are supposed to exercise.

You should find an appropriate time when to exercise. This will help you to establish a routine and get you great benefits. You can also schedule your exercise depending with your condition. For the people who have morning stiffness, exercising in the morning can be helpful. For people who have fatigue breaking up the exercise time into several bouts can help you manage the exercise. If you experience symptoms during the night you should avoid exercising less than two hours before sleep time. Stretching and relaxation exercises can help you to get sleep.

You should also be aware of the changes of your symptoms. You will need more rest during the times when you experience more joint pain and stiffness.

You can do your exercises at your preferred place. Some people will prefer doing their exercises in places where they are alone while others will prefer having it in a community gym. A community gym can be a better place because you can get support from an instructor.

Starting a regular exercise program can be challenging but understanding the benefits of the exercise can be helpful in motivating you to do the exercises. You should also set goals. These goals should be realistic. You can also reward yourself when you achieve them. Keeping a chart to check your progress can also be helpful. Exercises you are involved in should be convenient, fun and relatively inexpensive.

References

Agarwal RB, Rangari VD. Phytochemical investigation and evaluation of anti-inflammatory and anti-arthritic activities of essential oil of Strobilanthus ixiocephala Benth. Indian J Exp Biol. 2003;41(8):890–4. [PubMed]

Aho K, Kaipiainen-Seppanen O, Heliovaara M, Klaukka T: Epidemiology of rheumatoid arthritis in Finland. Semin Arthritis Rheum. 1998, 27: 325-334.PubMedView ArticleGoogle Scholar

Ala, S., Shokrzadeh, M., Shoja, A. M. and Saravi, S. S., 2009. Pak. J. biol. Sci., 12: 1041-1044. Alegre, C., Baro, J. and Obach, J., 1984. Arthritis Rheum., 27: 1073-1074.

Baka Z, Buzás E, Nagy G (2009) Rheumatoid arthritis and smoking: putting the pieces together. Arthritis Res Ther 11: 238.

Balbir-Gurman, A; Bianca Fuhrman, Yolanda Braun-Moscovici, Doron Markovits, Michael Aviram. Consumption of pomegranate decreases serum oxidative stress and reduces disease activity in patients with active rheumatoid arthritis: a pilot study. Isr Med Assoc J. *2011 Aug ;13(8):474-9.* PMID: 21910371

Binu Chandran, Ajay Goel. A randomized, pilot study to assess the efficacy and safety of curcumin in patients with active rheumatoid arthritis. Phytother Res. 2012 Nov;26(11):1719-25. doi: 10.1002/ptr.4639. Epub 2012 Mar 9.

Blain EJ, Ali AY, Duance VC. Boswellia frereana (frankincense) suppresses cytokine-induced matrix metalloproteinase expression and production of pro-inflammatory molecules in articular cartilage. Phytother Res. 2010 Jun;24(6):905-12.

Brighton SW, de la Harpe AL, van Staden DJ, Badenhorst JH, Myers OL: The prevalence of rheumatoid arthritis in a rural African population. J Rheumatol. 1988, 15: 405-408.PubMedGoogle Scholar

Burt S. Essential oils: their antibacterial properties and potential applications in foods--a review. Int J Food Microbiol. 2004;94(3):223–53. [PubMed]

Carmona L, Villaverde V, Hernandez-Garcia C, Ballina J, Gabriel R, Laffon A: The prevalence of rheumatoid arthritis in the general population of Spain. Rheumatology. 2002, 41: 88-95. 10.1093/rheumatology/41.1.88.PubMedView ArticleGoogle Scholar

Cecchetti, S; Zuzana Tatar, Pilar Galan, Bruno Pereira, Céline Lambert, Gael Mouterde, Angela Sutton, Martin Soubrier, Maxime Dougados. Prevalence of vitamin D deficiency in rheumatoid arthritis and association with disease activity and cardiovascular risk factors: data from the COMEDRA study. Clin Exp Rheumatol. *2016 Sep 30. Epub 2016 Aug 30.* PMID: 27749232

Chandrashekara, S; Anand Patted. Role of vitamin D supplementation in improving disease activity in rheumatoid arthritis: An exploratory study. Int J Rheum Dis. *2015 Oct 20. Epub 2015 Oct 20.* PMID: 26481198

Dans LF, TankehTorres S, Amante CM, Penserga EG: The prevalence of rheumatic diseases in a Filipino urban population: a WHO-ILAR COPCORD study. J Rheumatol. 1997, 24: 1814-1819.PubMedGoogle Scholar

Darlington LG, Ramsey NW. Review of dietary therapy for rheumatoid arthritis. Br J Rheumatol. 1993 Jun;32(6):507-14.

Dawczynski, C; M Dittrich, T Neumann, K Goetze, A Welzel, P Oelzner, S Völker, A M Schaible, F Troisi, L Thomas, S Pace, A Koeberle, O Werz, P Schlattmann, S Lorkowski, G Jahreis. Docosahexaenoic acid in the treatment of rheumatoid arthritis: A double-blind, placebo-controlled, randomized cross-over study with microalgae vs. sunflower oil. Clin Nutr. *2017 Mar 6. Epub 2017 Mar 6.* PMID: 28302406

DeChristopher, LR; J Uribarri, K L Tucker. Intake of high-fructose corn syrup sweetened soft drinks, fruit drinks and apple juice is associated with prevalent arthritis in US adults, aged 20-30 years. Nutr Diabetes. *2016 ;6:e199. Epub 2016 Mar 7.* PMID: 26950480

de Jong, H J I; O H Klungel, L van Dijk, R J Vandebriel, H G M Leufkens, Jw van der Laan, J W Cohen Tervaert, H van Loveren. Use of statins is associated with an increased risk of rheumatoid arthritis. Ann Rheum Dis. *2011 Oct 6. Epub 2011 Oct 6.* PMID: 21979000 del Puente A, Knowler WC, Pettit DJ, Bennett PH: High incidence and prevalence of rheumatoid arthritis in Pima Indians. Am J Epidemiol. 1989, 129: 1170-1178.PubMedGoogle Scholar

Doran MF, Pond GR, Crowson CS, O'Fallon WM, Gabriel SE. Trends in incidence and mortality in rheumatoid arthritis in Rochester, Minnesota, over a forty-year period. Arthritis Rheum 2002;46:625-31.3.

Deutsch, L; Evaluation of the effect of Neptune Krill Oil on chronic inflammation and arthritic symptoms. Am J Gastroenterol. *2005 Dec;100(12):2674-80.* PMID: 17353582

Drasar B S, Shiner M, McLeod G M. Studies on the intestinal flora. I. The bacterial flora of the gastrointestinal tract in healthy and achlorhydric persons. Gastroenterology 1969;56:71-9

Gabriel SE, Crowson CS, O'Fallon WM: The epidemiology of rheumatoid arthritis in Rochester, Minnesota, 1955–1985. Arthritis Rheum. 1999, 42: 415-420. 10.1002/1529-0131(199904)42:3<415::AID-ANR4>3.0.CO;2-Z.PubMedView ArticleGoogle Scholar

Gabriel SE: The epidemiology of rheumatoid arthritis. Rheum Dis Clin North Am. 2001, 27: 269-281.PubMedView ArticleGoogle Scholar

Geier, DA; Mark R Geier. A case-control study of serious autoimmune adverse events following hepatitis B immunization. Autoimmunity. *2005 Jun;38(4):295-301.* PMID: 16206512

George, MD; Joshua F. Bake. The Obesity Epidemic and Consequences for Rheumatoid Arthritis Care. Curr Rheumatol Rep. 2016 Jan; 18(1): 6.

Ghavipour, M; G Sotoudeh, E Tavakoli, K Mowla, J Hasanzadeh, Z Mazloom. Pomegranate extract alleviates disease activity and some blood biomarkers of inflammation and oxidative stress in Rheumatoid Arthritis patients. Eur J Clin Nutr. *2016 Aug 31. Epub 2016 Aug 31.* PMID: 27577177

Gibofsky A. Overview of epidemiology, pathophysiology, and diagnosis of rheumatoid arthritis. Am J Manag Care 2012;18:S295-302.

Gray J D A, Shiner M. Influence of gastric pH on gastric and jejunal flora. Gut 1967; 8: 574-81. 29 Giannella R A, Broitman S A, Zamcheck N. Gastric acid barrier to ingested microorganisms in man: studies in vivo and in vitro. Gut 1972; 13: 251-6.
Bennett J C. The infectious etiology of rheumatoid arthritis. Arthritis Rheum 1978; 21: 531-8.

Hakkinen, A. Arthritis and Rheumatism, March 2001; vol 44(3): pp 515-522.

Hakkinen, A. Current Opinion in Rheumatology, March 2004, 16(2): 132-137.

Hannson, L., Hunnan-Seppala, A. and Mattila, A., 1978. Scand. J. Rheumatol., 7: 237-240.

Harrison BJ, Silman AJ, Wiles NJ, Scott DG, Symmons DP: The association of cigarette smoking with disease outcome in patients with early inflammatory polyarthritis. Arthritis Rheum. 2001, 44: 323-330. 10.1002/1529-0131(200102)44:2<323::AID-ANR49>3.3.CO;2-3.PubMedView ArticleGoogle Scholar

Harvey J, Lotze M, Stevens MB, Lambert G, Jacobson D: Rheumatoid arthritis in a Chippewa band. I. Pilot screening study of disease prevalence. Arthritis Rheum. 1981, 24: 717-721.PubMedView ArticleGoogle Scholar

Hutchinson D, Shepstone L, Moots R, Lear JT, Lynch MP: Heavy cigarette smoking is strongly associated with rheumatoid arthritis (RA), particularly in patients without a family history of RA. Ann Rheum Dis. 2001, 60: 223-227. 10.1136/ard.60.3.223.PubMedPubMed CentralView ArticleGoogle Scholar

Helmick CG, Felson DT, Lawrence RC, et al. Estimates of the prevalence of arthritis and other rheumatic conditions in the United States. Part I. Arthritis Rheum 2008;58:15-25.

Jacobsson LT, Hanson RL, Knowler WC, Pillemer S, Pettitt DJ, McCance DR, Bennett PH: Decreasing incidence and prevalence of rheumatoid arthritis in Pima Indians over a 25 year period. Arthritis Rheum. 1994, 37: 1158-1165.PubMedView ArticleGoogle Scholar

Jaeger W. Horner's law. The first step in the history of the understanding of X-linked disorders. Ophthalmic Paediatr Genet. 1992;13(2):49–56. [PubMed]

Kernbauer, Yi Ding, Ken Cadwell.An enteric virus can replace the beneficial function of commensal bacteria Elisabeth. Nature, 2014.

Khojah, HM; Sameh Ahmed, Mahran S Abdel-Rahman, Al-Badr Hamza. Reactive oxygen and nitrogen species in patients with rheumatoid arthritis as potential biomarkers for disease activity and the role of antioxidants. Free Radic Biol Med. *2016 Jun 21 ;97:285-291. Epub 2016 Jun 21.* PMID: 27344969

Kordali S, Kotan R, Mavi A, Cakir A, Ala A, Yildirim A. Determination of the chemical composition and antioxidant activity of the essential oil of Artemisia dracunculus and of the antifungal and antibacterial activities of Turkish Artemisia absinthium, A. dracunculus, Artemisia santonicum, and Artemisia spicigera essential oils. J Agric Food Chem. 2005;53(24):9452–8.[PubMed]

Kremer JM: n-3 fatty acid supplements in rheumatoid arthritis. Am J Clin Nutr. 2000, 71 (Suppl): 349S-351S.PubMedGoogle Scholar

Lehmann, I., Sack, U. and Lahmann, J., 2011. Met. Ions Life Sci., 8: 157-185.

Leirisalo-Repo, M. Curr Opin Rheumatol. Early arthritis and infection. 2005 Jul;17(4):433-9.

MacGregor AJ, Snieder H, Rigby AS, et al. Characterizing the quantitative genetic contribution to rheumatoid arthritis using data from twins. Arthritis Rheum 2000;43:30-7.
Munneke, M., Arthritis and Rheumatism, June 15, 2005; vol 53(3): pp 410-417.

Marcolongo R, Bayeli P F, Montagnani M. Gastrointestinal involvement in rheumatoid arthritis: a biopsy study. _ Rheumatol 1979; 6: 163-73.

Naveh, Y., Schapira, D., Ravel, Y., Geller, E. and Scharf, Y., 1997. J. Rheumatol., 24: 643-646.

O'Connor M P, Nunes D P, Marin P, Keane C P, Weir D G, Casey E B. Small bowel flora in rheumatoid arthritis. Br Rheumatol 1989; 28 (suppl 2): 113.

Osborn CE, Barlas P, Baxter GD, Barlow JH. Aromatherapy: a survey of current practice in the management of rheumatic disease symptoms. Complement Ther Med. 2001;9(2):62–7. [PubMed]

Paffenbarger, R., New England Journal of Medicine, March 6, 1986; vol 314(10): pp 605-613.

Parks, CG; Jane A Hoppin, Anneclaire J DeRoos, Karen H Costenbader, Michael C Alavanja, Dale P Sandler. Rheumatoid Arthritis in Agricultural Health Study Spouses: Associations with Pesticides and Other Farm Exposures. Environ Health Perspect. *2016 Jun 10. Epub 2016 Jun 10.* PMID: 27285288

Peltonen, R; M Nenonen, T Helve, O Hänninen, P Toivanen, E Eerola. Faecal microbial flora and disease activity in rheumatoid arthritis during a vegan diet. Rheumatology (Oxford) (1997) 36 (1): 64-68.

Plenge RM. The genetic basis of rheumatoid arthritis. In: Hochberg MC, Silman AJ, Smolen JS, Weinblatt ME, Weisman MH, eds. Rheumatoid Arthritis. Philadelphia, Penn: Mosby Elsevier; 2009:23-27.

Rantzsch, U, G Vacca, R Dück, A Gillissen. Anti-inflammatory effects of myrtol standardized and other essential oils on alveolar macrophages from patients with chronic obstructive pulmonary disease. Eur J Med Res. 2009; 14(Suppl 4): 205–209.

de Jong, Z. Arthritis and Rheumatism, September 2003; vol 48(9): pp 2415-2424.

Riise T, Jacobsen BK, Gran JT: Incidence and prevalence of rheumatoid arthritis in the county of Troms, northern Norway. J Rheumatol. 2000, 27: 1386-1389.PubMedGoogle Scholar

Scudder, P. R., Al-Timimi, D., Zoob, B. C. and Dormandy, D. L., 1978. Ann. Rheum. Dis., 37: 67-70.

Shichikawa K, Inoue K, Hirota S, Maeda A, Ota H, Kimura M, Ushiyama T, Tsujimoto M: Changes in the incidence and prevalence of rheumatoid arthritis in Kamitonda, Wakayama, Japan, 1965–1996. Ann Rheum Dis. 1999, 58: 751-756.PubMedPubMed CentralView ArticleGoogle Scholar

Scher JU, Sczesnak A, Longman RS, Segata N, Ubeda C, Bielski C, Rostron T, Cerundolo V, Pamer EG, Abramson SB, Huttenhower C, Littman DR. Expansion of intestinal Prevotella copri correlates with enhanced susceptibility to arthritis. Elife. 2013 Nov 5;2:e01202. .

Silman AJ, Hochberg MC. Descriptive epidemiology of rheumatoid arthritis. In: Hochberg MC, Silman AJ, Smolen JS, Weinblatt ME, Weisman MH, eds. Rheumatoid Arthritis. Philadelphia, Penn: Mosby Elsevier; 2009:15-22.

Silman AJ, Pearson JE. Epidemiology and genetics of rheumatoid arthritis. Arthritis Res 2002;4 Suppl 3:S265-72.

Silman AJ, Ollier W, Holligan S, Birrell F, Adebajo A, Asuzu MC, Thomson W, Pepper L: Absence of rheumatoid arthritis in a rural Nigerian population. J Rheumatol. 1993, 20: 618-622.PubMedGoogle Scholar

Silman AJ, Enzer I, Knowler W, Dunn G, Jacobsson L: Strong influence of period of birth on the occurrence of rheumatoid factor: results from a 30 year follow-up study on Pima Indians [abstract]. Arthritis Rheum. 2000, 43 (Suppl): 605-Google Scholar

Silman AJ, Hochberg MC: Rheumatoid arthritis. In Epidemiology of the Rheumatic Diseases. Edited by: Edited by AJ Silman, MC Hochberg. 2001, Oxford: Oxford University Press;, 31-71.Google Scholar

Simopoulos AP (2008) The importance of the omega-6/omega-3 fatty acid ratio in cardiovascular disease and other chronic diseases. Exp Biol Med (Maywood) 233: 674-688.

Sorayya Kheirouri, Vahid Hadi, Mohammad Alizadeh. Immunomodulatory Effect of Nigella sativa Oil on T Lymphocytes in Patients with Rheumatoid Arthritis. Immunol Invest. *2016 May ;45(4):271-83. Epub 2016 Apr 21.* PMID: 27100726

Steva A. Komeh-Nkrumah, Siddaraju M. Nanjundaiah, Rajesh Rajaiah, Hua Yu, Kamal D. Moudgil. Topical dermal application of essential oils attenuates the severity of adjuvant arthritis in Lewis rats. Published online 2011. Phytother Res. 2012 Jan; 26(1): 54–59.

Svetlana Fischer, Nancy Agmon-Levin, Yinon Shapira, Bat-Sheva Porat Katz, Eduard Graell, Ricard Cervera, Ljudmila Stojanovich, Jose A Gómez Puerta, Raimon Sanmartí, Yehuda Shoenfeld. Toxoplasma gondii: bystander or cofactor in rheumatoid arthritis. Immunol Res. *2013 Jul ;56(2-3):287-92.* PMID: 23553228

Symmons DPM, Bankhead CR, Harrison BJ, Brennan P, Barrett EM, Scott DGI, Silman AJ: Blood transfusion, smoking, and obesity as risk factors for the development of rheumatoid arthritis: results from a primary care-based incident case-control study in Norfolk, England. Arthritis Rheum. 1997, 40: 1955-1961.PubMedView ArticleGoogle Scholar

Symmons, DP; K Chakravarty. Can immunisation trigger rheumatoid arthritis? Ann Rheum Dis. 1993 Dec; 52(12): 843–844.

Shulan Su, Jinao Duan, Ting Chen, Xiaochen Huang, Erxin Shang, Li Yu, Kaifeng Wei, Yue Zhu, Jianming Guo, Sheng Guo, Pei Liu, Dawei Qian, Yuping Tang. Frankincense and myrrh suppress inflammation via regulation of the metabolic profiling and the MAPK signalling pathway. Sci Rep. 2015; 5: 13668.

Stenstrom, C., Arthritis Care Research, December 1994; vol 7(4): pp 190-197.
van Vugt RM, Rijken PJ, et al. Antioxidant intervention in rheumatoid arthritis: results of an open pilot study,", Clin Rheumatol, 2008 Feb 15.

Tekeoglu I, Dogan A, Ediz L, Budancamanak M, Demirel A. Effects of thymoquinone (volatile oil of black cumin) on rheumatoid arthritis in rat models. Phytother Res. 2007;21(9):895–7. [PubMed]

Volker D, Fitzgerald P, Major G, Garg M: Efficacy of fish oil concentrate in the treatment of rheumatoid arthritis. J Rheumatol. 2000, 27: 2343-2346.PubMedGoogle Scholar

Vieira VM, Hart JE, Webster TF, Weinberg J, Puett R, Laden F, Costenbader KH, Karlson EW. Association between residences in U.S. northern latitudes and rheumatoid arthritis: A spatial analysis of the Nurses' Health Study. Environ Health Perspect. 2010 Jul;118(7):957-61.

Wada TT, Araki Y, Sato K, Aizaki Y, Yokota K, Kim YT, Oda H, Kurokawa R, Mimura T. Aberrant histone acetylation contributes to elevated interleukin-6 production in rheumatoid arthritis synovial fibroblasts. Biochem Biophys Res Commun. 2014 Feb 21;444(4):682-6

Yazar, M., Sarban, S., Kocyigit, A. and Isikan, U. E., 2005. Biol. Trace Elem. Res., 106:123- 132.

Yip YB, Tam AC. An experimental study on the effectiveness of massage with aromatic ginger and orange essential oil for moderate-to-severe knee pain among the elderly in Hong Kong. Complement Ther Med. 2008;16(3):131–8. [PubMed]

Zeng Q, Huang S, Chen R: 10-year epidemiological study on rheumatic diseases in Shantou area. Zhonghua Nei Ke Za Zhi. 1997, 36: 193-197.PubMedGoogle Scholar

Chapter 2

The Holistic Model of Health

I am certain that everybody reading this book will have come across the term "Holistic medicine" at some point in time. There is considerable confusion about the meaning of holistic. If you have ever entered a discussion about Holistic medicine, you will see that everybody has their own opinion. This is not surprising, since there are no accepted standard definitions for Holistic medicine. Most people use the term as a synonym for alternative therapies; basically, meaning that they are turning away from any conventional medical options and using alternative treatment exclusively. This is incorrect.

Holistic medicine means taking into consideration the complete person - physically, psychologically, socially, and spiritually - in the management and prevention of disease. It is underpinned by the concept that there is a link between our physical health and our more general 'well-being'. A Holistic approach means that the doctor is informed about a patient's whole life situation (Strandberg et al, 2007).

In the Holistic approach to medicine, there is the belief that our well-being relies not just on what is going on in our body physically in terms of illness or disease, but also on our psychological, emotional, social, spiritual and environmental state. These different states are equally important. They should be managed together so that a person is treated. In fact, some feel that the word holistic should really be spelt 'wholistic'.

Holistic medicine needs to look at the whole person; how they interact with their environment and the people around them. It needs diagnostic and therapeutic tools to examine and balance the physical, nutritional, environmental, psychological, emotional, social and spiritual levels of health. It therefore encompasses all modalities of diagnosis and treatment, including allopathic medicine using drugs and surgery if there are no other safer alternatives.

The goal of Holistic medicine is to use all diagnostic and treatment modalities available to optimize the health of the person on all levels of well-being, without doing harm to the person. It is the optimization of all resources to bring about a cure in the person, no matter what school or modality they belong to. Holistic medicine treats symptoms, but also looks for underlying causes of these symptoms.

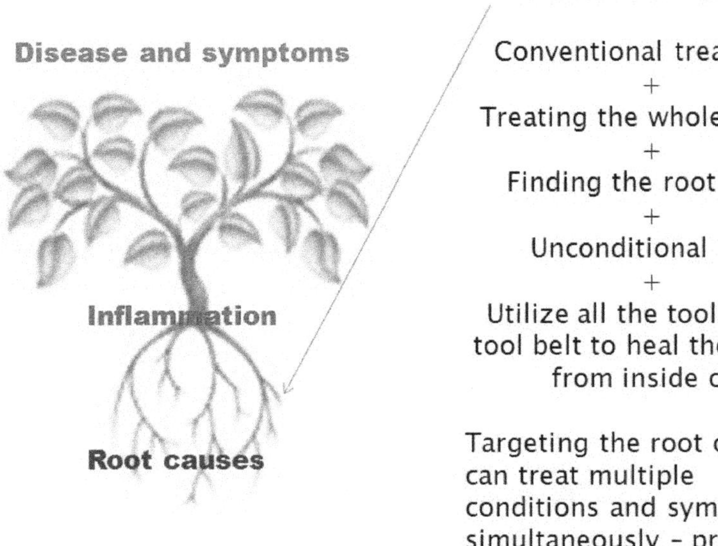

Research in Australia demonstrated that one of the reasons so many Australians seek out alternative and complementary medicine is because of the Holistic philosophy which guides their work. Conversely, it is also the reason why many Australians are becoming less enthusiastic about western or conventional medicine. They see it as non-holistic in nature (Hassed, 2004).

Holistic medicine is something that alternative medicine practitioners traditionally use as a basis for their treatments. However, it is a common misconception that holistic medicine is just 'alternative' or 'complementary' medicine. It is true though, that holistic medicine allows for a wider range of treatment approaches to be used together and encourages open-mindedness for these different approaches.

Some of these approaches may include the use of complementary and alternative medicine, but holistic medicine does not dismiss conventional medicine. It uses conventional medicine as part of the treatment approach. Nutrition, exercise, homeopathy, prayer, acupuncture and meditation are just a few other treatments that may be used together with conventional medicine as part of a Holistic approach.

There are several diagrams (Fig 1) that have tried to explain the multimodal approach of Holistic medicine. Perhaps one of the oldest was developed in the 1980's by Dr. Dietrich Klinghardt,[2] one of the leading proponents of Holistic medicine that has provided many tools for practitioners in this field.

The physical body is at the lowest level and is the foundation upon which everything else rests. This is the level that interests medical doctors as well as natural medicine practitioners such as herbal medicine, nutritionists and chiropractors.

On the second level is the electromagnetic body – it is the summation of all electric and magnetic events caused by the neuronal activity of the nervous system. This level is generally not examined by medical practitioners as it requires different tools to access this electromagnetic body. Acupuncturists tap into the meridians and chakras that are part of this second level.

The third-level body is called the "Mental body" and consists of our conscious and subconscious thoughts, attitudes and beliefs. This is where psychotherapists will work, but there are also other natural medicine healing modalities such as homeopathy, applied psychoneuro-biology and meditation that can access this level.

On the fourth level, the "Intuitive body", is the level beyond our level of consciousness; the level of the unconscious, meditative state and trance state. Hypnotherapy, regression therapy and Hellinger's Family Constellation therapy can access this level.

The fifth level, the "Soul", is perhaps the most profound level and the one that is least accessed by therapists of all kinds. It is the level where we are at one with a Higher Consciousness, a Higher Power, God. Prayer and the Spiritual aspects of religion can access this level.

It is generally believed that the first three levels belong to the personal realm, meaning the individual detached from others. The fourth and fifth levels belong to the transpersonal realm, meaning that these are levels that relate to our relationships with others. The lower levels generally supply energy to the higher levels, but the higher levels have an organizing influence on the lower levels.

---

2 http://www.klinghardtacademy.com

The premise of Holistic medicine is to attempt to treat the whole patient on all levels, as opposed to just the symptoms. Often a complaint such as migraines may have a myriad of different causes in each patient – so there is no standard therapy for migraines as the cause would be different in each person. Therefore, it is important to consider all the causative factors for each person, and ultimately treating the *patient* and not the *disease* per se. It appears that this wise statement made by Hippocrates, the Father of medicine, has been forgotten by modern medicine! Instead of looking at the person and trying to understand **WHY** they have the bunch of symptoms that make up their diagnosis, we consume ourselves with LABELLING the disease and suppressing its symptoms, when we should clearly be looking for its root causes.

"It is more important to know what sort of PERSON has the disease, than to know what sort of DISEASE a person has" (Hippocrates, 500 BC)

We can extrapolate from this that Holistic medicine is based on a "health-care system" and not a "disease-care system". It encompasses preventative medicine by attempting to catch developing health issues early on, instead of waiting until they reach pathological parameters. **Optimizing health should be the ultimate goal of all Holistic medicine practitioners.**

Often Holistic medicine is not interested in labelling the disease itself because this rarely gives information regarding the causes of the symptoms the person is suffering with. Holistic medicine should first identify the causes of the symptoms, which are the body's way of "talking" to the practitioner, without necessarily being overly concerned with the "diagnosis."

This can be clearly illustrated when a person goes to their medical doctor with bowel distension and pain after eating, as well as bouts of intermittent diarrhoea and constipation. The doctor diagnoses Irritable Bowel Syndrome (IBS) and usually gives antispasmodic medication to alleviate the symptoms.

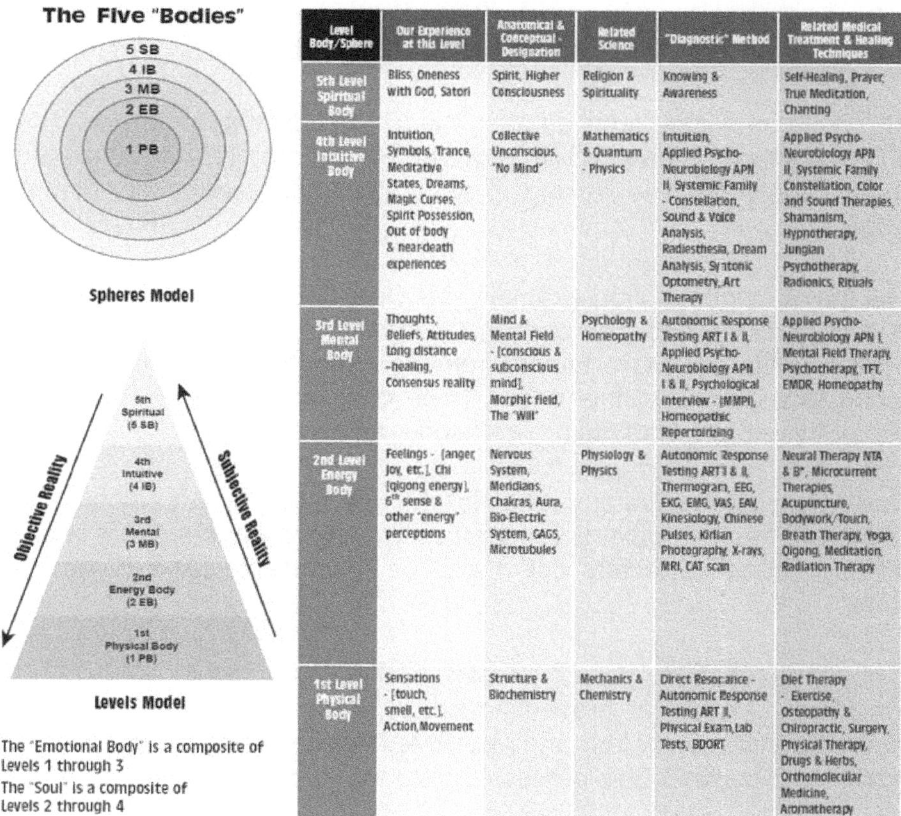

Level Body/Sphere	Our Experience at this Level	Anatomical & Conceptual - Designation	Related Science	"Diagnostic" Method	Related Medical Treatment & Healing Techniques
5th Level Spiritual Body	Bliss, Oneness with God, Satori	Spirit, Higher Consciousness	Religion & Spirituality	Knowing & Awareness	Self-Healing, Prayer, True Meditation, Chanting
4th Level Intuitive Body	Intuition, Symbols, Trance, Meditative States, Dreams, Magic Curses, Spirit Possession, Out of body & near-death experiences	Collective Unconscious, "No Mind"	Mathematics & Quantum - Physics	Intuition, Applied Psycho-Neurobiology APN II, Systemic Family - Constellation, Sound & Voice Analysis, Radiesthesia, Dream Analysis, Syntonic Optometry, Art Therapy	Applied Psycho-Neurobiology APN II, Systemic Family Constellation, Color and Sound Therapies, Shamanism, Hypnotherapy, Jungian Psychotherapy, Radionics, Rituals
3rd Level Mental Body	Thoughts, Beliefs, Attitudes, Long distance -healing, Consensus reality	Mind & Mental Field - [conscious & subconscious mind], Morphic field, The "Will"	Psychology & Homeopathy	Autonomic Response Testing ART I & II, Applied Psycho-Neurobiology APN I & II, Psychological interview - [MMPI], Homeopathic Repertorizing	Applied Psycho-Neurobiology APN I, Mental Field Therapy, Psychotherapy, TFT, EMDR, Homeopathy
2nd Level Energy Body	Feelings - [anger, joy, etc.], Chi [qigong energy], 6th sense & other "energy" perceptions	Nervous System, Meridians, Chakras, Aura, Bio-Electric System, GAGS, Microtubules	Physiology & Physics	Autonomic Response Testing ART I & II, Thermogram, EEG, EKG, EMG, VAS, EAV, Kinesiology, Chinese Pulses, Kirlian Photography, X-rays, MRI, CAT scan	Neural Therapy NTA & B", Microcurrent Therapies, Acupuncture, Bodywork/Touch, Breath Therapy, Yoga, Qigong, Meditation, Radiation Therapy
1st Level Physical Body	Sensations - [touch, smell, etc.], Action, Movement	Structure & Biochemistry	Mechanics & Chemistry	Direct Resonance - Autonomic Response Testing ART II, Physical Exam, Lab Tests, BDORT	Diet Therapy - Exercise, Osteopathy & Chiropractic, Surgery, Physical Therapy, Drugs & Herbs, Orthomolecular Medicine, Aromatherapy

Fig. 1. The 5-levels of healing as postulated by Dr. Klinghardt[3]

A Holistic medicine practitioner, however, would begin to investigate the causes of these symptoms such as:

- Lack of hydrochloric acid production in the stomach and deficiency in pancreatic enzymes, leading to poor digestion of food with resulting fermentation and bloating.
- Food intolerances to wheat, lactose, caffeine and eggs, causing the production of inflammatory chemicals such as cytokinines and COX-2's.
- Dehydration - the person only drinks 2-3 glasses of water daily, so is severely dehydrated and digestive processes suffer as a result.
- Eating a lot of junk food which is nutritionally deficient, resulting in a downward spiral of nutritional deficiencies.

---

[3] Klinghardt, D. Explore! Volume 14, November 4, 2005

- The patient is constantly stressed at home due to marital discord, poor communication with his wife and an autistic child.
- The patient is holding a grudge against a family member that hurt them many years ago and is simply not "letting go" by forgiving them.

Once all these causes are rectified, then the IBS will disappear forever. The IBS is the result of these causative factors provoking the symptoms and discomfort, and not because the person is lacking in anti-spasmodic medication, or any other medication.

Based on the abovementioned example, it is clear to see that there are no limits to the range of diseases and disorders that can be treated in a Holistic way; simply find all the potential causative factors, remove them, then help the body to repair, rebuild and rebalance. But this needs to be done on all levels – physical body, energetic body, etheric body, mind, emotions, and spirit.

Therefore, when an individual seeks Holistic treatment for a particular illness or condition, other health problems automatically improve without direct intervention, as the same causative factors could also be responsible for a myriad of other symptoms.

Holistic health teaches the person to reach and maintain higher levels of wellness, optimizing health as well as preventing illness. People generally enjoy the vitality and well-being that results from their positive lifestyle changes, and this provides the motivation to continue this process throughout their lives.

In Holistic medicine the healthcare professional and the patient work as partners. This is really the only way of succeeding, since healing is not really related to the practitioner's skill but the willingness of the patient to work with the practitioner and implement their bespoke healing programme.

Rather than just eliminating or masking symptoms, the symptom is used as a guide to look below the surface for the *root cause*. Whenever possible, treatments are selected that support the body's natural healing system.

HOLISTIC MEDICINE

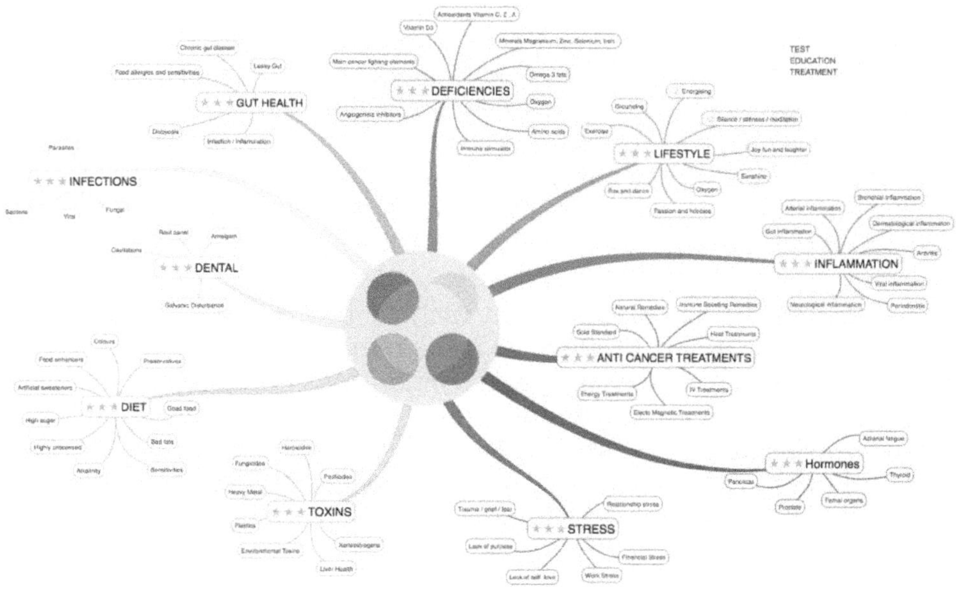

The Medical Model of Disease

Recently I have been discussing issues of Holistic medicine on national TV in Cyprus, where I work and live, in the presence of medical doctors. This has opened some interesting observations into how allopathic or medical doctors perceive and tackle diseases in their patients. Generally, with few exceptions, allopathic doctors perceive the body as a physical and chemical entity, much like a mechanic would view a machine. Using this "mechanistic" approach, their concern is to examine these structures using a variety of technologies such as X-rays, MRI's, CT scans, gastroscopy, colonoscopy, biochemical lab tests and the like.

These technologies and testing techniques are all measuring the physical and chemical structure of different body parts; the "physical body" which is on the first level of the five levels of healing. They will examine the body's organs, the various tissues, down to the cellular level, to determine pathology (disease) of their structure and the biochemical constituents of the blood, plasma and other body fluids.

Allopathic doctors are extremely well-trained in looking at the physical and chemical composition of the body, and they spend many years in medical school doing just this. However, this "mechanistic" perception of the body has many limitations. This only allows us to view one perspective of the human body, when in fact there are many different levels that are important in diagnosing and fully understanding the aetiology of disease.

When observing the allopathic profession examining a patient based on this mechanistic approach, it becomes obvious why they sometimes behave in rather irrational ways. Generally, the "Medical Model of Disease" or "Biomedical Model" is based on collating the symptoms, placing them into a diagnostic category with a specific label, and then using some form of drug, surgery or radiation to eliminate the symptoms. The assumption is made that all patients are homogenous. The Biomedical model is a "wait for illness" approach.

This is a "symptom suppression" approach to dealing with disease. It rarely identifies the real causes of disease, let alone removing the causes. The fact that a diagnosis has been placed on a diseased organ does not justify the rationale that the diseased organ is the CAUSE of the diagnosis. Tonsillitis, for example, is not the cause of inflamed tonsils; Irritable Bowel Syndrome (IBS) is not the cause of an irritable bowel. The diagnostic labels themselves may be important for the medical doctors themselves, but they do little to help understand the true causes of disease.

The label given to the symptoms of an illness is *not the illness itself*. It may surprise you to hear that a cancerous tumour is not the disease, it is merely a symptom. The disease itself is all the aetiological factors that caused the body to produce the tumour in the first place.

If you put yourself in the position of a medical doctor with this perception, then it is easy to understand why they behave as they do. For example, if there is a part of the gut that is ulcerated, and the symptoms cannot be eliminated using medicinal drugs, then the next "logical" step is to remove the organ itself. This may sound rather surprising to the objective onlooker, but personally I have heard from many patients who have been victims of this narrow-minded approach.

Let's Whip Out the Gut!

Late last year I was at the local general hospital seeing a young woman in her 20's who had ulcerative colitis. She was admitted to the hospital with a slight haemorrhage with diarrhoea, probably related to something that was irritating the gut. During her month's stay in the hospital, she had been taking IV cortisone with strong antibiotics (which will destroy all the protective bacteria in the gut and aggravate the inflammation), she had even had chemotherapy (what they give to cancer patients) – God knows what the logic was there – as well as a visit from the psychiatrist, who readily prescribed anti-depressants as he felt that her gut problems were related to her depression ,who would not be depressed in these circumstances?

Recently, her parents were invited to a round-table discussion by the head doctor who, with a solemn expression suggested that the gut should be removed immediately to stop the bleeding and irritation, as nothing else seems to be working!

The doctor added, in a final, desperate attempt, that they may instead decide to give Cyclosporine, a powerful immune-suppressing drug that is given to organ transplant patients to prevent rejection – this literally puts the immune system to sleep. Apart from the chances of catching a nasty bug in hospital which would be near impossible to combat without an immune system, the other side effects of this powerful drug are gum hyperplasia, convulsions, peptic ulcers, pancreatitis, fever, vomiting, diarrhoea, confusion, breathing difficulties, numbness and tingling, pruritus, high blood pressure, potassium retention and possibly hyperkalaemia, as well as kidney and liver dysfunction.[4]

I very recently saw another unfortunate tragedy, this time it was a 12-year old Swedish girl diagnosed with Crohn's Disease. She came to me about one month after the surgeons had removed a large part of her intestine and she had a colostomy bag on the side of her abdomen. If you had seen the psychological, emotional and spiritual devastation in this young teenage girl after the surgery it was a sight never to forget.

Yes, I know you are stunned, just as I was. It sounds unbelievable for a relatively simple case that is easy to bring under control simply by altering the diet (by identifying and removing food intolerances and using some healing herbs and homeopathics). Nutrition does not seem to be an issue that is of much concern to gastroenterologists, even though food is the primary material that travels through the entire gut many times per day.

The first patient in the hospital was told after querying the food she was eating, that it was a "controlled diet" that had been carefully planned by the hospital dietician – white bread, margarine, marmalade, hamburgers with spices, white macaroni and toxic chicken, as well as various dairy products and sweet foods – obviously, the hospital dietician needs to go back to school if she considers this to be a healthy diet!

---

[4] www.sideeffects.com

I made some quick suggestions to her so that she could change her diet immediately – to eat mostly steamed vegetables, vegetable juices and fruit, while taking Omega 3 and 6 fatty acids (which help the body produce natural anti-inflammatory prostaglandins), as well as a mixture of herbs known for their anti-inflammatory effects such as curcumin (turmeric) and boswelia, as well as aloe vera juice.

Three days after implementing this simple regime she began feeling a lot better. There is also a lot more that can be done, such as identifying and removing her food intolerances, as well as optimizing her diet based on her metabolic type – which will need to wait until she is discharged from the controlled hospital environment and her dietician.

Why the Blinkers?

So, why do all these intelligent doctors who were "A" grade students at school think in this narrow-minded, blinkered and insular way? In order to understand why they are so doctrinaire in their approach to disease, let's take a step back and look at an analogy of the human being as a whole entity – I will use the analogy of an iceberg to demonstrate the point: When we look at an iceberg, we normally see about 10% of the iceberg above the waterline, the remaining 90% is below it.

Most medical doctors are trained to observe only what is above the waterline – the 10% of causative factors that involve the physical and chemical structure of disease. This is the main part of the curriculum in most medical schools. Most of the funding for research comes from the pharmaceutical companies who want the budding doctors to prescribe their drugs! They therefore have a big say in what is included in the curriculum. Nutrition, environmental medicine, energy medicine and the psychoemotional and spiritual aspects of the person make up very little of this.

If we return to the iceberg analogy (Fig 2), we see that just like the iceberg is composed of the 10% above the waterline, PLUS the 90% below the waterline, so is the human being composed of many different levels. Some we can see and measure and some we cannot. However, they all interact to determine whether we are healthy or not – all these levels make up the HOLISTIC MODEL OF HEALTH that this book is all about. The tip of the iceberg where doctors spend most of their time looking is based on the Biomedical Model of Disease. Doctors tend to examine the physical body for pathology or disease and are not really trained in looking at the whole health spectrum from perfect health all the way through to pathology. Therefore, there is very little advice that you will obtain from your average medical doctor about preventative medicine.

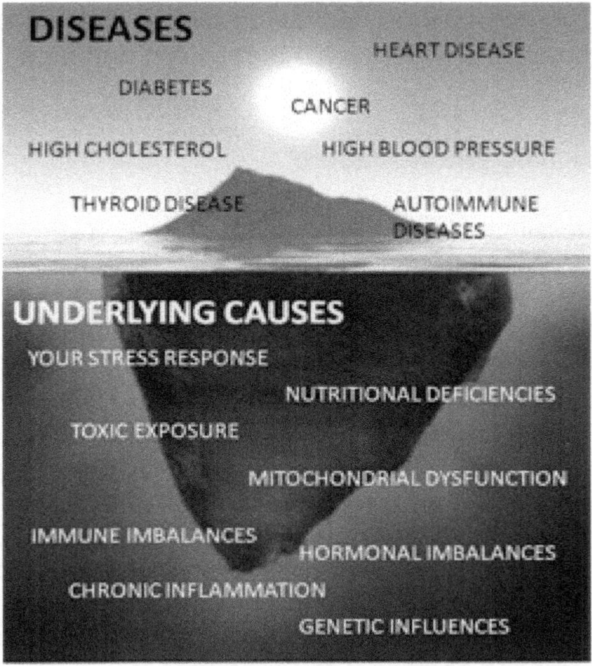

Fig 2. The iceberg analogy

It is important to note that this knowledge about the physical body, and all the medical technology that has emerged over the last 30-40 years has certainly played an important role in saving many lives, particularly in emergency medicine. This needs to be respected and honoured as it is a big contribution to the health of mankind.

However, it is when the medical profession has to deal with complex, chronic diseases that have taken years to develop and are multi-causal, that they freely admit defeat – there is really not much that they can do to cure these diseases, they can treat and manage them and provide palliative care only.

Why is this? It's simply that they are only looking at one level of the body - the physical level. They can identify and label most diseases known to man, but they will not be able to eradicate those that are related to a multitude of factors on the many different levels of health.

For example, many chronic diseases are now related to the accumulating toxicity from heavy metals and xenobiotics that are ubiquitous in today's world. It is rare that you will find a medical doctor looking for these – it is not really a part of their curriculum. It is also rare that the doctor examines the diet of the person and fully understands its implications – the field of clinical nutrition or orthomolecular nutrition is again not part of their curriculum. Nor is helping patients overcome psychoemotional issues that may remain unresolved and be a major cause of the illness.

Holistic Medicine – The Whole Iceberg

This completes the analogy of the iceberg. It's clear that modern medicine practitioners who have their perception fixed on the tip of the iceberg are not going to be able to identify and eliminate **ALL** the causative factors of chronic diseases. Instead, they will identify **ONLY** the structural and biochemical pathologies in the body and try to alleviate the symptoms using drugs, surgery or radiation.

This is one of the main reasons why modern medicine has such abysmal results in treating chronic diseases such as hypertension, diabetes, arthritis, cancer and asthma – diseases that normally have multiple causative factors. They never even look for poor nutrition which leads to gross deficiencies in nutrients, poor digestion and absorption; high levels of toxic metals and organic xenobiotics such as organochlorine pesticides, PCB's from plastics, Bisphenol-A, lead, mercury, arsenic, cadmium, as well as electromagnetic and geopathic stresses; not to mention psychological and emotional stresses from family, society and work.

If you were a patient with a chronic disease, would you not want to know what the causes of your disease were? Certainly, you would, but often we hear from medical doctors that the cause is "idiopathic" – another word for "unknown"! We also hear "psychosomatic" a lot, meaning that the causes are psychological and emotional. Genetic causes is another reason given to explain diseases that they do not know the causes of. This is not a scientific examination of the causes but guess work which is often the "dustbin" of modern medicine where all the "unknowns" are dumped. This would include all the patients who do not get better with drugs or surgery, mainly because the true causes of their problems have not been properly diagnosed.

Modern medicine rarely asks the patient what they eat or drink, let alone look at food intolerances and allergies. I was shocked to see a 33-year old man who was referred to me by his mother – he had a heart attack two months previously, with a serious diagnosis of "deep vein thrombosis" hanging over his head; with gross oedema (swelling) of the leg. He was being treated by the medical profession with Warfarin, a blood- thinning drug, for the last month, but generally was not getting better. What I found shocking was that no medical doctor, of the numerous that he had seen, had asked him about his lifestyle habits. He was smoking 2 packs of cigarettes per day, drinking large quantities of alcohol daily (he was a barman), eating lots of junk food and drinking only 2-3 glasses of water daily!

Within 4 days of drinking more water, cutting out the junk food, stopping smoking and drinking and beginning a detoxification diet of fruit and vegetables, his swelling had greatly reduced, and he was feeling so much better. This man could easily have died of his deep vein thrombosis: a very dangerous condition.

Another recent patient who was suffering from migraine attacks for 30 years, and had recently got worse, was symptom-free in one month after cutting her food intolerances, detoxifying and drinking more water. All the drugs she had been taking all those years were simply repressing symptoms – the real causes were elsewhere.

It's important to work in a holistic fashion with these chronic patients. The therapist must begin working through the levels of the potential causative factors. This is what we do at the Da Vinci Holistic Health Centre in Larnaca – the IDEL Diagnostic Programme is a 5-hour testing protocol that is designed to identify and eliminate the underlying causative factors. We often identify more than 15-20 possible causative factors in a chronically-ill patient. When these are eliminated, we see all sorts of degenerative diseases cured in amazingly short periods of time.

A Modern Paradigm

In 2004, Dr. Robison wrote a paper entitled, *"Towards a New Science"*. In the paper, he argues that Holistic medicine emphasizes the relationships among the spiritual, biological, psychological, and social dimensions of the human experience, and that these are critical to a true understanding of health and healing.

He writes, *"...therefore, rather than defining health in terms of the absence of biomedical risk factors for disease or the accumulation of some ideal list of healthy behaviours, we believe that: Health can be redefined as the way we live well despite our inescapable illnesses, disabilities, and trauma."*

He continues, *"The problem is, of course, that as human beings, we all live with varying amounts of physical, psychological, and spiritual baggage."*

How many people have ever experienced or ever known anyone in optimal health? What does that mean? David B. Morris suggests in his insightful book, *"Illness and Culture in the Postmodern Age":*

"Complete well-being is a fantasy. Health, whatever else it might be, is something that happens not so much in the absence of illness as in its presence" (Morris et al, 1998).

It is more than likely that we will all struggle with emotional, spiritual, and physical issues during our lifetimes, and it is inevitable that we will die. Understanding and living skilfully and compassionately with these struggles, rather than perpetually searching for the latest Holy Grail of optimal health, may come closer to what it truly means to be healthy.

The critical point in understanding health from a Holistic perspective is that health relates to the manner in which we deal with what we are given in life. The concept of health therefore becomes much less black and white; more a complex and dynamic dance that is not easily quantified, controlled, or predicted. Emerging research compels us to broaden our focus to consider a wide range of psychological, social, and spiritual factors that appear to have as much, if not more, influence on our health than the more traditional biomedical risk factors for disease.

This is an interesting perspective of health and allows the person who may come into the world with genetic predispositions, or who became toxic in the womb, or who has had accidents later in life, to use the holistic model to improve their health (even genes can change their expression with the correct lifestyle changes).

In the chapter on psychological, emotional and spiritual causes of disease, we will see how important it is to forgive those that hurt us and not carry grudges in order to gain optimal health. We will also see how people that pray are much healthier compared to those that do not.

In the next chapter we will examine how important toxins are in causing a myriad of disease processes in the body, and what we can do about it.

References

Hassed, C.S. (2004). Bringing holism into mainstream biomedical education. Journal of *Alternative & Complementary Medicine, 10*(2), 405-407.

Morris DB. Illness and Culture in The Postmodern Age. University of California Press, Berkeley, 1998.

Robison, J. (2004). Toward A New Science. WELCOA's Absolute. Advantage Magazine, 3(7), 2-5.

Strandberg EL, Ovhed I, Borgquist L, et al; The perceived meaning of a (w)holistic view among general practitioners and BMC Fam Pract. 2007 Mar 8;8:8.

Chapter 3

Toxicity: Underlying Cause of All Diseases

I first became interested in heavy metals, particularly mercury, back in 1997. After running a routine Hair Tissue Mineral Analysis (HTMA) on myself, I inadvertently discovered that I had severely high mercury levels in my system (see column 'Hg' in Fig 1 – it is off the scale)! In fact, they were about 10 times higher than the acceptable levels. That's 1,000% higher!

This had occurred after removing about 10 amalgam fillings with the help of a holistic dentist here in Cyprus, who gave me chlorella as part of the detoxification protocol. I have since realized how misinformed the dentist was concerning toxic metal chelation protocols. I learned many years later that chlorella is simply not enough to eliminate toxic metals from the body. There are many other dentists all over the world that are inadvertently poisoning people with mercury due to their ignorance. This chapter hopefully will highlight some of the adverse effects on health mercury toxicity has.

It was no surprise that I had many health problems in those days including hand tremors, memory loss, skin irritation, ataxia (poor balance), kidney pains and neurological disturbances. I was trying so hard to keep some sort of balance to maintain my busy work schedule, not to mention bringing up a demanding family.

It took me many years of study to discover how to remove this mercury from my body and regain my health. In the last few years, I have been actively involved in developing heavy metal detoxification protocols that have been scientifically proven to work. I will be discussing these, with case examples, towards the end of this chapter.

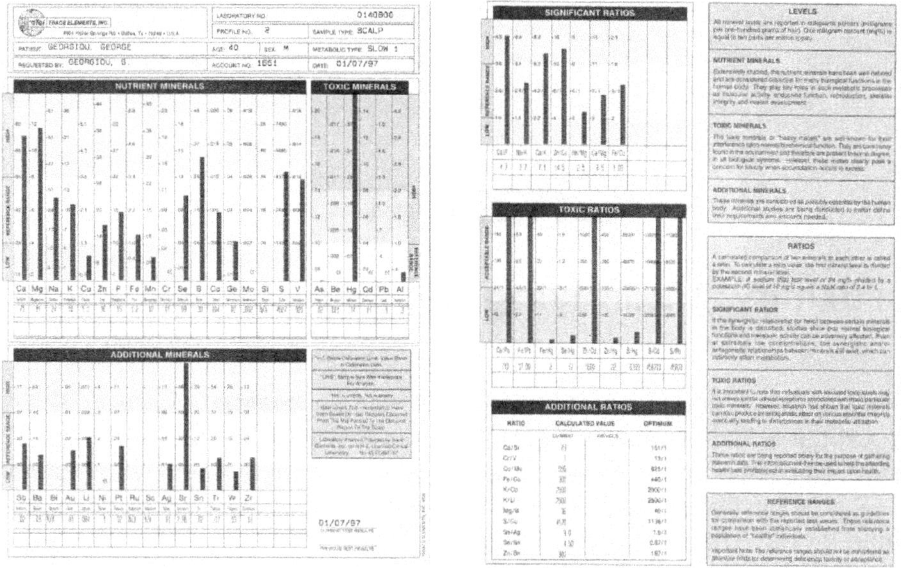

Fig 1. Dr. Georgiou's Hair Tissue Mineral Analysis results

Xenobiotics

Toxic chemicals, otherwise known as 'xenobiotics' (*Greek:* 'foreign to life') which are scattered all over our planet from the North Pole to the South Pole, are constantly being researched. The conclusion is that they are *extremely* toxic to humans as well as wildlife. Even though some chemicals have been taken off the market, those that remain are even more noxious than the ones already banned.

Bioaccumulation in soils, water supplies, and the tissues of animals and humans is a real problem. It results in these chemicals lingering for many, many years even after they have been banned. DDT, for example, has been banned for more than 25 years in the Western world, yet it is still being found in the tissues of wildlife in the arctic, as well as humans in many different countries.

One study noted that only five organochlorine compounds, as well as mercury, were found in marine mammals in the 1960's. Today over 265 organic pollutants and 50 inorganic chemicals have been found in the same species.[5]
Other recent research has focused on how chemicals affect the thyroid and pituitary systems. Some chemicals have been identified as endocrine disrupters

5 O'Shea, T.J., Tanabe, S., Persistent ocean contaminants and marine mammals: a retrospective overview. In: O'Shea, T.J. et al. (Eds.), 1999. Proceedings of the Marine Mammal Commission Workshop Marine Mammals and Persistent Ocean Contaminants, pp 87-92. (cited in Tanabe, S. Contamination and toxic effects of persistent endocrine disrupters in marine mammals and birds. *Mar Pollut Bull* 2002;45:69-77.)

because they can interfere with the body's own hormones, which are secreted by the endocrine glands.

It is also emerging that endocrine disrupters can have many physiological effects not directly associated with the primary system. For example, the thyroid system is well known for regulating metabolism, but it is also a crucial component in foetal brain development in mammals. Too much or too little thyroid hormone at crucial developmental points can cause permanent damage.

The immune system is also vulnerable to hormone-mediated disruption. Chemicals can cause neurological problems, reproductive and developmental abnormalities, as well as cancers. Researchers are only just beginning to disentangle the questions about the effects of chronic low-level exposure to chemicals (as opposed to brief high doses), combinations of chemicals, and interactions between chemicals and other physiological and environmental factors.

Low Dose Exposure

Toxicologists studying chemical toxicity usually have a reference range of values which indicate the 'safe levels' of toxic chemicals. New research is showing, however, that even low-dose exposure[6] of mercury is accumulative over time and can lead to children having decreased performance in areas of motor function and memory.

Similarly, disruption of attention, fine motor function and verbal memory has also been found in adults on exposure to low mercury levels. It is an occupational hazard for dental staff, chloralkali factory workers, gold miners and those of similar professions. Mercury has been found to be a causative agent of various sorts for disorders, including neurological[7], nephrological, immunological, cardiac, motor, reproductive and even genetic. Recently, heavy metal mediated toxicity has been linked to diseases like Alzheimer's, Parkinson's, Autism, Lupus, Amyotrophic lateral sclerosis, and even cancers. Besides this, it poses danger to wildlife. This low-dose toxicity and its effects on health will be the toxicologists' next goal for future research.

Let's look at some specific sources of toxins that we encounter daily:

- Cigarettes, alcohol, caffeine and drugs are all substances that the body cannot use for building and repair, so will add to the mounting waste. A lot of these toxic wastes are stored in the tissues and organs of the body.

---

6 Zahir, F., Rizwi, S.J., Haqb, S.K., Khanb, R.H. Low dose mercury toxicity and human health, *Environmental Toxicology and Pharmacology*, March 2005. http://www.detoxmetals.com/images/newsletter/Low%20dose%20Hg%20exposure.pdf

7 http://www.youtube.com/watch?v=VImCpWzXJ_w

- Heavy metals: mercury from fish and amalgam fillings; aluminium found in cheeses, baking powders, cake mixes, self-raising flour, cosmetics, toothpastes, antiperspirants and some drugs such as antacids; arsenic given to chickens as a growth promoter; cadmium found in tea and coffee, as well as cigarette smokers. Lead found in paints, fuels, rubber, plastics, inks, dyes, toys, building materials and hair restorers.

- Roxarsone - 4-hydroxy-3-nitrobenzenearsonic acid - is by far the most common arsenic-based additive used in chicken feed.[8] It is mixed in the diet of about 70% of the 9 billion broiler chickens produced annually in the U.S. In its original organic form, roxarsone is relatively benign. It is less toxic than the inorganic forms of arsenic-arsenite [As(III)] and arsenate [As(V)]. However, some of the 2.2 million lbs of roxarsone mixed in the nation's chicken feed each year converts into inorganic arsenic within the bird, and the rest is transformed into inorganic forms after the bird excretes it. Arsenic has been linked to bladder, lung, skin, kidney and colon cancer. Low-level exposures can lead to partial paralysis and diabetes.

- Plastics containing Bisphenol A, the building block of polycarbonate plastics, which are everywhere; in pesticides, antioxidants, flame retardants, rubber chemicals, a coating in metals, cans and food containers, refrigerator shelving, returnable containers for juice, milk and water, nail polish, compact discs, adhesives, microwave ovenware and eating utensils.

A diet that is high in animal fats will add to the waste. There are many different drugs and chemicals that are given to animals these days; antibiotics, hormones, feed concentrates, etc. All these chemicals will accumulate in the fat cells of the animals that we then eat. So, we slowly build up an accumulation of these chemicals over time.

Sluggish bowels can lead to a great deal of toxicity throughout the body. Try to imagine a 10-metre tube running from mouth to anus packed with meat, sausage, fish, fruit salad, beef burgers, sugars, milk and other goodies – all fermenting and putrefying for days on end. This fermentation produces highly toxic substances such as putrescine, neuracine, and cadaverine, which are so poisonous that a small amount injected into a laboratory animal will kill it in minutes. All these toxic substances, apart from causing disease in the body, will also act as metabolism

[8] Hileman, B. Arsenic in Chicken Production: A common feed additive adds arsenic to human food and endangers water supplies. *Chemical and Engineering News*. Volume 85, Number 15, pp. 34-35, April 9, 2007.

blockers, and will therefore have consequences on weight-loss too. This process of 'self-poisoning' by these putrefying foods in the gut is called 'autointoxication.'

Refined foods such as white sugar, white flour, white rice, etc. are all deficient in nutrients, but loaded with calories. They also help to create a lot of sludge and debris in the body. If you remember from your childhood days, you probably used white flour and water to make a glue to build a kite, or to glue your coloured paper in to your exercise book at school. When you eat white flour and its products, it becomes glue in the intestine and sticks to the internal wall. When mixed with sticky sugar and fat, it becomes a rubber-like substance that blocks absorption of foods through the intestine, as well as being a constant source of toxins. If you don't believe me, read Dr. Jensen's book entitled, *'Tissue cleansing through bowel management'*[9]. There are also plenty of photos of what comes out of the intestine if you do a proper detox – disgusting!

Thousands of new, toxic chemical compounds are produced each year by the chemical industry, most of which are approved by various so-called 'Environmental Protection Agencies' (EPA's) without any serious toxicological studies. The cumulative number of toxic chemicals polluting our planet today exceeds *100,000*.

Many claim that some of these chemicals, such as the flame retardants used in children's clothing, have potentially life-saving applications. But how many of these chemicals do we ingest or are absorbed by our bodies and those of our children? And at what cost to our health? What is the capacity of the human body to eliminate them? Has anyone conducted a general contracting cost-benefit analysis as to whether the benefits offered, for example, by fire hazard protection, truly outweigh the toxicity generated within us, our children and the environment? The answer is: No. There are *no* comprehensive, scientific answers, other than to confirm the obvious: toxicity levels in humans and animals across the globe are rising fast. Whether we realize it or not – we are all toxic.

In an article published in the October 2006, *National Geographic* entitled, '*The pollution within*', journalist David Ewing Duncan had himself tested for 320 synthetic chemicals and certain heavy metals at a cost of $16,000, paid for by the magazine. According to the article, Duncan was considered a healthy individual. Nevertheless, he had higher than average amounts of chemical toxins, such as flame-retardants (known as PDBE's), phthalates, Polychlorinated Biphenyls (PCBs), pesticides and dioxins, as well as heavy metals such as mercury.

Duncan's article alludes to some of the possible ways toxic chemicals may have accumulated in his body; some might have originated in childhood, while others

[9] Jensen, B. Dr. Jensen's guide to better bowel care: A complete program for tissue cleansing through bowel management. USA: Avery Publishers, 1999.

may have been picked up in airplanes due to his extensive work-related travel. However, he and his doctors were merely speculating. Duncan also describes his pre- and post-mercury toxicity results after a fresh fish dinner and breakfast. Duncan had fresh halibut for dinner and fresh swordfish for breakfast (cooked in his toxic non-stick pan), both of which were caught in the ocean just outside the Golden Gate Bridge in the San Francisco Bay area.

He tested himself for serum mercury before and after the meals and found that his blood mercury levels had shot up from five micrograms per litre to *over twelve*. The doctors conducting the tests advised him not to repeat that experiment ever again, yet I'm sure this dangerous diet is adhered to by thousands, unaware of the impact of toxicity on their health. After all, fish is promoted as a health food. Nevertheless, drawing conclusions on the experience of only one healthy adult is not robust, toxicological science. So, let's review the research…

It is difficult to fathom how we can live in houses that make us sick, but the term "sick building syndrome" (SBS),[10] first employed in the 1970s, describes a situation in which reported symptoms among a population of building occupants can be temporally associated with their presence in that building. Typically, though not always, the structure is an office building.

Typical complaints may include eye and/or nasopharyngeal irritation, rhinitis or nasal congestion, inability to concentrate, and general malaise-complaints suggestive of a host of common ailments, some ubiquitous and easily communicable. The key factors are commonality of symptoms and absence of symptoms among building occupants when the individuals are not in the building.

There has been extensive speculation about the cause or causes of SBS. Poor design, maintenance, and/or operation of the structure's ventilation system may be at fault. The ventilation system itself can be a source of irritants. Interior redesign, such as the rearrangement of offices or installation of partitions, may also interfere with efficient functioning of such systems. Low levels of specific pollutants found in new furniture, carpeting and other furniture and fittings may also be one of the causes.

A 1984 World Health Organization report suggested that as many as 30 percent of new and remodeled buildings worldwide may generate excessive complaints related to indoor air quality.[11]

---

10 Burge, S. et al. Sick Building Syndrome: A Study of 4373 Office Workers. *Ann. Occupational Hygiene*. 31: 493-504, 1987.

11 U.S. Environmental Protection Agency, Office of Air and Radiation. Indoor Air Facts No. 4: Sick Building Syndrome. revised, 1991.

In a nationwide, random sampling of U.S. office workers, 24 percent perceived air quality problems in their work environments. 20 percent believed their work performance was hampered because of this.[12]

Toxic from Birth

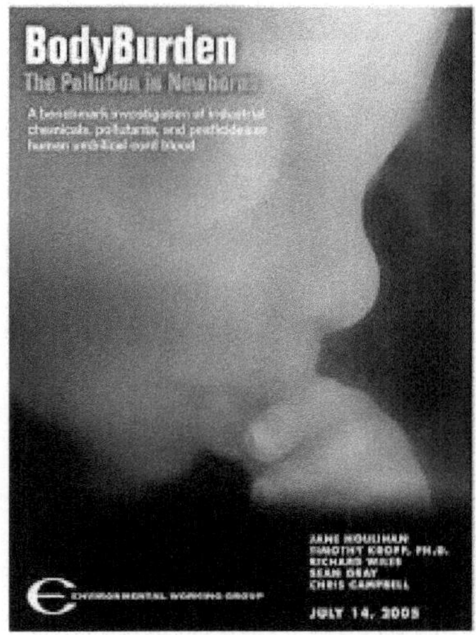

In September 2005, Greenpeace International, in tandem with the World Wildlife Fund, published a document entitled, *'A Present for Life: Hazardous chemicals in umbilical cord blood.'*[13] The research showed convincingly that new-borns tested for hundreds of different xenobiotics[14] showed high levels of these toxins.

Specifically, the blood tests demonstrated that these infants had an average of 287 toxins in their bodies – 180 of these, known carcinogens. Some of these chemicals included the commonly-used artificial musk HHCB, which was found in almost all blood samples at higher levels than the other artificial musk's. Musk ambrette, a chemical banned from use in cosmetics in the EU since 1995, was still found in 15 maternal and 12 cord blood samples.

Other banned alkylphenol compounds, extensively used in industrial cleaning agents, were also found. Additionally, the study quantified the antibacterial agent triclosan in human blood, which was found in almost 50% of the samples. DDT, the notorious pesticide banned from agricultural use worldwide, was found in all blood samples. Similarly, the organochlorine by-product and pesticide hexachlorobenzene – also subject to a global ban – was found in the samples. Perfluorinated compounds like PFOS and PFOA, used to make non-stick pans and water-repelling coatings, were present in all but one maternal sample. PFOS was detected in all cord blood samples; PFOA in half of them.

12 Kreiss, K. The Sick Building Syndrome: Where Is the Epidemiologic Basis? *American Journal of Public Health* 1990; 80:1172-73.

13 Schuiling, J., van der Naald, W. A Present for Life: Hazardous chemicals in umbilical cord blood. Greenpeace International and WWF-UK, Sept. 2005.

14 A xenobiotic is an artificial or natural substance found in an organism that simply should not be present. The term covers chemicals, medical drugs, naturally occurring heavy metals and all the pollutants released into the environment from human activity.

Another US-based study, *'Baby care products: possible sources of infant phthalate exposure,'* published in *Paediatrics*, February 2008,[15] concluded that phthalate toxicity is widespread in infants. Babies coming into contact with lotions, powders and shampoos had increased urinary concentrations of phthalates, in direct proportion to the number of products they had been exposed to. This association was strongest in young infants, who are more vulnerable to the developmental and reproductive toxicity of phthalates, given their immature metabolic capability and increased dosage per unit of body surface area. Thus, babies become heavily polluted with toxic and carcinogenic substances by their unsuspecting, well-meaning parents. Essentially, *we are unwittingly poisoning our own children*.

One could argue that these studies conducted in the United States – where the toxicity levels are perhaps higher than in other countries – exaggerate the problem. Perhaps in poorer parts of the world, parents use fewer of the culprit lotions and powders, or do without them. Yet, does general environmental toxicity have boundaries?

To address this question, let's examine a similar study conducted on pregnant women living well within the Arctic Circle, which most people feel is a pristine part of Earth. The research was published as an article in *The Science of the Total Environment* entitled, *'Organochlorines and heavy metals in pregnant women from the Disko Bay area in Greenland.'*[16] The study showed high concentrations of heavy metals, such as mercury, and organochlorines in the blood and fatty tissue of the Inuit population. This was attributed to their high consumption of the meat and blubber of marine mammals, which are clearly toxic.

In this study, 180 pregnant women and 178 new-born babies were sampled, amounting to 36% of the total number of births in the Disko Bay area during 1994–1996. What this study showed was that the main food supply of the native population in Greenland, that is, marine mammals, is heavily toxic. It is therefore obvious that pollution has no boundaries. While not within the scope of this book, the fact that the Inuit's were unlikely to have been the main polluters of their coastal waters raises serious additional questions of global ethics, politics and economics.

A further study published in the journal, *Environmental Research* has shown there is a correlation between the levels of methylmercury in a pregnant or lactating woman's blood and urine and that of her yet-to-be-born or new-born baby, with toxins passing from the mother to the foetus through the placenta. There has since

---

15 Sathyanarayana, S. Karr, CJ., Lozano, P., Brown, E., Calafat, AM., Liu, F., and Swan, SH. Baby Care Products: Possible Sources of Infant Phthalate Exposure. *Pediatrics*, Vol. 121 No. 2, pp. e260-e268, Feb 2008.

16 Bjerregaard, P., and Hansen, JC. Organochlorines and heavy metals in pregnant women from the Disko Bay area in Greenland. The Science of the Total Environment 245, 2000.

been much research indicating the grave effects on the health of children of high mercury levels, for instance, autism and developmental delays.

The University of Cincinnati published a study in February 2008, entitled: *'Plastic bottles release potentially harmful chemicals (Bisphenol A or BPA) after contact with hot liquids.'* BPA is another synthetic chemical classified as an endocrine disruptor, widely used in plastics. The study concluded that the most important factor regarding exposure to BPA from plastic bottles is not whether the container is new or old, rather, it is the temperature of the liquid contained, that is crucial to the amount of BPA that is released. Hot liquids such as tea, coffee or milk increase the release of BPA up to *55 times*! Other similar studies have shown that if you repeatedly scrub, dish-wash, and boil polycarbonate baby bottles, these also release significant amounts of BPA.

BPA is widely used in products such as reusable water bottles, tin linings, water pipes, dental sealants and baby bottles, and has been shown to affect reproduction and brain development. Consider a baby bottle – it is supposed to be scrubbed clean and steam-sterilized before a hot liquid, such as formula milk, is poured into it and left to cool ahead of feeding a baby. The whole procedure amounts to unintentional infant poisoning! Will these infants be given the chance to naturally detoxify themselves into adulthood? The evidence indicates that this is not the case.

Mercury is a well-established, cumulative neurotoxic agent that can have serious adverse effects on the development and functioning of the human central nervous system, especially when exposure occurs prenatally.[17] Given the potential threat that methylmercury poses to the optimal development of cognitive function, clinicians and regulatory agencies are concerned about the levels of methylmercury that a pregnant women regularly ingests, as well as the levels organic mercury in diets, especially from fish containing methylmercury, which is a major source of mercury exposure to the general population. While cases in which treatment with dental amalgam resulting in elevated blood mercury concentration have been reported, other clinicians have indicated this is not the case.[18] Therefore, this issue remains controversial.

In one study conducted by a Korean research group[19], they showed that the amount of mercury (from eating fish) in the mother's blood correlated with levels found in cord blood. Blood mercury levels in the group who ate fish more than four times per month was significantly higher than that of the group who did not

---

17 Methylmercury. Geneva: World Health Organization; Environment Health Criteria 101, 1990.
18 Behrman RE, Kliegman R, Jenson HB. Nelson Textbook of Pediatrics. 17th ed. Elsevier Science Saunders; 2004. Heavy metal intoxification; pp. 702–703.
19 Kim, EH., Kim, IK., Kwon, JY., Kim, SW., and Park, YW. The Effect of Fish Consumption on Blood Mercury Levels of Pregnant Women. *Yonsei Med J.* 31; 47(5): 626–633, Oct 2006.

consume fish ($p = 0.02$). In follow-up studies, blood mercury levels were decreased in the study group but slightly increased in the control group ($p = 0.014$). The maternal blood mercury levels in late pregnancy was positively correlated with mercury levels of cord blood ($r = 0.58$, $p = 0.047$), which was almost *twice* the level found in maternal blood. So, pregnant women who consume a large amount of fish may have high blood mercury levels.

North Americans are also Toxic

In July 2005, the US Department of Health and Human Services, Centers for Disease Control and Prevention, published a 475-page document entitled, *'Third national report on human exposure to environmental chemicals'*[20], which clearly indicates the growing number of chemical toxins present in all age groups in North America.

A Canada-based study has also compared heavy metal intake in different age groups and their corresponding intake guidelines. The report: *'Metallic lunch: an analysis of heavy metals in the Canadian diet'*[21], showed that Canadians young and old are ingesting unhealthy levels of toxic substances, such as cadmium and lead. In addition, Canadian children are also being exposed to potentially unsafe levels of copper, manganese, molybdenum and nickel.

Europeans of All Age Groups are Toxic

A study conducted by the World Wildlife Fund set out to explore whether there was any link between the types and levels of contamination found in three generations of families. They wanted to examine possible links between contamination and a family's lifestyle, consumption patterns and use of everyday products.

The study entitled, *'Contamination: the next generation - Results of the family chemical contamination survey'*[22], summarizes the findings of an analysis of 104 different chemicals in the blood of 33 volunteers from 7 families living in England, Scotland, and Wales. The volunteers in each family spanned 3 generations, comprising a grandmother, mother, and 2 children. In all, 14 children, 13 adults, and 6 grandmothers took part in the study. The ages of the volunteers ranged from 9 to 88. On analysing the results, all 3 generations were shown to be contaminated by a cocktail of hazardous artificial chemicals, some of them every day domestic products. Every child carried in his or her body the same range of toxic substances: organochlorine pesticides, PCB's, brominated flame-retardants, phthalates and

20 A full colour report can be downloaded from http://www.cdc.gov/exposurereport/pdf/thirdreport.pdf
21 Download the full report at http://www.environmentaldefence.ca/reports/Metallic%20Lunch%20Report_final.pdf
22 WWF-UK. Contamination: the next generation. Results of the family chemical contamination survey. October 2004.

perfluorinated ('non-stick') chemicals. Five such substances found in each parent and grandparent, were also found in every child.

While it might be expected that the chemical load increases with age, the study demonstrated that this is not always true. Children can be more contaminated by higher levels of certain newer chemicals than their parents or even their grandparents, despite being exposed to these chemicals for only a fraction of the time.

Another interesting report compiled by the World Wildlife Fund UK (2005), *'Still dirty: a review of action against toxic products in Europe,'* highlights the occurrence of hazardous chemicals in everyday products and notes which EU member states have taken measures to help protect their citizens and wildlife. One of the report's observations is that phthalates used in plastics and cosmetics have been linked to reduced sperm counts. The report also documents that lead is still in use in the EU, despite its proven toxicity to children and wildlife.

Other chemicals found, such as alkyl phenols and alkyl phenol ethoxylates – industrial chemicals used in plastics, pesticides, and detergents – are toxic and mimic the female hormone oestrogen, causing feminization of male fish. Brominated flame-retardants - chemicals widely used in electronic equipment, fabrics and plastics - are now found in human breast milk and wildlife, even in remote areas.

Cosmetics Beautify but They Also Poison

Are hair dyes worth perishing for? Is your lipstick making you sick? What about beauty creams and other cosmetics? Over 50% of women of all ages colour their hair. Men increasingly dye their hair, too. Research shows a connection between the use of commercial hair dyes and various diseases, including cancer.[23] Newer studies state that because of the prevalence of hair dye use, further studies are necessary to address the effects of specific colours and types of hair dyes with the possible role of individual susceptibility. So, are *you* susceptible?

I have seen and tested several patients who were suffering from many serious, inexplicable symptoms whose doctors were mystified as to the reasons for their deteriorating health. One 34-year-old lady came up high on tin toxicity, with all the accompanying symptoms – skin rash, stomach complaints, nausea, vomiting, diarrhoea, abdominal pain, headaches and palpitations. As she was not eating

23 Ames, BN, Kammen, HO and Yamasaki, E. Hair dyes are mutagenic: identification of a variety of mutagenic ingredients, 1975. See also Watanabe T, Hirayama T, Fukui S, Mutagenicity of commercial hair dyes and detection of 2,7-diaminophenazine, Kyoto Pharmaceutical University, Japan, 1990.

anything from tin cans, but she investigated and found it in her lipstick. Stannous fluoride or tin fluoride is also found in some toothpastes.

Independent laboratory testing initiated by the 'Campaign for Safe Cosmetics' in 2007, found that lipsticks from top brands contain lead also. *Two-thirds* of the 33 cosmetics samples tested contained detectable levels of lead.[24] It was lucky that this lady's lipstick only contained tin, which was eliminated using the heavy metal detox agent HMD™[3].

Almost all cosmetics can cause allergic reactions in certain individuals. Nearly one quarter of the people questioned in the FDA's 1994 cosmetics survey responded 'Yes' to having suffered an allergic reaction to personal care products including moisturizers, foundations, and eye shadows. In the book, *'Drop dead gorgeous: protecting yourself from the hidden dangers of cosmetics'*[25], Kim Erickson, with a forward by Dr Samuel Epstein, reveals how manufacturers exploit loopholes in legislation designed to protect the public. So, cosmetic users: beware.[26]

Given that just about everything you put on your skin gets absorbed into your bloodstream, it is interesting that there is such a lack of regulation of carcinogenic ingredients in skin care products. There are over 150 toxic, cancer-causing ingredients currently used in cosmetic products alone. Sunscreens are particularly suspect given that they are recommended, without serious research, as cancer prevention products, whereas in fact they contain many chemicals that *promote* cancer. Another book worth reading that describes the consequences of many of these chemicals on cosmetics is Judi Vance's book entitled, *"Beauty to Die For: The Cosmetic Consequence."*[27]

Mercury is Everywhere

One of the causative factors that led to my health saga (which I discussed in chapter one), was the extraction of over 10 mercury amalgam fillings several years back. My holistic dentist and I at the time were not so knowledgeable, and we proceeded to remove all the amalgams as quickly as possible. THIS IS A CRITICAL MISTAKE! Notice that this is CAPITALIZED! Removing mercury amalgams quickly, particularly when not using a chelation protocol to remove the mercury released, is the best way of making you so toxic with mercury that the chances of developing a chronic disorder such as cancer or multiple sclerosis

---

24 For more details see: http://www.safecosmetics.org
3 See www.detoxmetals.com
25 Erickson, K. Drop-Dead Gorgeous: Protecting Yourself from the Hidden Dangers of Cosmetics, McGraw Hill, 2002.
26 In response to the toxic onslaught from cosmetics, the Environmental Working Group began an initiative to register the fairly safe cosmetics, which can be accessed at: http://www.cosmeticdatabase.com.
27 Vance, J. Beauty to Die For: The Cosmetic Consequence. USA: iuniverse.com, 1999.

increases exponentially. After poisoning my own self out of ignorance, I have consequently spent many years studying and developing natural products for detoxification that also work for mercury – one of the products is the above mentioned, **HMD™**, that we will discuss a little later.

Mercury in Amalgam Fillings

Mercury used in amalgam tooth fillings remains a big issue of dispute. Amalgam was found to be a cheap and long-lasting substance to fill teeth with, but the danger of mercury poisoning was overlooked and ignored. The use of amalgams is now prohibited in many countries. Norway recently announced a ban on the use of mercury, including dental amalgam, that took effect on January 1, 2008. Sweden announced a similar ban and dentists in Denmark will no longer be allowed to use mercury in fillings after April 1, 2008.[28]

The biomedical literature contains numerous articles on the adverse health impact before and after amalgam removal. The International Academy of Oral Medicine and Toxicology[29] has even produced video evidence showing mercury vapour released from amalgam fillings, even though they may be over 30 years old.

Chewing gum, drinking hot beverages, brushing teeth and dental polishing increase the methylmercury released from amalgam fillings.[30] If you doubt how lethal mercury can be, particularly for the nervous system and the brain, a video produced by the University of Calgary Faculty of Medicine, entitled *'How mercury causes brain neuron degeneration'*[31] may persuade you. It clearly shows how mercury degrades neural fibres in a petri dish in zero time. Despite all this damning evidence, in the USA alone around 180 million mercury amalgams are placed in peoples' mouths every year.

Before we leave the topic of mercury amalgams, I would like to broadcast a loud warning AGAIN to all those reading this – PLEASE DO NOT REMOVE YOUR AMALGAMS UNLESS YOU ARE FOLLOWING AN ADEQUATE CHELATING PROTOCOL!! There is research which clearly shows that once the dentist's drill is on the amalgams, there are huge mercury deposits released into the blood – up to *100 times* the initial level before the dentist starts working on your amalgams.[32]

---

28 www.mercurypolicy.org

29 www.iaomt.org

30 Gebel T, Dunkelberg H. Influence of chewing gum consumption and dental contact of amalgam fillings to different metal restorations on urine mercury content. Zentralbl Hyg Umweltmed. 199(1):69-75, Nov 1996.

31 http://commons.ucalgary.ca/mercury

32 Bjorkman, L, Sandborgh-Englund, G, Ekstrand, J: Mercury in saliva and faeces after removal of amalgam fillings. Toxicol Appl Pharmacol 144(1): 156-162, 1997.

Mercury in Vaccines

Many adult vaccines and inoculations use Thimerosal as a preservative. Following a 1999 recommendation in the US, this is generally being phased out, though it remains in use in several countries. Thimerosol contains around 50% toxic mercury; often linked to Autism. There is an interesting article published in *Medical Hypotheses*: *'Autism: a novel form of mercury poisoning'*[33], showing how exposure to mercury can cause immune, sensory, neurological, motor and behavioural dysfunctions, like traits defining or associated with Autism.

The authors of this paper conclude: *"A review of medical literature and U.S. government data suggests that: (i) many cases of idiopathic autism are induced by early mercury exposure from thimerosal; (ii) this type of autism represents an unrecognized mercurial syndrome; and (iii) genetic and non-genetic factors establish a predisposition whereby thimerosal's adverse effects occur only in some children."*

The similarities extend to neuroanatomy, neurotransmitters and biochemistry. By the age of 10, a child may be many hundreds of times over what is considered a 'safe' dose of mercury poisoning from injections. <u>There is no safe dose of mercury.</u>

There are a variety of chemicals that have been found in vaccinations such as:

- Mercury - the heavy metal used in the disinfectant and preservative, Thimerosal, known to cause brain injury, Autism, attention deficit hyperactivity disorder (ADHD) and autoimmune diseases.
- Aluminium - a toxic metal additive used to promote antibody response, associated with Alzheimer's disease, brain damage, seizures and cancer.
- Formaldehyde - a preservative, as well as a nerve-damaging and cancer-causing agent.
- Ethylene glycol - (antifreeze).
- Monosodium glutamate (MSG) - a breakdown product of protein, and common flavour enhancer well known for poisoning brain cells.
- Sulphites - cause genetic damage.
- Neomycin - an antibiotic, also previously registered for use in US pesticides, known to cause reproductive and developmental harm such as birth defects, infertility, sterility and impairment of normal growth and development.

Servicemen and women who are subjected to many different injections during their tours of duty are at risk of toxic poisoning. Most fish are contaminated with mercury

33 Bernard, S., Enayati, A., Redwood, L., Roger, H., Binstock, T. Autism: a novel form of mercury poisoning. *Medical Hypotheses* 56(4), 462–471, 2001.

and other toxic substances, as the *National Geographic* reporter (mentioned above) easily discovered. Even polar bears living in the Arctic, thousands of miles away from any industry, have been found in poor health and even dying because of toxic poisoning.[34,35] No animal or human living on planet Earth is free from the risk of contamination.

Toxins accumulate in the body over time. Some people experience toxicity symptoms from birth, while others experience symptoms gradually. Children with Autism, Attention Deficit Disorder and similar neurological problems are usually found to have high levels of mercury, which is thought to be a major contributory factor in these conditions. Disruptions of the endocrine system and other metabolic functions develop over time, leading to chronic diseases, including multiple sclerosis and cancer.

Toxicity and the Fertility Threat

In 1992, a study in the *British Medical Journal* entitled, *'Evidence for decreasing quality of semen during the past 50 years'*[36], reported that semen quality is seriously declining. In 1997, Dianne Dumanoski and others published a book entitled, *'Our stolen future: are we threatening our fertility, intelligence and survival?'*[37] This ground-breaking book revealed that chemicals in the environment have affected human reproductive patterns in ways that may threaten the survival of the species. Yueliang Guo and others in 2000 published a study in the *Lancet*: *'Semen quality after prenatal exposure to polychlorinated biphenyls and dibenzofurans.'*[38] The study reported that boys prenatally exposed to such chemicals have sperm with abnormal morphology, reduced motility and reduced strength. These results are consistent with studies on animals exposed in the womb to such toxic chemicals.

---

34 Brown, V. Toxic Chemicals: A Threat to Wildlife and Humans. WWF. December 2003.

35 WWF International Arctic Programme. The Tip of the Iceberg: Chemical Contamination in the Arctic. 2006.

36 Carlsen E, Giwercman A, Keiding N, Skakkebaek NE. Evidence for decreasing quality of semen during past 50 years. *BMJ.* 12;305(6854):609-13, Sept 1992.

37 Theo, C., Dumanoski, D., Myers, JP. Our stolen future: are we threatening our fertility, intelligence and survival? Penguin, USA: 1999.

38 Guo YL, Hsu PC, Hsu CC, Lambert GH. Semen quality after prenatal exposure to polychlorinated biphenyls and dibenzofurans. *Lancet.* 7;356(9237):1240-1, Oct 2000.

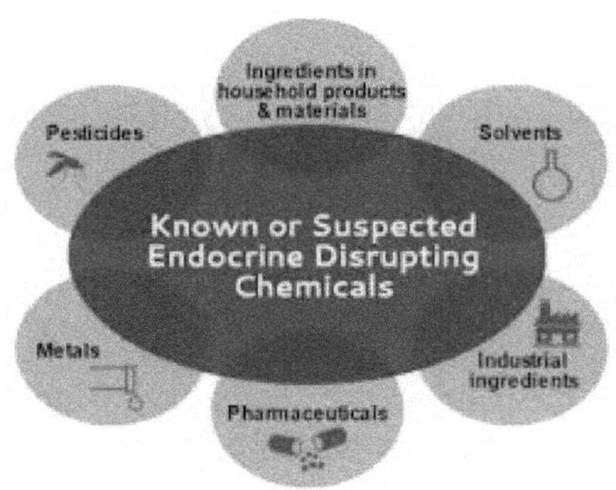

Another study entitled, *'Chlorinated pesticides and heavy metals in human semen'*[39], published in 2000, measured concentrations of chlorinated pesticides and heavy metals (lead and cadmium) respectively, in semen samples collected from men amongst the normal population in India. The study concluded that the presence of these xenobiotics in human semen related to the use of pesticides, emissions of exhausts from motor vehicles and industrial operations.

A 2006 study entitled, *'Persistent pesticides in human breast milk and cryptorchidism'*[40] investigated a possible association between maternal exposure to 27 organochlorine compounds used as pesticides and cryptorchidism among male children. The study concluded that the link between congenital cryptorchidism and certain persistent pesticides in breast milk, as a proxy for maternal exposure, suggests that testicular descent in the male foetus may be adversely affected.

There are, of course, other concurrent reasons for human reproductive decline, but the toxicity explanation is the most compelling. And yet, most of these women and men could reclaim their lost fertility simply by removing toxins. It is a cheaper and less risky solution and offers other health benefits as well – just think about it.

The Toxic Onslaught in a Nutshell

There are countless toxicological studies on pregnant and lactating women, infants, as well as young and old members of both genders confirming that we are all toxic. How much more scientific evidence do we need to be convinced of the obvious? The problem has been well identified. In a nutshell, it can be stated as follows:

We have converted our world into a toxic waste dump.

Even before we are born, we accumulate several toxins, which are passed on to us in the womb. After our birth, our bodies keep on accumulating and storing up all types of toxins. From the food we eat, the water we drink, the air we breathe and nearly everything we put in and on our bodies.

---

39 Kumar R; Pant N; Srivastava S P. Chlorinated pesticides and heavy metals in human semen. *International journal of andrology* 23(3):145-9, 2000.

40 Damgaard, IN., Skakkebæk, NE., Toppari, J., Virtanen, HE., Shen, H. Schramm, K., Petersen, JH., Jensen, TK., Main, KM. Persistent Pesticides in Human Breast Milk and Cryptorchidism. *Environmental Health Perspectives* Volume 114, Number 7, July 2006.

This includes cigarettes, caffeine, medical drugs including over-the-counter drugs, alcohol, deodorants, shampoos, tap water, plastic-bottled water, plastic food containers, insecticides, pesticides, herbicides, ordinary food, junk food, fast food, processed food, gourmet food, 'Health' food, beauty creams, shaving creams, tin and lead-contaminated lipsticks; nickel ear/nose/nipple rings, artificial cleaning materials, swimming pools loaded with chemicals, dental mercury amalgams, other toxic dental restoration materials, root canals, dental implants and dentures, childhood vaccinations, adult vaccinations, food additives, flavour-enhancers, food preservatives, hormones, antibiotics and God-only-knows what else.

Unfortunately, there is a lot of medical ignorance that could be exacerbating the situation. Despite the growing number of press reports linking chemicals with disease, and the increasing number of urgent warnings from scientists specializing in environmental medicine, the medical world appears to be oblivious to these warnings.

The problem begins in medical schools. Few doctors are taught about modern-day chemicals and their sources, let alone their health effects. Therefore, during the taking of a medical history, the aspect of toxicity that often manifests itself in the patient's symptoms, and the reporting of it, are completely ignored. Maybe one of the reasons why none of this is taught in medical school is that there is no drug they can give to remove these toxins; not to mention this is not good for the profits of the pharmaceutical companies who have a strong influence within the medical faculties. In addition, many of these chemicals are present in foods, cosmetics, vaccinations, herbicides and the like – which involve large international corporations. The topic is controversial if one does not want to stir the waters.

Toxins Versus Nutrients: The Uneven Battle

The body puts up a good fight for survival against the toxic onslaught. But the capacity of the body to deal with and eliminate these toxins is limited. It has several primary and secondary defence lines; namely its excretory and immune systems. These systems need 'ammunition' to keep up the fight, that is, a continuous intake of high-quality nutrients. Sadly, while the amount and varieties of toxins are increasing, the nutrient intake in humans is declining. The nutrient content of the average modern meal has been on the decline for some decades now.

Only a small part of the globe's population has access to – and the inclination for – wholesome, nutrient dense, organic products. The rest of us struggle to survive on the conventional produce available in the typical grocery store. Even worse, a large percentage of the population feeds on junk, toxic, denatured and heavily-processed food – a recipe for a health catastrophe. And the toxins are rising fast, while the nutrients (or antitoxins) are declining equally swiftly. Chronic degenerative diseases are largely the direct outcome of this uneven battle between nutrients and toxins.

The least you can do to help the imbalance is to try to eat a much organic food as possible, while supplementing with a good quality, high-potency multivitamin and mineral formula.

New 21st Century Theory of Disease

Dr. Miller, of the Department of Family Practice, University of Texas Health Science Center at San Antonio, USA, believes that we are on the threshold of the new theory of disease that is based on the toxicity of chemicals. She states in one of her papers,[41] *"In the late 1800's, physicians observed that certain illnesses spread from sick, feverish individuals to those contacting them, paving the way for the germ theory of disease. The germ theory served as a crude but elegant formulation that explained dozens of seemingly unrelated illnesses affecting literally every organ system."*

She continues: *"Today we are witnessing another medical anomaly – the unique pattern of illness involving chemically exposed people who subsequently report multisystem symptoms and new-onset chemical and food intolerances. These intolerances may be the hallmark for a new disease process, just as fever is a hallmark for infection."*

I strongly agree with Dr Miller and believe that many of the new diseases that we are seeing today such as Gulf War Syndrome,[42] Chronic Fatigue Syndrome, Myalgic Encephalomyelitis (ME), fibromyalgia, childhood diabetes, attention deficit hyperactivity disorder and others are all chemically related disorders.[43]

How exposed are you to these chemicals?

Check out below how prone you are to develop a chemically-triggered, 21st century disease, by checking off the various categories – the more of these that apply to you, the higher your risk if you:

- work with chemicals

---

[41] Miller C. Are We on the Threshold of a New Theory of Disease? Toxicant-induced Loss of Tolerance and its Relationship to Addiction and Abdiction. *Tox. Ind. Health.* 15:284-294, 1999.

[42] Miller, C. and Prihoda, TA Controlled Comparison of Symptoms and Chemical Intolerances Reported by Gulf War Veterans, Implant Recipients and Persons with Multiple Chemical Sensitivity. *Tox. Ind. Health* 15:386-397, 1999.

[43] Miller, C. Prihoda, T. The Environmental Exposure and Sensitivity Inventory (EESI): A Standardized approach for measuring Chemical Intolerances for Research and Clinical Applications. *Tox. Ind. Health* 15:370-385, 1999.

- use pesticides around the house and garden such as fly spray, weed killer or flea powder
- use non-environmentally friendly cosmetics, toiletries and household cleaners
- you are responsible for disposal of chemicals used in medicines such as mercury preservatives in vaccines and flea shampoo
- eat nonorganic fruit, vegetables and meat products
- eat contaminated seafood, usually containing mercury
- eat too many processed foods, full of preservatives, colourings, flavourings and other additives
- drink unfiltered tap water containing aluminium and fluoride
- consume soft drinks from aluminium cans
- have mercury amalgam fillings in your mouth
- live in a major city with air pollution

These chemicals are accumulative, so do not think that a little exposure will do you no harm – it simply takes longer to reach critical levels in the body before symptoms appear.

Mercury: 'The Big One'

Let us take a closer look at mercury – which I refer to as the 'Big One' as it is omnipotent and ubiquitous. There is probably not a living person on this planet or living animal – whether domesticated or wild – that does not have their share of mercury toxicity. Mercury is a very toxic substance; more toxic than lead, cadmium, or arsenic.[44]

Mercury is listed as one of the top six most poisonous metals on Earth, with known human toxicity occurring at minimal doses, producing urine levels of 5 mcg/l – which is another way of saying 5 millionths of one gram.

44 Sharma, RP; Obersteiner, EJ., Metals and Neurotoxic Effects: Cytotoxicity of Selected Metallic Compounds on Chick Ganglia Cultures, *J Comp Pathol*, 91(2):235-44 (1981).

Many Forms of Mercury

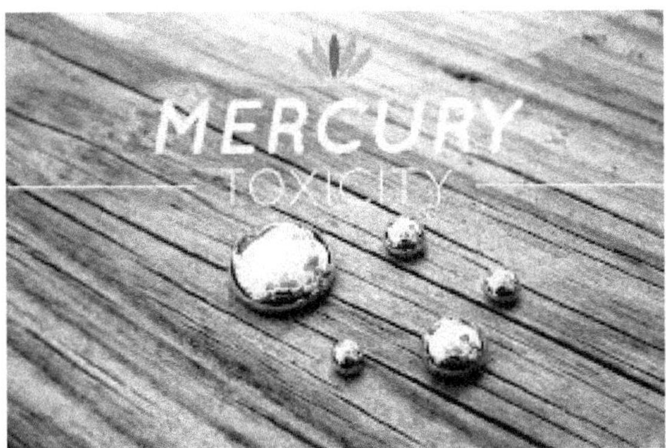

Mercury's elemental symbol is *Hg*, which is derived from the Greek word *hydrargyrias*, meaning 'water silver.' As stated above, mercury is found in organic and inorganic forms. The inorganic form can be further divided into elemental mercury and mercuric salts. Mercury in any form is toxic. The difference lies in how it is absorbed, the clinical signs and symptoms and the response to treatment modalities. Mercury poisoning can result from vapour inhalation, ingestion, injection or absorption through the skin.

Elemental mercury is found in liquid form, which easily vaporizes at room temperature (the only metal to do so) and is well absorbed through inhalation. Its lipid (fat)-soluble property allows for easy passage through the alveoli into the bloodstream and red blood cells. This inorganic form has similar properties to organic mercury. Small amounts of non-oxidized elemental mercury continue to persist and account for CNS toxicity.

Mercury in Surprising Places

The use of mercury in Medicine predates its use in dentistry by centuries. Mercury has been found in Egyptian tombs, indicating that it was used as early as 1500 BC. As far back as 500 BC there is evidence that India was using mercury as a drug.

However, Arabic physicians first studied mercury as a drug and introduced the use of a mercurial ointment in the 10th century AD. It was towards the end of the 18th century that mercury found its way into medical practice in the US as a prescription item. In the late 18th century, antisyphlitic agents contained mercury. For centuries, mercury was an essential part of many different medicines such as diuretics, antibacterial agents, antiseptics and laxatives.

The number one source of human contamination of *inorganic* mercury today is coal-burning plants. However, the primary source of *organic* mercury contamination is right in your mouth – dental fillings composed of an amalgam, which about 50% of is the metallic form of mercury. A small, tenth-of-a-gram mercury filling would release enough organic mercury to last *27 years*, which is pretty much a consistent chronic toxic exposure for the life of most fillings.

At least seventeen separate studies have confirmed that dental patients absorb a daily dose of mercury derived from their mercury fillings.[45] Mercury poisoning is usually misdiagnosed because of its insidious onset, nonspecific symptoms and lack of knowledge within the medical profession. In medicine today, mercury is still used in various antiseptic agents as well as amalgams.

Mercury is found in many industries such as the manufacture of batteries, thermometers and barometers. It can also be found in fungicides used in the agricultural industry. Before 1990, paints contained mercury as an antimildew agent. On July 7, 1999, a joint statement by the American Academy of Paediatrics and the US Public Health Service was issued, alerting clinicians and the public to the dangers of *thimerosal*, a methylmercury[46]-containing preservative used in vaccines.

Although several sources contributing to the domestic mercury concentrations have been identified, human waste (faeces and urine) from individuals with dental amalgam fillings is believed to be the most significant source – greater than 80 percent.

Mercury is also in many of the foods we eat and it is contained many over-the-counter drugs and cosmetics; e.g. mascara, contact lens solution, haemorrhoid preparations, etc. The mercury ingredients used are *thimerosal, phenylmercuric acetate, phenylmercuric nitrate, mercuric acetate, mercuric nitrate, MB for merbromin* and *mercuric oxide yellow.*

Mercury Toxicity in Fish

About 95% of methylmercury ingested in fish is absorbed into the gastro-intestinal tract, although the exact site of absorption is not known. It is distributed to all tissues in a process completed in about 30 hours. About 5% is found in the blood components and about 10% in the brain. The concentration in red blood cells is about 20 times the concentration in the plasma.

Guidelines for Minimizing Mercury Exposure from Fish and Shellfish

Fish and shellfish are an important part of a healthy diet. Fish and shellfish contain high-quality protein and other essential nutrients, are low in saturated fat, and contain omega-3 fatty acids. A well-balanced diet that includes a variety of fish and shellfish can contribute to heart health and children's proper growth and

45 Richardson, G.M., Inhalation of Mercury-Contaminated Particulate Matter by Dentists: An Overlooked Occupational Risk, *Human and Ecological Risk Assessment,* 9:1519-1531 (2003).

46 Ethylmercury – an organic form of mercury widely used as an antifungal agent

development. So, women and young children should include fish or shellfish in their diets due to the many nutritional benefits.

By following these 3 recommendations for selecting and eating fish or shellfish, women and young children will receive the benefits and be confident that they have reduced their exposure to the harmful effects of mercury:

- Do not eat shark, swordfish, king mackerel, or tilefish because they contain high levels of mercury.
- Eat up to 12 ounces (2 average meals) a week of a variety of fish and shellfish that are lower in mercury.
- Five of the most commonly eaten fish that are low in mercury are shrimp, canned light tuna, salmon, pollock and catfish.
- Another commonly eaten fish – albacore ('white') tuna - has more mercury than canned light tuna. So, when choosing your two meals of fish and shellfish, you may eat up to 6 ounces (one average meal) of albacore tuna per week.
- Check local advisories about the safety of fish caught by family and friends in your local lakes, rivers, and coastal areas. If no advice is available, eat up to 6 ounces (one average meal) per week of fish you catch from local waters, but don't consume any other fish during that week.

<u>Follow these same recommendations when feeding fish and shellfish to your young child but serve smaller portions.</u>

On January 12, 2001, government health officials issued new advisories warning women to limit fish consumption during pregnancy to avoid exposing their unborn children to unsafe levels of methylmercury.

In February 2009, the Zero-Mercury Working Group[47] published a report entitled *"Mercury in Fish is a Global Health concern.*[48]*"*

"Mercury contamination of fish and mammals is a global public health concern," said Michael Bender, co-author and member of the Zero Mercury Working Group. *"Our study of fish tested in different locations around the world shows that internationally accepted exposure levels for methylmercury are exceeded, often by wide margins, in each country and area covered."*

47 The Zero Mercury Working Group is an international coalition of more than 75 public-interest non-governmental organizations from around the world, formed in 2005 by the European Environmental Bureau and the Mercury Policy Project/Ban Mercury Working Group. The aim of the group is to continually reduce emissions, demand and supply of mercury from all sources we can control, with the goal of eliminating mercury in the environment at EU level and globally. See www.zeromercury.org

48 http://www.zeromercury.org/press/090210-MercuryFishRelease.pdf

The Food and Drug Administration (FDA), which regulates commercially sold fish, recommends that pregnant and nursing women and young children don't eat any shark, swordfish, tilefish, or king mackerel; but does recommend 12 ounces per week of any other fish.

The Environmental Protection Agency (EPA), which makes recommendations to states about safe mercury levels in sport fish, allows up to 8 ounces of any fish per week for pregnant women with no prohibitions on consumption of any individual fish caught recreationally.
These restrictions are steps in the right direction, but they need to be tightened significantly to adequately protect women and their unborn children from the toxic effects of methylmercury.

The nutritional benefits of fish complicate the task faced by health officials when protecting the public from methylmercury. Protein, omega-3 fatty acids, Vitamin D, and other nutrients make fish an otherwise exceptionally good food for pregnant mothers and their developing babies.

Some research suggests that the risk of cardiovascular disease increases with methylmercury exposure.[49] In extreme cases, methylmercury poisoning can lead to paralysis, coma and even death.

A new Mercury Policy Project (MPP) report recently published entitled, Mercury in Fish: An Urgent Global Health Concern,[50] explains that the mercury risk is greatest for populations whose per capita fish consumption is high, as well as in areas where pollution has elevated the average mercury content of fish. But methylmercury hazards also exist where per capita fish consumption and average mercury levels in fish are comparatively low. In cultures where fish-eating marine mammals are part of the traditional diet, mercury in these animals can add substantially to total dietary exposure.

Toxicity caused by excessive mercury exposure is now becoming recognized as a widespread environmental problem and is continuing to attract a great deal of public attention. A National Academy of Sciences study [51] published in July 2001 estimates that up to 60, 000 children born in the US each year may be affected by mercury toxicity. In March of 2002, an environmental group charged the FDA with failing to warn the public of the dangers of mercury contamination from eating tuna, which contains high levels of mercury.

49 Konig, A., et al. (2005), A Quantitative Analysis of Fish Consumption and Coronary Heart Disease Mortality. *Am J Prev Med* 29 (4): 355-346.

50 Mercury in Fish: A Global Health Hazard, Zero Mercury Working Group, *Mercury Policy Project*, Feb. 2009.

51 NAS (2000). National Academy of Sciences Report: Toxicological Effects of Methylmercury. C. R.A. Goyer, National Academy Press: pp. 344.

The World Health Organization reports that the amount of mercury absorbed daily by the average human body is 0.3 micrograms (mcg) from water and air; 2.61 mcg from fish; and 17 mcg from dental amalgams (silver fillings). Uptake of up to 100 µg daily has been observed in extreme cases. Research points out that mercury vapour is 80% absorbed into the blood, and that in animal studies, mercury vapour goes directly from the nose to the brain, following nasal nerve pathways. Amalgam fillings release mercury for as long as *70 years*. Someone with 8 amalgams could release 120 mcg into the saliva per day.

The maximum mercury exposure allowable by the US Environmental Protection Agency (EPA) is less than 0.1mcg per kilogram of body weight per day to be absorbed.

Dental Amalgams: A Closer Look

"The mercury uptake from amalgams is the dominating source for inorganic mercury in the central nervous system and is the major source of total mercury uptake in the population" (Maths Berlin, a leading Swedish toxicologist)

So, what is an amalgam? It was dentists who, over 150 years ago, discovered a new, less expensive way to fill cavities in teeth, rather than using gold and silver alone. This was a mixture of an assortment of metals such as mercury (45% - 52%),[52] silver (30%) and small amounts of copper, zinc and tin. Mercury causes adverse health effects in dentists and dental personnel[53,54,55,56]. Dentists have 4 times as much of a body burden of mercury as an average non-dentist. Dental workers show 50-300% more mercury in hair and fingernails than the average population.

Denying the Truth About the Dangers of Amalgam Toxicity

Initially, back in the early days, the American Society of Dental Surgeons opposed its use because they knew that mercury was so toxic. However, so many dentists were using it that the original society collapsed, and the rogue dentists replaced it with a new one: the American Dental Association (ADA), which is still in existence. This has now grown to be a powerful lobby in Washington and other states. After 150 years, the ADA is still allowing over 180

52 Sandra Denton MD : Proceedings of the First International Conference on Biocompatibility 1988.

53 Ngim, CH; et al., Chronic Neurobehavioral Effects of Elemental Mercury in Dentists, *Brit J Indust Med*, 49:782-90, 1992.

54 Echeverria, D; et al., Behavioral Effects of Low-Level Exposure to HgE Among Dentists. *Neurotoxicol Teratol*, 17(2):161-8 (1995).

55 Shapiro, I.M., et al., Neurophysiological and neuropsychological function in mercury-exposed dentists. *The Lancet* 1, 1147-1150 (1982).

56 Uzzell, B.P., et al., Chronic low-level mercury exposure and neuropsychological functioning. *J of Clin and Exper Neuropsych.* 8, 581-593.

million mercury-containing amalgam fillings to be placed in people's mouths, including young children!

The ADA has been covering up the danger by saying that the mercury is 'locked in' to the tooth and is not released from the filling itself. The scientific evidence is now so overwhelmingly against this lie, that the ADA had to eventually admit that mercury is released from amalgam fillings (as a vapour) and that over 80% of this is absorbed into the body.

Amalgams release mercury even quicker when a person chews or drinks hot liquids. This is a shocking realisation given that everyone alive today will chew and drink hot liquids on occasions![57]

Consumers aren't being told the truth: Amalgam fillings contain 50% mercury – a known neurotoxin. Worse, they are deceived. The ADA still uses the deceptive word 'silver' to describe a product that is mainly mercury, thus hiding the product's main ingredient.

In previous years, the ADA had managed to de-license various dentists who proclaimed amalgams to be dangerous, and strictly enforced a Gag Rule[58]. In response, these dentists have taken the issue to court, protecting their right, among others, to Free Speech. And yet today, member dentists of the ADA who talk against mercury, or even mention that mercury 'might' be toxic, run a high risk of being expelled as well as having their licenses revoked. The ADA even calls it 'unethical and unprofessional conduct' to inform patients of the potential dangers of the most hazardous metal known to mankind. Yet European countries like Sweden[59] have legislated a total ban on all amalgams and other products containing mercury, after spending years reviewing the scientific research.

Yielding to scientific pressures, the ADA now admits that mercury is indeed released from amalgam fillings, even after placement, but state that it is perfectly safe and still support the use of amalgam fillings. They claim their use is safe, based on over 150 years of use, and that no scientific evidence shows mercury exposure from dental fillings causes any known diseases. Yet the ADA does admit there is a potential hazard for dental office personnel with the handling of dental amalgam and recommend that dentists use a 'no-touch' technique, because dentists and their staff might become contaminated. They admit that the 'scrap' amalgam – the excess amalgam left over after filling a tooth – also constitutes a hazardous threat because of continuous vapour release.

57 http://www.iaomt.org/videos/

58 The Gag Rule is a pillar of the ADA's agenda to block consumers from learning that the major component of amalgam is Mercury. The Gag Rule instructs dentists to abandon their allegiance to patient health care - to remain silent or face disciplinary action.

59 http://www.sweden.gov.se/sb/d/11459/a/118550

There is no scientific evidence showing amalgam's safety, and mixed dental amalgam has never had US Food and Drug Administration (FDA) research or approval. If it were to be classified as a *class II* medical device and made to undergo the rigorous testing needed to prove safety, it would *never* pass.

After filing petitions, testifying at Congressional hearings, providing state fact sheet laws, testifying at Scientific Advisory Committee hearings, and writing hundreds of letters, the Consumers for Dental Choice (CDC)[60] eventually won their ten-year battle to get the FDA to comply with the law and recently (2008) reclassify mercury amalgam. The FDA website[61] now states:

> *"Dental amalgams contain mercury, which may have neurotoxic effects on the nervous systems of developing children and fetuses.[62] ... Pregnant women and people who may have a health condition that makes them more sensitive to mercury exposure, including individuals with existing high levels of mercury bio burden, should not avoid seeking dental care, but should discuss options with their health practitioner."*

Each amalgam filling has as much mercury as a thermometer, and its poisonous vapours are constantly emitted from the teeth to the brain. A particular risk, according to the US government, to the developing brain of the child. As mentioned earlier, the foetus is at the greatest risk of all if the pregnant woman has dental fillings drilled out or implanted, because of the proven transport of mercury through the placenta. So too is the nursing infant of a woman with amalgam dental fillings, because of the transport of mercury into the breast milk.

Confirmation of the escape of mercury vapour and ions from amalgam dental fillings is provided by The World Health Organization (WHO) Environmental Health Criteria 118 document (EHC 118) on inorganic mercury. It clearly states that the largest estimated average daily intake and retention of mercury and mercury compounds in the general population is from dental amalgams, not from food or air.

---

60 www.toxicteeth.org

61 www.fda.gov

62 Mercury has been removed from thermometers and vaccines, controls have been tightened on mercury emissions from coal power plants, and pregnant women have been warned about consuming fish tainted by mercury.

The Nuts and Bolts of Mercury Vapour Inhalation from Amalgams

Mercury vapour inhaled into the lungs is absorbed almost 100 percent and immediately passes into the bloodstream. It takes approximately four minutes before mercury is converted or oxidized into an ionic state from its elemental vapour state. While in its elemental form, mercury vapour is lipid (fat) soluble and readily passes through the blood-brain barrier or the placental membrane.

"Worldwide there are over 4,000 research papers indicating that mercury is a highly toxic substance. How can dentists be so thoughtless as to place one of the deadliest toxins in existence two inches from our brains?"

Mercury vapour inhaled into the lungs is absorbed almost 100 percent and immediately passes into the bloodstream. It takes approximately four minutes before mercury is converted or oxidized into an ionic state from its elemental vapour state. While in its elemental form, mercury vapour is lipid (fat) soluble and readily passes through the blood-brain barrier or the placental membrane.

It can also accumulate in other organs and tissues of the body. The estimated average daily intake of mercury from dental amalgams is 3.8 - 21 micrograms per day. Two-thirds of the body burden of mercury is derived from the mercury vapour released from amalgams. The static release of mercury vapour from amalgam fillings that is not being stimulated, which goes on 24 hours a day, 365 days a year, is a major contributor to the total mercury body burden. A large amount of mercury vapour is released during chewing. After only ten minutes of gum chewing, there is an average increase in mercury release of 15.6 times more than during the resting state in test subjects. That converts to a *1,560% increase* in mercury release.

Increased amounts of mercury are excreted in the faeces of individuals with amalgam fillings. Engqvist et al.[63] found that only 25% of the total mercury in fecal samples was in the form of amalgam particles, in samples taken from six adults with a moderate load of amalgam fillings. About 80% of an oral dose of amalgam particles or mercuric mercury attached to sulfhydryl groups was excreted in the faeces. Interestingly, 60% of an oral dose of vapor dissolved in water was retained. Previously it had been assumed that intake of vapor was due solely to inhalation.

Mercury readily mixes with food and is swallowed with it. The body uptake from inorganic mercury, swallowed with saliva, can be as much as hundreds of micrograms per day for individuals with many amalgam fillings. Urinary excretion

63 Engqvist A, Colmsjo A, Skare I. Speciation of mercury in faeces from individuals with amalgam fillings. Arch Environ Health 53:205–213 (1998).

is a common indicator of mercury toxicity, even though faecal excretion of mercury is twenty times greater than the corresponding urinary excretion.
There is a statistical correlation between the mercury concentration in saliva and the number of amalgam fillings. The United States government has determined and ruled that the continual exposure to mercury from amalgam fillings is not without risk to patients.

"You wouldn't take a leaky thermometer, put it in your mouth, and leave it there 24 hours a day, 365 days a year. Yet that's exactly what happens when an amalgam filling is installed in your mouth" Dr Michael Ziff

If other dental work is also present in the mouth, such as gold crowns, nickel crowns and removable bridges or braces, the mercury emission further increases from the amalgam. This is due to the electrical current generated by the presence of dissimilar metals in an electrolyte medium such as saliva.

Chronic inhalation of mercury vapour from amalgam fillings for twenty years or more can result in the accumulation of pathologic quantities of mercury in the brain and other critical organs and tissues. Human autopsy studies of accident victims have shown a positive correlation between the numbers of mercury amalgam dental fillings and the concentration of mercury in the brain. The onset of clinically observable signs or symptoms of mercury toxicity may take as long as 20-30 years to appear, depending on a person's biochemical individuality.

Several recent reviews have discussed in detail the uptake, distribution, excretion, metabolism, and kinetics of inhaled mercury vapour.[64,65,66] About 80% of inhaled mercury vapour is retained in the body. However, approximately 7-14% is exhaled within a week after exposure.

Diagnosis of Heavy Metal Toxicity

The diagnosis of heavy metal toxicity must consider the exposure history, clinical signs and symptoms and laboratory tests. While the US Centers for Disease Control has steadily dropped the 'allowable level' of lead in the blood over the last fifteen years, there remains a problem with using blood levels to evaluate toxicity in the first place. Blood levels may not accurately reflect the *total* body burden of toxic metals. High blood levels are usually only found in acute toxic metal exposure, or in people exposed to high levels of toxins over a long period. In chronic low-level exposure, however, the blood levels may actually be low, due to redistribution of the toxins throughout the body, while bone and other tissue levels remain high.

---

64 U.S. EPA. Mercury Report to Congress Office of Air Quality and Standards. Washington, DC:U.S. Environmental Protection Agency, 1997.

65 ATSDR. Toxicological Profile for Mercury. Atlanta, GA:Agency for Toxic Substances and Disease Registry, 1999.

66 WHO. Environmental Health Criteria 118. Inorganic Mecury. International Program on Chemical Safety. Geneva: World Health Organization, 1991.

Hair Tissue Mineral Analysis (HTMA)

Hair analysis[67] is a method of determining toxin exposure which is popular with many clinicians. The amount of mercury in the hair is determined by first digesting the hair in acids and then using a spectrometer such as ICP-MS to measure accurately, to parts per billion, the levels of mercury.

What are we measuring from hair, and why? When the body has toxic metals circulating in the blood, the first thing that it tries to do is remove them from circulation. This is because the toxic metals are prone to do a lot of damage to different cells of the body through their vicious free radical activity. The first place that the body stores these metals is in inert tissues, such as the hair and nails, which are situated outside the body and therefore would do the least harm. When these storage sites are full, the body will start distributing and storing the metals in other less inert tissues and organs, such as fat, liver, kidneys, thyroid, brain and other organs.

The hair sample taken represents about a two month 'history' of what has been circulating in the blood – the typical sample of hair is about 1 inch long, which takes about two months to grow. Therefore, the levels of metals in the hair correlate quite well with the levels in the circulating blood. If there are no metals circulating in the blood during the last two months, then there is a good probability that none will appear in the hair either.

This is a far more clinically significant test that facilitates the practitioner's clinical decision-making, which shows a timeline or history of progress, not simply a snapshot. There are also many advantages to using this over the urine pre-post provocation test using chemical provocation agents:

- It is a 'gentle' way to proceed as there is no aggressive mobilization and release of large quantities of metals – as with the chemical chelators[68] – which can greatly exacerbate symptoms of neurological problems such as MS, cancer, autism, cardiovascular diseases and others.
- The history of progress can be mapped over time. The decline in toxic metals shown on the HTMA is an indication that the storage sites in the body are also diminishing. If the levels are still high on the HTMA, then this is an indication that the storage sites are still loaded and that HMD™ chelation should be continued for longer. HMD™ is a natural, heavy metal chelator that we will talk about more below.

---

67 https://www.detoxmetals.com/hmd-hair-test-testing/

68 The word 'chelation' comes from the Greek word 'chelos' which stands for 'claw' – these are chemical or natural substances that attach to toxic metals and help in their removal from the body.

- It is not a 'snap-shot' picture provided by urine tests, which are difficult to interpret over time.
- The HTMA is far more cost effective than the urine tests – costing the patient about $120 every two months.[69]
- The HTMA is very quick, and easily implemented by an assistant in any clinical setting. It also negates the compliance problems often faced by practitioners when they ask the patient to collect urine over a 24-hour period.

Urine and Faeces Testing

Urine and faeces testing can also be used, but as we have already mentioned, these are only 'snapshots' of metabolic activity in the body at the time of collection, which usually runs over a 24-hour period. The differences between the baseline sample and the post-provocation sample when a provocation agent such as EDTA or DMSA is used are not comparable; they are arbitrary figures. These tests are fine for research purposes but don't really help the practitioner make clinical judgements for the best interest of the patient.

What Can We Do to Protect Ourselves?

The answer to this question is two-fold. Firstly, we can push for legislation to ban a lot of the harmful chemicals which are known to be detrimental to animals and humans. Secondly, we need to be able to detoxify our bodies to eliminate many of these chemicals. Given that we are exposed to these literally *daily*, this process must be an ongoing one.

Treating Heavy Metal Toxicity Using Conventional Chelators

Many health practitioners use synthetic chelating agents such as DMPS, DMSA, EDTA and others to mobilize and eliminate heavy metals from the body. One advantage of these is the power of their mobilizing activity. They are quick to mobilize and eliminate certain metals in the body. However, this may place a huge burden on the body's detoxification systems. Furthermore, symptoms have been reported by natural medical physicians throughout the US, such as intractable seizures in paediatric patients and multiple sclerosis in adult patients, due to taking high doses of DMSA, (also known as Succimer), over extended periods of time.[70,71,72]

69 http://www.worldwidehealthcenter.net/product-category/hair-mineral-analysis/

70 Smith, D.R., et al, Succimer and the urinary excretion of essential elements in a primate model of childhood lead exposure, *Toxicological Sciences*, 2000, Apr, 54 [2] 473-80.

71 Mann, KV. and Travers, JD., Succimer, an oral lead chelator, Clinical Pharmacology, 1991, 10 [12] 914-22.

72 Jorgensen, FM., Succimer: the first approved oral lead chelator, *American Family Physician*, 1993, 48 [8] 1495-1502.

The above are valid reasons to at least be cautious of using DMSA for the treatment of mercury-toxic paediatric patients. The fragile brains and nervous systems of children, and particularly those with autism, PDD and seizure disorders, should be handled with considerable care so as not to increase the damage. As of March 2009, as I write, the Federal Drug Administration (FDA) in the USA is considering removing DMSA from the market, but the motives for this move remain unclear.

DMSA and DMPS can certainly be life-saving drugs in cases of ACUTE metal poisoning. Toxicologists have noted that synthetic chelators should only be used in cases of ACUTE metal poisoning, or as a last resort for intractable chronic poisoning. Natural methods are preferable and should be exhausted first.

Natural Heavy Metal Chelators: Do They Work?

It is not safe to use chemical chelators on an ongoing basis. Natural ones can be used instead, much like a supplement, daily. There are several purported natural heavy metal chelators on the market, but literally none of these have been investigated in depth using double blind, placebo-controlled trials; except one.

The natural product called HMD™,[73,74,75] has undergone a 'gold standard' double blind, placebo-controlled study using 350 people, at a cost of over one million US Dollars.

It can be used safely over long periods of time with no side effects and is presently being tested to see its efficacy in eliminating some of the xenobiotics mentioned in this chapter.

HMD™ is a Patent-Pending, proprietary synergistic blend of three natural ingredients:

- Chlorella Growth Factor (CGF)
- Organic Coriandrum sativum leaf tincture
- Homaccord of cell-decimated, energized Chlorella

Research on HMD™

The research initially began as a health impact study to determine the levels of heavy metals in 374 metal foundry workers in Russia. These were randomly

73 Georgiou, GJ. Scientific research on natural heavy metal chelators: testing what works. International Journal of Complementary & Alternative Medicine. Volume 11 Issue 5 - 2018

74 Georgiou, G.J. Natural Heavy Metal Chelators. Explore! Volume 16, Number 6, 2007.

75 Georgiou, G.J. A Natural Heavy Metal Chelator Is Born: It's Use With Paediatric Cases. Volume 24, Number 1, 2007.

chosen from a workforce of 2,000 people and screened using Hair Tissue Mineral Analysis (HTMA) in a reputable US laboratory specializing in this type of analysis, using Inductively Coupled Plasma–Mass Spectrometer (ICP-MS) technology. There were four major heavy metals identified in this sample that were present at very high levels and were common to the entire workforce (they were by-products of the production process): lead, antimony, cadmium and arsenic.

The research design was a double blind, placebo-controlled study. Neither the participants, researchers, nor the analytical chemists doing the spectrometry analysis knew which treatment protocol each participant belonged to. The coding was stored in the co-ordinator's safe until it was time to interpret the statistical data. All participants signed an Informed Consent Form after discussion of the research protocols. There was a medical team on 24-hour standby to deal with any potential side-effects.

Each participant had to acquire a baseline sample of urine (24-hour collection) and faeces before taking HMD™. Both urine and faeces samples were taken to determine the excretory route used by the various substances tested. These samples were returned to the research team and circumspectly recorded in preparation for spectrometry, using the foundry's in-house instrument. Further ICP-MS analyses were conducted using two independent laboratories in Russia and the USA.

Table 1 below shows the summarized results of several different trials over a 3-year period. To make sense of the data, there was a group of people who were in the placebo group; these people took an initial urine and faeces sample, then they began taking a weak solution of chlorella (the same dosage used for the experimental group mentioned below). The chlorella solution had been shown in previous trials to not mobilize metals in any way.

After a 24-hour period, another urine sample was taken, and after 48-hours another faeces sample was taken. The difference between the baseline sample and the final sample is expressed in Table 1 below as the mean percentage increase of toxic metals after provocation – this is given for both the placebo group that took the inert chlorella as well as the experimental group that took the HMD™. 'U' denotes the Urine samples and 'F' the Faeces samples. The Mercury results are from a recent independent trial which is discussed in more detail below.

The experimental group followed the same protocol as the chlorella group, as mentioned above, but they took the HMD™ - 40 drops in the morning, 50 drops at lunch and 60 drops in the evening; all taken in a little water before food for both groups. Further research showed that similar results were achieved when taking 50 drops x 3 daily which is the present dosage recommended.

The mean percentage increase of heavy metals after provocation with HMD™ is compared with the elimination while using a placebo (a mild chlorella tincture).

METALS	Mean % increase after provocation (Experimental group)	Mean % increase after provocation (Placebo group)	Number in sample	t-test results	Degrees of Freedom	Sig. (p =)
ARSENIC-U	7,409.00	11.16	84	-	-	p<0.0005
ARSENIC-F	59.83	61.13	84	-	-	p<0.05
LEAD-U	466.47	-16.95	84	-	-	p<0.005
LEAD-F	142.16	-6.012	84	-	-	p<0.05
CADMIUM-U	67	-27.91	84	-	-	p<0.05
CADMIUM-F	43.13	22.62	84	-	-	p<0.05
ANTIMONY-U	59.16	14.91	84	-	-	p<0.05
ANTIMONY-F	50	6.61	84	-	-	p<0.05
NICKEL-U	80	5.52	77	t = 1.425	76	p<0.158
BISMUTH-U	564	7.95	19	t = 2.109	18	p<0.04
URANIUM-U	707	18.23	76	t = 1.015	75	p<0.03
MERCURY-U *	448	0.799	56	t = 5.395	55	p<0.0005

Table 1: HMD™ data over several trials conducted over a 3-year period

* Mercury trial was conducted separately and the results of this are discussed below.

There were no serious side effects during the trials. Two people complained of a minor, transitory headache. Kidney, heart, liver and electrolyte blood tests showed that there were no pathological parameters in the post urine and faeces samples in all people tested, suggesting that HMD™ is a 'gentle' chelator that does not place undue stress on the kidneys and liver.

Moreover, Heart Rate Variability Testing (HRV), a measure of the functioning of all the physiological systems of the body, showed a significant increase in 40% of the people tested, only 48 hours after provocation with the HMD™. It is predicted that HRV scores would be greatly improved if the HMD™ were taken for much longer periods of time.

Independent Mercury Trial Using HMD™

Over the last year, a voluntary group of clinical patients from the Da Vinci Holistic Health Centre in Cyprus were used to test the efficacy of HMD™ on mercury. All urine analyses were conducted on a mercury-dedicated PSA Atomic Fluorescence Spectrometer, measuring levels of parts per billion. This involved a total of 56 patients who participated in a 24-hour provocation trial using HMD™ at dosages of 40, 50 and 60 drops throughout the day. Initial 6-hour baseline pre-urine samples were collected, along with a 24-hour collection for the post-urine sample.

There was a 448% increase in eliminated mercury in the post-test after 24-hour provocation with HMD™ in the 56 people tested, as compared with the pre-test baseline sample. Moreover, there was a negligible increase in mercury in the control group that were given only powdered chlorella in a little alcohol as a placebo. There was a statistically significant difference between the percentage increase of mercury in the post-sample as compared with the controls ($t = 5.395$, $df = 55$, $p<.0005$).

Percentage Increase of Mercury in

Pre-Post Test and Controls

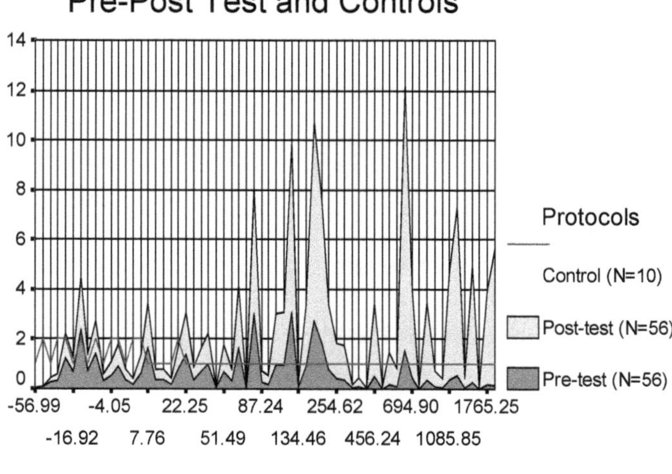

Liver and kidney serum test results during the HMD™ pre-post provocation trials:

During the HMD™ research trials, blood samples were taken from a small group of people (N=16) to determine the effects of the HMD™ provocation on liver and kidney function. The average percentage increase was calculated from the pre- and post-sample figures of these biochemical tests.

Table 2 below shows the percentage increase of these biochemical parameters in the post-serum samples when taking of HMD™, as compared with the baseline serum sample before HMD™ was taken. Overall, there are small average increases in creatinine, bilirubin, urea, ALT and AST, but nothing that surpassed pathological parameters. The minimum and maximum levels are also shown, but generally the higher levels were present in one individual only.

LEVELS OF LIVER & KIDNEY FUNCTION TESTS DURING HMD™ PROVOCATION					
	CREATININE	**BILIRUBIN**	**UREA**	**ALT**	**AST**
% INCREASE	11.95	3.15	25.35	16.74	5.25
MINIMUM	0	0	0	0	0
MAXIMUM	42.80	20.19	53.73	75.00	38.46
N=	16	16	16	16	16

Table 2: Details of the liver and kidney function tests

It can be concluded from these tests that HMD™ is a gentle chelator that does not adversely affect liver and kidney function tests and is tolerated by most people of all ages.

However, based on clinical use of HMD™ over the last 5 years, it would be advisable for the practitioner to use a universal drainage remedy that can work concomitantly on all detoxification systems including the liver, kidney, skin, lymph and blood. I have formulated such a natural herbal drainage remedy called Organic Lavage.[76]

Natural Heavy Metal Chelation Protocol

I have been working on a natural, heavy metal chelating protocol based on scientific and clinical evidence for over five years now. This is what I suggest can

76 See http://www.detoxmetals.com *for more details*

be used for most cases of heavy metal toxicity – I have called it the HMD ULTIMATE DETOX PROTOCOL and it consists of the following:

- **HMD™** – 45 drops x 3 daily for adults[77] – sensitive adults who have chronic diseases or compensated detoxification organs, as well as people with neurological diseases such as multiple sclerosis and the like, as well as autistic people, should begin with half this dose or less, and increase by one drop x 3 daily, every day until they reach a comfortable level.

- **ORGANIC LAVAGE** – this is a herbal formula of wild-crafted and organic herbs such as Silybum marianum (Milk Thistle Seed), Taraxacum officinale (Dandelion Root), Arctium lappa (Burdock Root), Trifolium pratense (Red Clover Tops), Curcuma longa (Turmeric Root), Hydrangea arborescens (Hydrangea Root) and Arctostaphylos uva ursi (Bearberry Leaf). This herbal formula is designed to facilitate detoxification of the liver, kidneys, lymphatics and skin, as well as cleanse the blood and act as a natural anti-inflammatory. Adult dosage: 25 drops x 3 daily for adults, or more as directed by a practitioner.

- **ORGANIC CHLORELLA** – there are many concerns about finding good quality, clean Chlorella that is void of heavy metals and xenobiotics. We have searched and travelled far and wide and found an excellent source that is provided with a Certificates of Analysis with each pot. This chlorella comes from the western coast of Hai-Nan Island, China's southernmost island. Hai-Nan Island is a tropical island with an excellent climate and lies on the same latitude as Hawaii. The non-industrialized, pollution-free, tropical island offers favorable growth conditions for chlorella, including intense sunlight, pure water, and clean air. Available in 475 mg tabs, adult dosage should be 2 tabs x 2 daily.

- **A-LIPOIC ACID** – I believe that when metals and other xenobiotics are mobilized in the body, there should be some protection against free radical damage. Lipoic acid is that extraordinary antioxidant which is both water and fat soluble, able to penetrate the brain and other nervous tissues, and is therefore able to protect all parts of the body against free radical damage.

- **MINERALS** – flushing the body with high levels of most of the minerals and trace elements will prevent the metals from re-entering the cell, as well as providing the raw materials for enzyme systems to reactivate, including detoxification systems. The easiest way is to take a colloidal multi-mineral

77 See http://www.worldwidehealthcenter.net/hmd-dosage-guidelines/ for full details

formula in solution. Otherwise, a good-quality, high-potency, multi-mineral capsule will suffice.

I will often fine-tune this protocol depending on the needs of the patient, but generally this works well for most cases as a basic protocol.

Further Research

During the 10 years of experience with HMD™ we have had many reports from women of all ages who have suffered from chronic endocrine problems coming back into balance while using HMD™ for 2-3 months. Many of these women suffered from irregular periods, heavy bleeding, PMS and other hormonal imbalances.

Based on this anecdotal evidence, we believe that HMD™ is eliminating other chemicals (xenobiotics) such as Bisphenyl A and Phthalates which are known endocrine-disrupting chemicals, as described above.

Preliminary trials have already been done which have shown that indeed this is the case – HMD™ is eliminating the xenobiotics through the urine. However, the sample of people tested is small, so further trials need to be conducted in this area before any scientific papers can be written.

Conclusion

There is an overwhelming amount of scientific evidence to support the relationship between heavy metal toxicity and chronic diseases in general.

This is why these toxic metal detoxification protocols detailed in this chapter are relevant to ALL diseases, without exception. So, these protocols need to be assimilated and practiced regularly. We are continuously accumulating toxins; it doesn't matter where we live these days, toxins are *everywhere!*

If you wish to see the progress of your own toxicity, then a good starting point is to run a Hair Mineral Analysis on yourself to determine the amount of toxic metals in circulation, and begin taking the HMD ULTIMATE DETOX PACK for 2 months, before running the hair test again.

If there is a percentage increase of toxic metals in the second test, then you will know that you have accumulated a number of toxic metals and will need to continue detoxing.

All these supplements can be obtained from www.worldwidehealthcenter.net and www.detoxmetals.com

In the next chapter we will look at the important topic of detoxification in order to rid the body of these toxins in order to optimise health.

Chapter 4

Detoxification: The Health Secret of all Time

Earlier on, I talked about the importance of detoxification in regaining my own health – this was a critical step to my recovery and I have consequently learned that it should be the foundation of all healing protocols.

Because of my healing journey and new-found health, I have developed several detoxification protocols which I am now implementing with hundreds of my patients every year at the Da Vinci Holistic Health Centre in Cyprus (www.naturaltherapycenter.com).

I am certain that the topic of detoxification will one day become a true science; all the biochemical pathways mapped out showing how the body cleanses itself when the detox protocols mentioned here are used.

Do not underestimate the power of these simple protocols. As a clinician, I have seen miraculous changes in many chronically ill patients after detoxifying. In fact, there is an academically oriented clinical course entitled *"Detoxification and Toxicology"* that has been written for the Bachelor and Doctor of Science in Holistic Medicine.[78]

We will concentrate on talking about detoxification protocols, or different ways to detoxify, in this chapter.

Many diseases in our society are related to toxicity. Here are just some of the diseases that are linked to toxicity:

1. Parkinson's
2. Alzheimer's
3. Dementia
4. Heart disease
5. Chronic fatigue syndrome
6. Fibromyalgia syndrome

[78] www.collegenaturalmedicine.com

7. Cancers
8. Autoimmune diseases
9. Food allergies and intolerances
10. Arthritis
11. Digestive diseases like Crohn's disease, ulcers, colitis, and inflammatory bowel
12. Menstrual problems like heavy bleeding, cramps, PMS, menopausal symptoms, mood changes, and hot flashes

It might seem that everyone is toxic. This may be true to differing degrees.

What are Toxins?

A toxin is anything that is harmful or detrimental to the body.
Toxins can be internal (created by the biological processes of the body) or external (something that is introduced to the body, ingested, absorbed or inhaled).

The immune system, gastrointestinal (GI) system and skin are designed to protect you from toxins. However, you are exposed to toxic substances daily via what you apply to your skin, what you breathe and what you ingest.

Within your lifetime, you will consume up to 50 tonnes of food. Your GI system is responsible for breaking down these foods, digesting and absorbing components which are useful and eliminating the rest.

The liver works to remove toxins from the food you eat as well as toxins produced by your body. When the GI tract is not functioning well, the liver must do more work due to the additional burden placed upon it.

What Do Toxins Do to the Body?

When toxins build up, the ability for your body to remove them is quickly impaired. The body's self-regulation systems go out of balance, digestion becomes impaired and the liver and immune system become overwhelmed and cannot keep up.

The function of the large intestine slows down which in turn leads to congestion in the lymphatic system - which is designed to drain waste products from blood and tissues - thus forcing waste to re-circulate within the body.

When the liver is clogged, it allows toxins to travel into the body, instead of filtering them out. Toxins then get into the bloodstream and cause inflammation in other parts of the body. Thus, the body resorts to using the skin to purge the waste. Acne, rashes and eczema are signs that the body is trying to rid itself of toxins.

Toxins are also stored in body fat, causing weight gain and preventing the body from fully detoxifying itself.

How do you know that you are toxic?

Do you suffer from tiredness, lethargy, a 'heavy' feeling, digestive problems, bowel distension, headaches, muscle aches, poor concentration and memory, insomnia and many other symptoms too numerous to list? Well, all these symptoms can be related to toxins in your body that have accumulated over time.

Table 1 below shows some common signs and symptoms of toxicity:

Headaches	Backache	Runny nose	Fatigue
Joint pains	Itchy nose	Nervousness	Skin rashes
Cough	Frequent colds	Sleepiness	Hives
Wheezing	Irritated eyes	Insomnia	Nausea
Sore throat	Immune weakness	Dizziness	Indigestion
Tight or stiff neck	Environmental sensitivity	Mood changes	Anorexia
Angina Pectoris	Sinus congestion	Anxiety	Bad breath
Circulatory deficits	Fever	Depression	Constipation
High blood fats	Unexplained irritability	Chronic fatigue	Muscle twitching

Table 1. Signs and symptoms of toxicity

Signs and Symptoms of Toxicity

Life is toxic! There are toxins in the food you eat, the water you drink and the air you breathe. Even your own body produces toxins as a result of its many metabolic processes that keep you alive.

Signs that detoxification is needed if you have:

- Unexplained headaches or back pain
- Joint pain or arthritis
- Memory failure
- Depression or lack of energy
- Brittle nails and hair

- Abnormal body odour, coated tongue or bad breath
- Unexplained weight gain
- Psoriasis
- Frequent allergies
- A history of heavy alcohol use
- A history of natural and synthetic steroid hormone use
- An exposure to cleaning solvents, pesticides, diuretics and certain drugs.

Benefits of Detoxification

There are several benefits of detoxification such as:

- The digestive tract is cleansed of accumulated waste and fermenting bacteria.
- Liver, kidney and blood purification can take place, which is not possible during regular eating patterns.
- Mental clarity is enhanced as chemical and food additive overload is reduced.
- Reduced dependency on habit-forming substances such as sugar, caffeine, nicotine, alcohol and drugs.
- The stomach size is returned to normal as bad eating habits are stopped.
- The hormonal system is enhanced which is especially true for growth hormones.
- The immune system is stimulated.

It never ceases to amaze me that most symptoms, if not all, can disappear in less than 15 days! After detoxifying on an alkaline diet for 15 days, patients report high energy levels; clear and glowing skin with a brilliance that is obvious (I have said on many occasions that I should take before-detox and after-detox photos of patients - the change is striking!); weight loss of several pounds, which is an excellent motivating factor to continue with a detox programme; clear-headedness; higher thresholds for stress and tension; reduced cellulite; good body tone and a great feeling of being relaxed.

"How do you achieve this?" you may ask. Well, the secret lies in using a variety of detoxification protocols, which I will share with you below.
Detoxification has become a household word and a colloquialism that could mean anything from drinking a glass of carrot juice to entering a detoxification centre if you are an alcoholic or drug addict.

The term has now become a misnomer for many things that it is not. In the context that we are using the term, detoxification is the process of removing the toxins that have been accumulating in the body tissues and organs throughout a person's life.

These toxins will have been acting as metabolism blockers by literally poisoning the cells and not allowing them to function correctly.

You can have toxins stored in your body for years without experiencing any negative symptoms. It is only when the toxin levels become too high that you start to feel ill.

Sources of Toxins

So where do toxins come from? There are many sources, some of which I will mention here.

The three main sources are:

a) **<u>Exogenous toxins</u>:**

Exogenous toxins (Greek: 'from outside') are those that enter our bodies from the outside, i.e. food additives, pesticides, herbicides, fungi from food, industrial pollutants, viruses, bacteria, parasites and electromagnetic pollution such as X-rays, electromagnetic radiation and geopathic stress.

These external toxins may also come from other sources such as water, beverages, alcohol, medicines, accidents and injuries. Various industries have polluted our environment with an array of toxic heavy metals such as aluminium, antimony, arsenic, beryllium, bismuth, cadmium, lead, mercury, nickel, thallium and uranium.

Bisphenol A and Phthalates, commonly referred to as BPA, are toxic substances that exist in cheap plastic drinking bottles. While most bottles with BPA have been phased out, some still use them and should be avoided. A 2015 study confirmed that about 44% of canned food producers still use BPA-lined cans.

Amalgam teeth fillings contain 50% mercury, which is a potent neurotoxin. We will discuss this later when we talk about toxicity and heavy metals.

Processed foods contain artificial food additives, colours, flavours and preservatives.

Meat often contains hormones and antibiotics, which can cause hormonal disruption.

Caffeine and other stimulants, sedatives, alcohol, tobacco and illegal drugs, all must be filtered out of the body through the liver and kidneys.

Household chemicals are also guilty of introducing toxins into indoor living spaces. Common surface cleaners can emit dangerous fumes that may concentrate in small, enclosed areas. Even pet products may contain toxic elements that can harm both you and your pet.

In the past 100 years, around 75,000 new chemicals have been released into the environment. Chemicals that your body was never designed to cope with.

On top of all that, people are not getting the proper amount of sleep and exercise needed to stay healthy. Sleep and exercise play a critical role in relieving stress and eliminating harmful toxins.

b) **Endogenous toxins:**

Endogenous (Greek: 'from within') are toxins that are found or generated within the human body. This can occur when the body's normal metabolic mechanisms function inefficiently. For example, it typically takes several steps to convert the amino acid methionine into cysteine. If one step is sluggish, an intermediate called homocysteine accumulates in tissues. Accumulation of homocysteine can damage the vascular system and contribute to heart disease.[79]

Other toxins are associated with tuberculosis, syphilis or other diseases due to microbes; excess hormone secretions; constipation, producing toxins in the gut; pathogenic bacteria, causing food to putrefy and produce toxins in the gut;[80].

Hormones, such as oestrogen and androgen, get broken down and excreted in the liver after they are used. If the hormones are not properly taken care of by the liver, then hormonal imbalances and symptoms occur. Toxic build-up can occur when elimination mechanisms are inadequate due to poor nutrient intake or malabsorption of key detoxification nutrients.

Emotional stress is also a large contributor to toxins in the body. Research has shown that there is a connection between your emotions and well-being. When experiencing a traumatic or stressful event, it is common to react with anger, fear, grief, resentment etc. Repeated cycles of emotional stresses have a direct effect on the nervous and hormonal systems, which can indirectly affect our body's ability to detoxify.

---

[79] Graham, I, Daly, L, Refsum H, et al. Plasma homocysteine as a risk factor for vascular disease. *JAMA*. 277;1775-1781, 1997.

[80] Donovan P. Bowel toxemia, permeability and disease: new information to support an old concept. In: Pizzorno JE, Murray MT. Textbook of Natural Medicine. St. Louis, MO: Elsevier Ltd; 1993.

Not dealing with your issues, and the emotions that get triggered by them, does not make the issue go away and only adds to the damaging effects on the body.

c) **Autogenous toxins:**

Autogenous toxins (Greek: 'Born within') are generated within the body from miasmic influences, which are inherited tendencies that can pass through up to seven generations. Examples of these are psora, sycosis, tuberculosis, syphilinum and others. There is no detection of these pathogens with scientific testing, but their deep presence can affect the body's organs, primarily by inhibiting a good immune response and lowering its resistance.
Let's look at some specific sources of toxins that we encounter daily:
Cigarettes, alcohol, caffeine and drugs are all substances that the body cannot use for building and repair, so will add to the mounting waste. A lot of these toxic wastes are stored in the tissues and organs of the body.

Heavy metals such as mercury from fish and amalgam fillings; aluminium found in cheeses, baking powders, cake mixes, self-raising flour, cosmetics, toothpastes, antiperspirants and some drugs such as antacids. Cadmium is found in tea and coffee, as well as cigarette smoke. Lead is found in paints, fuels, rubber, plastics, inks, dyes, toys, building materials and hair restorers.

Arsenic is given to chickens as a growth promoter. Roxarsone - 4-hydroxy-3-nitrobenzenearsonic acid - is by far the most common arsenic-based additive used in chicken feed.[81] It is mixed in the diet of about 70% of the 9 billion broiler chickens produced annually in the U.S. In its original organic form, roxarsone is relatively benign. It is less toxic than the inorganic forms of arsenic-arsenite.

However, some of the 2.2 million lbs of roxarsone mixed in the nation's chicken feed each year converts into inorganic arsenic within the bird, and the rest is transformed into inorganic forms after the bird excretes it. Arsenic has been linked to bladder, lung, skin, kidney and colon cancer, while low-level exposures can lead to partial paralysis and diabetes.

Plastics containing Bisphenol A, the building block of polycarbonate plastics, which are everywhere: in pesticides as fungicides, antioxidants, flame retardants, rubber chemicals, a coating in metals, cans and food containers, refrigerator shelving, returnable containers for juice, milk and water, nail polish, compact discs, adhesives, microwave ovenware and eating utensils.

---

[81] Hileman, B. Arsenic in Chicken Production: A common feed additive adds arsenic to human food and endangers water supplies. *Chemical and Engineering News*. Volume 85, Number 15, pp. 34-35, April 9, 2007.

A diet that is high in animal fats will add to the waste. There are many different drugs and chemicals that are given to animals these days, ranging from antibiotics, hormones, feed concentrates, etc. All these chemicals will accumulate in the fat cells of the animals that we then eat – so we slowly build up an accumulation of these chemicals over time.

Sluggish bowels can lead to a great deal of toxicity throughout the body.

Try to imagine a 10-metre tube running from mouth to anus packed with meat, sausage, fish, fruit salad, beef burgers, sugars, milk and other goodies – all fermenting and putrefying for days on end.

This fermentation produces highly toxic substances such as putrescine, neuracine and cadaverine. These are so poisonous that a small amount injected into a laboratory animal will kill it in minutes. All these toxic substances, apart from causing disease in the body, will also act as metabolism blockers, and will therefore have consequences on weight-loss too.

This process of 'self-poisoning' by these putrefying foods in the gut is called 'autointoxication.'

Refined foods such as white sugar, white flour, white rice, etc. are all deficient in nutrients, but calorie loaded. Apart from this, they also help to create a lot of sludge and debris in the body. If you remember from your childhood days, you probably used white flour and water to make a glue to make your kite, or to glue your coloured paper in your exercise book at school.

When eaten, white flour and its products become glue in the intestine and stick to the internal walls. When mixed with sticky sugar and fat, it becomes a rubber-like substance that blocks absorption of foods through the intestine, as well as being a constant source of toxins. If you don't believe me, read Dr. Jensen's book entitled, *'Tissue cleansing through bowel management'*[82]. There are also plenty of photos of what comes out of the intestine if you do a proper detox – disgusting!

Thousands of new, toxic chemical compounds are produced each year by the chemical industry, most of which are approved by various so-called 'Environmental Protection Agencies' (EPA's) without any serious toxicological studies. The cumulative number of toxic chemicals polluting our planet today exceeds 100,000.

Many claim that some of these chemicals, such as the flame retardants used in children's clothing, have potentially life-saving applications. But how many of these

[82] Jensen, B. Dr. Jensen's guide to better bowel care: A complete program for tissue cleansing through bowel management. USA: Avery Publishers, 1999.

chemicals do we ingest or are absorbed by our bodies and those of our children? And at what cost to our health? What is the capacity of the human body to eliminate them?

Has anyone conducted a general contracting cost-benefit analysis as to whether the benefits offered, for example, by fire hazard protection, truly outweigh the toxicity generated within us, our children and the environment? The answer is: *No.* There are no comprehensive, scientific answers, other than to confirm the obvious: toxicity levels in humans and animals across the globe are rising fast. Whether we realize it or not – *we are all toxic.*

In an article published in the October 2006 *National Geographic* entitled, *'The Pollution Within,'* journalist David Ewing Duncan had himself tested for 320 synthetic chemicals and certain heavy metals at a cost of $16,000, paid for by the magazine.

According to the article, Duncan was considered a healthy individual. Nevertheless, he had higher than average amounts of chemical toxins, such as flame-retardants (known as PDBE's), phthalates, Polychlorinated Biphenyls (PCBs), pesticides and dioxins, as well as heavy metals such as mercury.

Duncan's article alludes to some of the possible ways toxic chemicals may have accumulated in his body: some might have originated in childhood, while others may have been picked up in airplanes due to his extensive work-related travel. However, he and his doctors were merely speculating…

Duncan also describes his pre- and post-mercury toxicity results after a fresh fish dinner and breakfast. Duncan had fresh halibut for dinner and fresh swordfish for breakfast (cooked in his toxic non-stick pan), both of which were caught in the ocean just outside the Golden Gate Bridge in the San Francisco Bay area.

He tested himself for serum mercury before and after the meals and found that his blood mercury levels had shot up from five micrograms per litre to over 12. The doctors conducting the tests advised him not to repeat that experiment ever again, yet I'm sure this dangerous diet is adhered to by thousands, unaware of the impact of toxicity on their health. After all, fish is promoted as a health food! Nevertheless, drawing conclusions on the experience of only one healthy adult is not robust, toxicological science. So, let us review the research.

New 21st Century Theory of Disease

Dr. Miller, of the Department of Family Practice, University of Texas Health Science Center at San Antonio, USA, believes that we are on the threshold of the new theory of disease that is triggered by toxic chemicals. She states in one of her papers[83]:

"In the late 1800's, physicians observed that certain illnesses spread from sick, feverish individuals to those contacting them, paving the way for the germ theory of disease. The germ theory served as a crude but elegant formulation that explained dozens of seemingly unrelated illnesses affecting literally every organ system."

She continues:

"Today we are witnessing another medical anomaly – the unique pattern of illness involving chemically exposed people who subsequently report multisystem symptoms and new-onset chemical and food intolerances. These intolerances may be the hallmark for a new disease process, just as fever is a hallmark for infection."

I strongly agree with Dr Miller and believe that many of the new diseases that we are seeing today such as Gulf War Syndrome,[84] Chronic Fatigue Syndrome, Myalgic Encephalomyelitis (ME), fibromyalgia, childhood diabetes, attention deficit hyperactivity disorder and others are all chemically related disorders.[85]

How exposed are you to these chemicals?

Check out below how prone you are to develop a chemically-triggered 21st century disease, by checking off the various categories. The more of these that apply to you, the higher your risk. Do you:

- ✓ Work with chemicals
- ✓ Use pesticides around the house and garden such as fly spray, weed killer or flea powder
- ✓ Use non-environmentally friendly cosmetics, toiletries and household cleaners
- ✓ You are responsible for disposal of chemicals used in medicines such as mercury preservatives in vaccines and flea shampoo
- ✓ Eat nonorganic fruit, vegetables and meat products

---

[83] Miller C. Are We on the Threshold of a New Theory of Disease? Toxicant-induced Loss of Tolerance and its Relationship to Addiction and Abdiction. *Tox. Ind. Health*. 15:284-294, 1999.

[84] Miller, C. and Prihoda, TA Controlled Comparison of Symptoms and Chemical Intolerances Reported by Gulf War Veterans, Implant Recipients and Persons with Multiple Chemical Sensitivity. *Tox. Ind. Health* 15:386-397, 1999.

[85] Miller, C. Prihoda, T. The Environmental Exposure and Sensitivity Inventory (EESI): A Standardized approach for measuring Chemical Intolerances for Research and Clinical Applications. *Tox. Ind. Health* 15:370-385, 1999.

- ✓ Eat contaminated seafood, usually containing mercury
- ✓ Eat too many processed foods, full of preservatives, colourings, flavourings and other additives
- ✓ Drink unfiltered tap water containing aluminium and fluoride
- ✓ Consume soft drinks from aluminium cans
- ✓ Have mercury amalgam fillings in your mouth
- ✓ Live in a major city with all the air pollution.

These chemicals are accumulative, so do not think that a little exposure will do you no harm – it simply takes longer to reach critical levels in the body before symptoms appear.

Signs and Symptoms of Chemical Poisoning

In clinical practice, I am often very vigilant in trying to detect symptoms that are related to chemical sensitivity and other toxicity issues. If the patient suddenly develops the following symptoms, then chemical exposure should be suspected:

- ✓ Dark blue, black or pink circles under the eyes
- ✓ Wrinkles or abnormally puffy bags under the eyes, as well as wrinkles on hands and knuckles
- ✓ Bright red cheeks, nose tips or ear lobes
- ✓ Unstable legs
- ✓ A spaced-out look and feeling
- ✓ Itchy nose
- ✓ Licking lips frequently
- ✓ Fuzzy thinking, confusion; difficulty in concentrating, thinking clearly or remembering
- ✓ Joint or arthritic pains
- ✓ Runny nose or nasal congestion causing sinusitis and blocked nose
- ✓ Extreme fatigue, even when rising in the morning
- ✓ Headaches

One study that tried to assess exposure to Bisphenol A (BPA) and 4-tertiary-octylphenol (tOP) in the American population found 92.6% and 57.4% of the persons, respectively had these chemicals in their urine.[86] These are industrial chemicals used in the manufacture of polycarbonate plastics and epoxy resins (BPA) and non-ionic surfactants (tOP). These products are in widespread use in the United States and the rest of the world.

---

[86] Calafat AM, Ye X, Wong LY, Reidy JA, Needham LL. Exposure of the U.S. Population to Bisphenol A and 4-*tertiary*-Octylphenol: 2003-2004. *Environ Health Perspect* Jan;116(1):39-44, 2008.

Ways to Address Toxicity: The good, the bad and the ugly

Let's start with the ugly first: the typical misguided response to the toxicity onslaught is to visit the average doctor, who will note a few toxicity-induced symptoms, and come up with a superficial diagnosis.

At first, a diagnosis appears simple: flu, sinusitis, eczema, tonsillitis, or otitis. Over time, diagnoses get complicated: asthma, arthritis, sacroiliatis, heart disease, renal disease, liver disease, cancer or any of the currently labelled chronic degenerative diseases which can strike.
This ugly, symptom-based approach amounts to a classically wrong diagnosis.

The main causative factor, TOXICITY, remains undetected. Hardly anyone is searching for it, let alone finding it! Tragically, the ugly approach has become the norm, instead of the exception. Depending on the wrong diagnosis, which is typically a mere description of the symptom, the typical physician will prescribe chemical drugs to ingest, or refer you to other specialists who may contemplate removal of body parts (pardon the cynicism here, but this is the truth, as I experienced it from allopathic doctors – hopefully there will always be the exception among such practitioners).

With the ugly approach, the worse the disease, the worse the treatment gets. Cancer, the dreaded disease, is the perfect example.

The reasoning goes: many toxins are proven carcinogens, so they could well be the cause of a person's cancer, right? Wrong! The ugly approach sees the world differently. Even at this advanced stage of body toxicity, when the body's immunity and vitality has been seriously compromised by carcinogens, the default medical intervention is to load the body with even more toxins: potent chemotherapeutic agents that are super-toxic, or cancer-causing radiation treatments to remove the original cancer.

You also need additional drugs (Erythropoietin Stimulating Agents) to counter the decrease in red blood cell production caused by chemotherapy, which add their own serious side-effects. By then, the tumour is reduced, the cancer has metastasized, and the patient is either dead or bankrupt – or likely both. 'Common sense' at its best!

What we should be doing, medics and patients alike, is exactly the opposite. Should we not be addressing the cause of the problem - the toxins - instead of chasing and suppressing the symptoms? We should be reducing the toxic load, not increasing it.

We should be improving the tissue integrity, not cutting it apart. It seems evident to me that the common-sense approach would dictate addressing the safe removal of the toxins. Assuming our interest lies in achieving real, long-term relief for the patient.

Indeed, between the ugly and the good approach, there is also a bad way to address toxicity-caused illnesses.

If you try to release toxins from the body too fast, or too clumsily, the body may be tipped over the edge. This is an issue that many well-meaning practitioners underestimate – either because of inadequate technical know-how, insufficient experience or poor judgment – with disastrous results vis-à-vis the recovery prospects of their patients.

Unfortunately, there are plenty of bad ways out there to deal with toxicity-induced diseases. Therefore, sound and continuous research by the patient and practitioners to minimize such a risk is integral.

Meanwhile, a growing group of medical practitioners have 'jumped on the bandwagon' so to speak, using their medical licenses to chelate people with various heavy metals – using more drugs such as EDTA, DMSA, DMPS and the like. This can often lead to disastrous consequences as these drugs mobilize metals quicker than the body can eliminate them, while stripping the body of the good minerals.

In other words, the typical MD's knowledge of toxicology needs improvement, to say the least. There are natural, gentler ways of detoxifying the body of heavy metals and other xenobiotics.

I hope that this book, based on extensive research, will provide food-for-thought to the many out there that are lost and confused about these complex issues.

Let's move now to the main detoxification treatments and protocols that I use at the Da Vinci Centre, which effectively deal with the toxicity within my patients' bodies and are instrumental to the recovery of many diseases, including chronic degenerative disorders.

The Da Vinci Centre Detoxification Diet – clean, clean, clean!

The 15-day Alkaline Detoxification Diet (15-DADD)

Most of the patients that come to me for a wide variety of health problems will be placed on the Da Vinci Centre's 15-day Alkaline Detoxification Diet (15-DADD). This is a diet that I have put together through clinical experience, as well as studying the work of other practitioners[87,88,89,90] who are very well versed in the field of detoxification.

Most of my patients can safely follow this 15-day detoxification programme, except for a few who have other diseases such as diabetes, cancer, heart conditions, low blood pressure and some neurological diseases. There are modified protocols for all the aforementioned, but these should be supervised by a qualified health practitioner.

These more complex patients need more thought and each detoxification regime can be tailored to suit each patient. Therefore, I take a careful history from each one, as well as examining all their clinical findings. These include blood tests, blood pressure, conducting an Iridology examination (looking at the iris, the coloured part of the eye, using an iris microscope which gives me further health information), as well as other diagnostic instruments that I have at my disposal such as Live Blood Analysis, VEGA testing, Biological Terrain Analysis, heavy metal testing, Autonomic Response Testing, Thermography and more[91].

Generally, most patients will be able to tell me what their problem is and its severity, as they have usually received a medical diagnosis before arriving on my doorstep.

Given that all is OK to begin the 15-day detox diet, I suggest that they eat only fresh fruit, salads, freshly squeezed juices, steamed vegetables and vegetable soups for 15 consecutive days. This means that they ONLY eat these foods for the duration, most of which will be rich in the live enzymes, which are the tools required to flush out the toxins from the body. You must be patient and put your mind to it.

I cannot emphasize just how important the detoxification diet is to your success!

---

[87] Ballie-Hamilton, P. The Detox diet. UK: Penguin, 2002.

[88] Scrivner, J. Detox Yourself. UK: Judy Piatkus (Publishers) Ltd., 1998.

[89] Wade, C. Inner Cleansing: How to Free Yourself from the Joint-Muscle-Artery-Circulation Sludge. New York: Parker Publishing Co., 1992.

[90] Cabot, S. Juice Fasting Detoxification. USA: The Sprout House, 1992.

[91] www.naturaltherapycenter.com

What will I be eating during the 15-DADD?

I strongly suggest that you try to eat as many raw fruits and vegetables as possible, including at least 1-3 fruit and vegetable juices daily. Carrot juice has a strong effect on the digestive system, provides energy, serves as an important source of minerals, promotes normal elimination, has diuretic properties and helps to build healthy tissue, skin and teeth. So, I recommend as many carrot juices as they can handle, mixed with beetroot juice (about 1/3rd of a glass), which are powerful cleansing agents of the body. Beets are said to really cleanse the blood and kidneys. In nature, homogenous colours do not occur by accident – it is no coincidence that the red beetroot affects the blood!

I also encourage the use of a little 'green juice' mixed with each carrot juice. This can be anything from fresh parsley, lettuce, kale, collard greens, Swiss chard, alfalfa, cabbage, spinach, turnip greens, watercress, celery, cucumber, green pepper, scallions, coriander, or any other green vegetable in season. You can place a couple of inches of the green juice in the glass and top up with carrot juice. All green vegetables contain chlorophyll, which is very oxygenating for the body. It is also an effective antiseptic, cell stimulator, red blood builder and rejuvenator – therefore helping to remove toxic sludge faster. Greens are also super-rich in live enzymes.

I also suggest that each meal should begin with raw fruit or vegetables, seasoned with a little lemon, ginger, garlic, coconut or desired herbs. This way, they are available for digesting the fat, protein, and carbohydrates from the meal that follows. The enzymes in vegetables control or restrict the amount of waste deposited on your adipocytes. Remember to chew all foods thoroughly.

These are the foods that I allow during the detoxification phase – no other family of foods is allowed. You may eat as many of the following foods as you wish, but it is best to eat only when you feel hungry. Wash all fruit and vegetables in a bowl of water with 4-5 tablespoons of grape vinegar added (not apple cider vinegar), to help wash away any pesticide/herbicide residues. Rinse afterwards with clean water. Here are the foods that you can eat in plenty – in fact, the more you eat and drink, the quicker you detoxify:

• **SALADS** – use any type of fresh vegetables you like, in any combination. Use organic vegetables when available and include bean sprouts when in season. Salad dressings should be kept simple – a little virgin olive oil with fresh lemon or lime juice, or cider vinegar. Add plenty of fresh onion and garlic – these are very detoxifying!

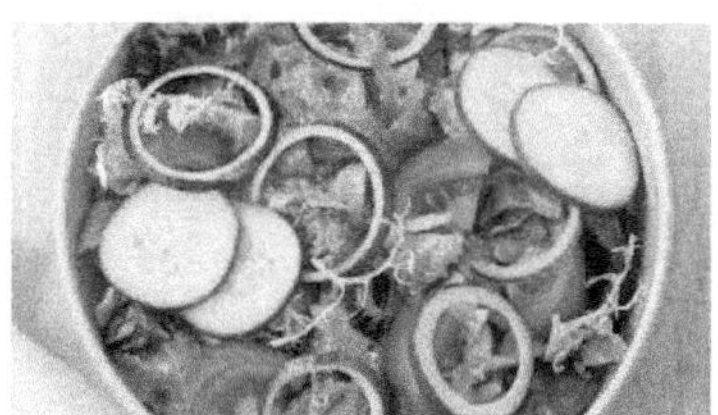

• **STEAMED VEGETABLES** – eat any variety you like, including broccoli, cauliflower, potatoes, beetroot, carrots, etc. Steam as opposed to boil, and eat with a little herbal salt, lemon and a little virgin olive oil, with plenty of garlic. You may also have jacket potatoes with a little olive oil, garlic and parsley dressing.

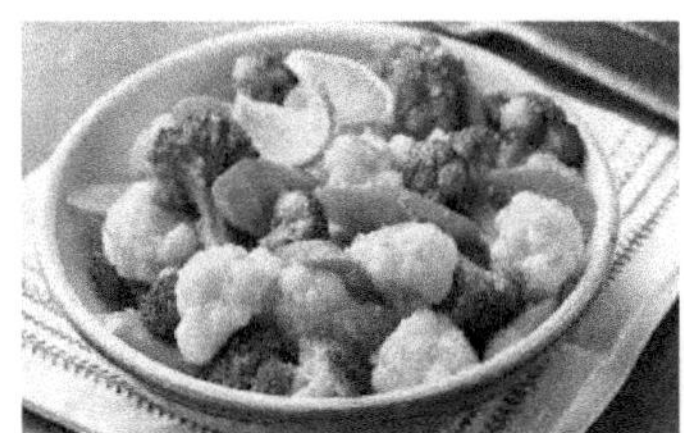

• **STIR-FRIED VEGETABLES** – this is a quick, easy way of cooking vegetables healthily. Use no more than four cups of chopped, hard or medium-hard vegetables or eight to twelve cups chopped leafy greens in a 14-inch wok to avoid crowding the pan. It's important that the vegetables are very dry, otherwise, the vegetables will steam and braise in the pan and lose their crisp texture. Giving the vegetables a whirl in a salad spinner is the easiest solution, but you can also pat them thoroughly with kitchen towels.

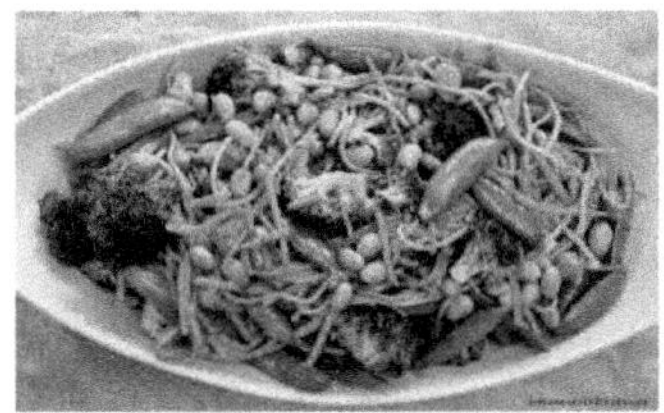

• **VEGETABLE SOUPS** – again quick and easy to make, and very nutritious, providing all the vegetables that our bodies require. It is easy to digest and is generally low in calories. Studies have shown that we tend to eat 20% less calories overall when we eat soups before a main meal. You can make nutritious leak and broccoli soups, as well as tomato and clear soups with various vegetables, adding onion and garlic for their detoxification benefits too.

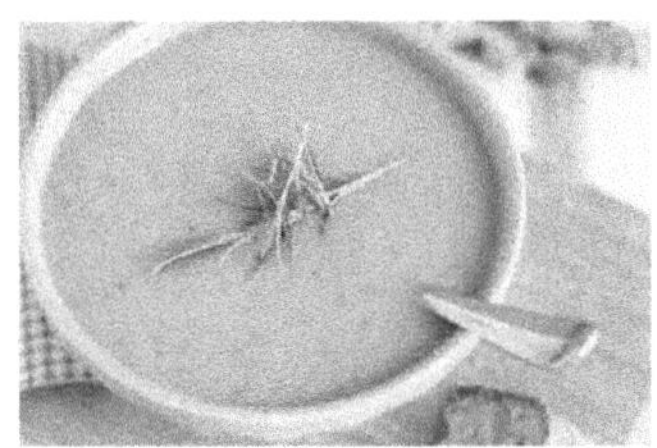

• **VEGETABLE/FRUIT JUICES** – drink a minimum of 1-3 per day and try to include one cocktail comprising one-third of a glass of raw, green juice (spinach, parsley, cabbage and any other green vegetables), topped up with carrot juice. There is no limit to the amount of fresh vegetable and fruit juices that you may drink in a day.

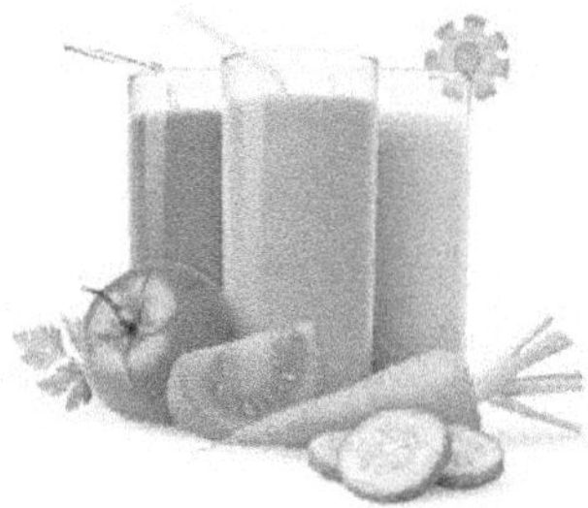

• **FRESH FRUIT** – choose the fruit of your choice (preferably organic) and eat as much as you like, whenever you like. You could begin the day with 2-3 pieces of fruit, which are gentle on the digestive system. Make a tasty fruit salad and eat it in the morning as this helps to detoxify. Fruit is rich in antioxidant phytonutrients which are beneficial to the body in many ways; protecting us from chronic diseases.

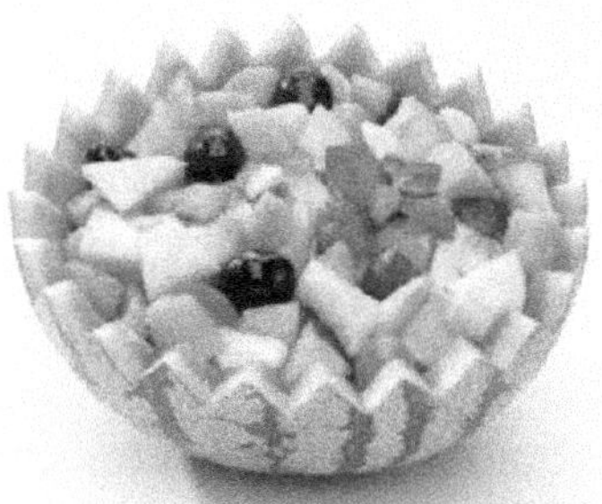

• **HERBAL TEAS** – choose any of your choice. Chamomile is a good relaxant; aniseed and mint is good for the digestive system; Kombucha; dandelion tea or 'coffee' (which is excellent for purifying the blood and detoxifying and stimulating liver function); Sage tea, (which is a blood cleanser); or Nettle tea, (which is excellent for driving away excess fluid out of the tissues and is a wonderful cleanser for all the detoxification organs). Drink as many as you like, with a little honey on the tip of a teaspoon if you like, but plain is best.

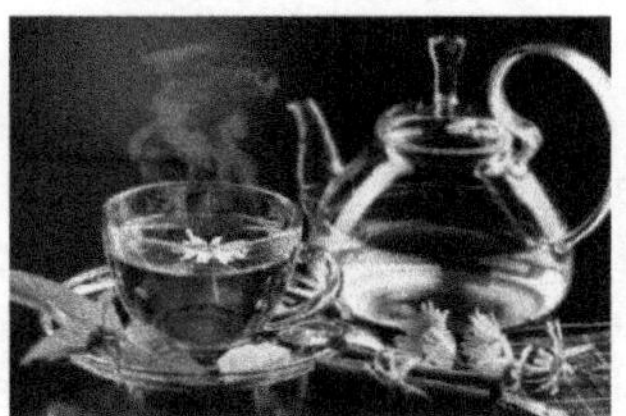

You will also need to drink at least 8-10 glasses per day of still mineral water to flush out the toxins – this is VERY IMPORTANT, so please take note!

When the 15 days are over, you should carry on eating the above for a couple more days while gently adding a little protein such as fresh steamed or grilled fish, organic chicken, pulses, a soft-boiled organic egg or a little cheese. Go gently on the protein for a couple of days before you begin eating normally again so that you do not overload your digestive system.

Lots of Food and Calories

This may appear to be an awful lot of calories, since there are no restrictions on the amount of such foods consumed over the 15-day period. The purpose of this diet, however, is to DETOXIFY – to remove the toxins from the fat cells and tissues as well as the organs, so that the body can return to its optimum level of functionality. I have yet to see anyone going through the 15-DADD put on any weight, so don't worry about counting calories – most people lose one or more kilos (2-4 lbs) over the 15-day period.

I had one gentleman weighing 150 kg (nearly 24 stone) who lost 10 kg (22 lbs) in 15 days, but I believe that most of this was accumulated fluid due to a drinking problem. On a biochemical and microbiological level, there is much going on during the detoxification.

The pH or acidity/alkalinity of the body is being adjusted back to normal, and any nasty pathogens in the body are encouraged to reverse their course. This is based on the work of Enderlein, Neissens and Beauchamp who were proponents of pleomorphism as opposed to monomorphism.
With our bad eating, smoking and drinking habits, body chemistry is unbalanced in most people. This unbalanced body chemistry will be another metabolism blocker that will not allow the body to digest, assimilate, eliminate or get rid of fatty deposits optimally.

Detoxification Symptoms: "The healing crisis"

When the body detoxifies, it goes through various biochemical and physiological changes.[92] Generally, on the first day of fasting the blood sugar level is likely to drop below 65-70 mg/dl. The liver immediately compensates by converting glycogen to glucose and releasing it in the blood. After a few hours, the basal metabolic rate is likely to fall to conserve energy. This means that the heart, pulse and blood pressure will drop. More glycogen may be used from muscles, causing some weakness.

As the body requires more energy, some fat and fatty acids are broken down to release glycerol from the glyceride molecules and are converted to glucose. You may notice the skin becoming quite oily as these fatty acids and glycerol increase in the blood. The skin is one of the largest detoxification organs, so you may get some skin problems such as pimples, acnes or a pussy boil – this is all part of the body trying to cleanse. The complexion may become pallid for a day or two as the wastes accumulate in the blood.

The incomplete oxidation of fats may result in the formation of Ketones resulting in ketoacidosis. Combined with high levels of urea, resulting from protein metabolism, this state can cause several symptoms which may suppress appetite; they affect the satiety centre in the hypothalamus.

Generally, this takes a few days to happen and you may notice your appetite dwindling. You may get pains in different joints, or organs such as the lungs. There may be a considerable amount of yellow mucus released from the throat and expelled. The sinuses may also begin clearing with more mucus secreted.

Given that the body is releasing these toxins quickly during the first few days of the detoxification process, it should not surprise you to experience some changes in your body that may cause certain symptoms. Initially, for the first 2-3 days these symptoms can be a little unpleasant, SO BE WARNED!

A fair number of people will have headaches, nervousness, diarrhoea, upset stomach, energy loss, furry tongue, halitosis (bad breath), as well as acne or other skin rashes, a general feeling of malaise, frequent urination due to the toxins irritating the bladder and some of their existing symptoms may be exacerbated. When the toxic residues enter the blood, they affect mind and body functions.

These may be unpleasant symptoms for the first couple of days, but they are a NORMAL part of the detoxification process, and in natural medicine we call this

92 Salloum, TK. Fasting Signs and Symptoms: A Clinical Guide. USA: Buckeye Naturopathic Press, 1992.

the HEALING CRISIS. All these symptoms indicate that the DETOX IS WORKING! This is a temporary and transient crisis, it will pass – so hang on in there and don't worry that there is something wrong with you.

There was always something wrong with you, and now you are doing something about it – you are reversing this toxic process that your body has adapted to.

If you are a coffee drinker, then the symptoms will be more pronounced, as your body will be in a state of withdrawal. Yes, coffee is a drug and when you come off it you go into withdrawal, meaning that your body will start asking for a dose of what it is addicted to. When it doesn't get it, then it screams for it louder and louder, usually in the form of headaches, migraines, muscle pains, general weakness and lack of concentration.

Enduring a cleansing crisis is the hardest part of the healing process. To stop feeling bad, most people want to eat, but do not eat during a cleansing crisis! The body is overloaded with the work of removing toxins. Digestion makes matters worse. Drinking one or two glasses of sodium bicarbonate (baking soda) – one teaspoon in each glass drunk twice daily - will help to neutralize the ketoacidosis.

Helter-skelter rides are common – the 'downward slope' is when the body is vigorously cleansing, and the blood gets swamped with toxins causing you to feel down, moody, depressed and achy, like having a bad cold. You feel weak and lethargic. The mind rationalizes: 'I feel horrible: this can't be working.' You can maintain a normal routine of work on a dip but it requires willpower and determination. It also helps to know that the longer the down period, the greater the fasting high.

Phases of Detoxification

There is a lot going on in the body during the detoxification process – most of the work is happening in the largest detoxification organ of the body – the liver. The detoxification phases in the liver are composed of two phases, known as Phase I and Phase II. These phases chemically biotransform toxins into progressively more water-soluble substances through a series of chemical reactions so that they can be excreted from the body.

Phase I: Detoxification

This phase of detoxification usually involves oxidation, reduction, or hydrolysis. A family of enzymes commonly referred to as cytochrome P450 mixed-function oxidases perform the most important processes – detoxifying xenobiotics and endogenous substances.[93]

At least 50 enzymes in 10 families governed by 35 different genes allow Phase I to take place. Many forms of cytochrome P-450 enzymes are involved in Phase I reactions. The highest concentration of cytochrome P-450 occurs in the liver, which is the most active site of metabolism. The lungs and the kidneys are secondary organs of biotransformation, with about one-third of the liver's detoxification capacity. Cytochrome P-450 has also been found in the intestines, adrenal cortex, testes, spleen, heart, muscles, brain, and skin.

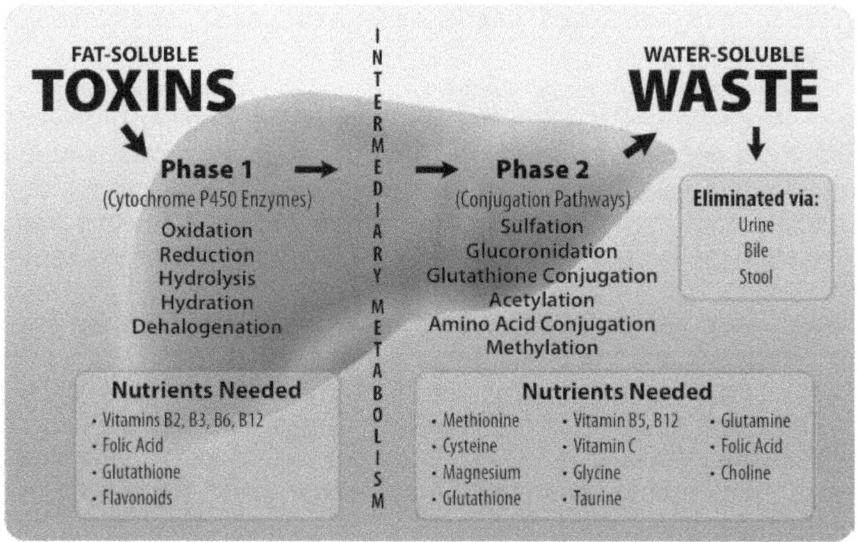

Our understanding of these detoxification pathways over the last couple of decades has helped clinicians understand how they can help patients overcome toxic effects.[94] Sluggish, imbalanced, or impaired detoxification systems can result in the accumulation and deposition of metabolic toxins, increased free radical production and its ensuing pathology, impaired oxidative phosphorylation, and reduced energy.

93 Grant DM. Detoxification pathways of the liver. *J Inher Metab Dis*. 14;421-430, 1991.
94 Davies MH, Gough A, Sorhi RS, Hassel A, Warning R, Emery P. Sulphoxidation and sulphation capacity in patients with primary biliary cirrhosis. *J Hepatol*. 22(5):551-560, May 1995.

Nutrients Required for Detoxification Phase

The action of detoxification enzymes in both Phase I and Phase II detoxification pathways depends on the presence of various nutrients.[95,96] For example, alcohol dehydrogenase, an enzyme that converts alcohols (such as ethanol) to aldehydes in an oxidation reaction, depends on an adequate supply of zinc to function properly.

In the next metabolic step, the enzyme aldehyde oxidase changes the aldehyde into an acid that can be excreted in the urine. Aldehyde oxidase depends on an adequate supply of molybdenum and iron. Other minerals that are required by enzymes include manganese, magnesium, sulfur, selenium, and copper.

Other supporting nutrients involved in cytochrome P-450 enzymes include vitamins B2, B3, B6, B12 and folic acid. The tripeptide glutathione and the branched-chain amino acids leucine, glycine, isoleucine, and valine are also required. Flavonoids and phospholipids are supportive as well.

Protective antioxidant support is required for handling reactive oxygen intermediates produced during Phase I activity. Antioxidant support requires the carotenoids, including beta-carotene, vitamin C and E and coenzyme Q10.

To summarize, the nutrients required during Phase I and Phase II detoxification are:

- B-complex vitamins: necessary co-factors used in Phase 1 detoxification
- Digestive enzymes: may be necessary to ensure that protein is adequately digested and glycine is readily available
- Essential fatty acids
- N-acetyl cysteine (NAC): an immediate precursor to glutathione, a potent antioxidant and among the most import detoxification nutrients for the liver
- Reduced glutathione
- Selenium, zinc, magnesium and manganese; possibly iron and copper if used with caution
- Taurine
- Vitamins C and E and beta carotene
- Inositol & Methionine: lipotropic agents (help with the breakdown of fat in metabolism) that work to transport fat out of the liver
- High ORAC vegetable extract blend with polyphenols (a phytonutrient)

---

95 Anderson KE, Kappas A. Dietary regulation of cytochrome P-450. *Annu Rev Nutr*. 11:141-167, 1991.

96 Bland JS, Bralley JA. Nutritoinal upregulation of hepatic detoxification enzymes. *J Appl Nutr*. 44(3&4):2-15, 1992.

Most of these are available in one high-potency multivitamin/mineral formula that we use called HMD MULTIS. The fatty acids can be obtained from KRILL OIL. All supplements mentioned here are obtainable from www.worldwidehealthcenter.net.

In addition, liver herbs can be used to aid detoxification (traditionally known as 'blood cleansing' herbs):

- ❖ Dandelion root, beet leaf & Yellow Dock: cholagogue (stimulates liver secretions and bile flow)
- ❖ Artichoke leaf: promotes regeneration of the liver and promotes blood flow in that organ; stimulates bile flow
- ❖ Silymarin (bioflavonoid found in Milk Thistle): according to research, this herbal extract stabilizes the membranes of liver cells, preventing the entry of virus toxins and other toxic compounds including drugs and supports the protection of the liver and promotes its regeneration
- ❖ Turmeric: a cholagogue like dandelion.
- ❖ Caraway, dill seeds, sassafras tea

Most of these can be found in the herbal formula that we use called HEPATO PLUS.

Usually, the enzymatic reactions in Phase I decrease chemical toxicity. However, toxic or reactive chemicals can form during Phase I that are more toxic than the original compound. This is known as bioactivation. When Phase II detoxification proceeds normally, these chemicals are then rendered harmless and excreted. However, if there is an imbalance in the active levels of Phase I and II detoxifications, these toxins will remain in the body. Imbalance between Phase I and Phase II is associated with increased symptoms of nervous, immune, and endocrine system toxicity.

Toxic chemicals produced during Phase I include teratogens (causing fetus malformation), mutagens (causing cell mutation), and carcinogens (causing cancer). For example, benzo[a]pyrene, a chemical found in coal tar and cigarette smoke, is biologically inert until it is converted by the mixed-function amine oxidase system into a metabolite that can then initiate cancer causing activity. During Phase I, many compounds also form dangerous reactive free radicals - chemicals with an unpaired electron that can cause tissue damage. A buildup of free radicals can increase the risk of cancer.

Here is a more detailed diagram showing these important nutrients:

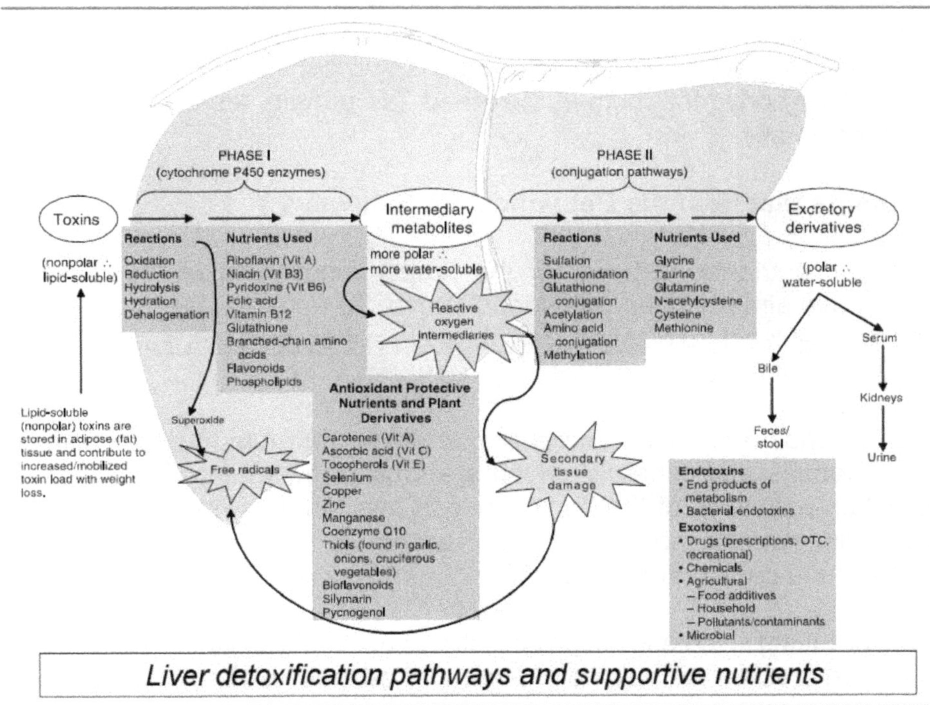

Liver detoxification pathways and supportive nutrients

The level of functioning of Phase I can be measured with a simple caffeine metabolism test. A known quantity of caffeine is ingested, and saliva samples are taken twice at specified intervals. The efficiency of caffeine clearance is directly related to the efficiency of Phase I detoxification. Rapid clearance of caffeine shows enzyme induction (increased production), either from xenobiotic exposure or toxins within the body. A slow rate of caffeine clearance indicates that cytochrome P-450 activity in the liver is abnormal. Patients with slow caffeine clearance have difficulty eliminating xenobiotics and other toxins.

The function of Phase II can be evaluated through the ingestion of both acetaminophen and aspirin. This test measures the recovery of the products of glutathione conjugation, sulfur conjugation, glucuronidation, and glycine conjugation (acylation) in the urine. Comparison to normal values allows evaluation of the efficiency of Phase II. A high ratio between Phase I and any of the Phase II pathways implies imbalanced detoxification in the body.

The detoxification process requires large amounts of caloric energy, which comes mainly from the food we eat. If we do not eat enough protein, the body breaks down vital tissue protein to produce the energy it needs. This decreases the available amounts of Phase I and Phase II enzymes, amino acids, and peptides, because the body breaks down protein to amino acids and peptides. The greater the toxic burden of the body, the higher the need for protein, carbohydrate, fat, and micronutrient intake.

Supplements that Help the Detoxification Pathways

Some of the nutrients required for the proper functioning of the detoxification pathways have already been mentioned above. To reiterate, it is strongly advised that you drink at least 10 glasses of mineral or reverse osmosis water daily, so that you can flush out the toxins quicker.

We have already mentioned taking a multivitamin formula to help optimize your levels of vitamins and minerals, which are crucial raw materials for many of the detoxification pathways of the body. Choose one that has high levels of vitamins and minerals, not just the RDA levels – at the Da Vinci Center we use a high-potency formula called HMD MULTIS.

In addition, taking a couple of grams of vitamin C three times daily during the detoxification process will also help. Vitamin C will help to absorb certain toxins, as well as helping the immune system cope with a heavy burden of toxins that it needs to get rid of. I usually recommend a Calcium/Magnesium Ascorbate in powder form, which is an alkaline form of vitamin C, and is much gentler on the stomach and gut than plain ascorbic acid.

At the Da Vinci Center we use one in capsule form called VITAMIN C (Mixed Blend). Take 2 caps x 3 times daily, or you can open these up and place them in some juice or water.

Other supplements that we recommend include the following:

HEPATO PLUS - this is a herbal combination, specifically designed to provide extra support to the detoxification organs and systems of the body – particularly during periods of over-indulgence in food, alcohol or smoking.

Beneficial for...

- Liver cleansing
- A sluggish liver and gallbladder
- Body cleansing and detoxification
- Blood purifying support
- High energy levels
- Cholesterol levels
- Body odour
- Digestive health
- Indigestion
- Relieving symptoms of occasional over-indulgence in food and drink
- A colon cleansing program
- Those with a poor diet
- Those with a high toxic load

You can take one capsule x 3 times daily. Each capsule contains:

- Artichoke extract (40:1), 2.5% cynarin (equivalent to 4800mg of fresh artichoke)
- Parsley powder
- Beetroot extract (5:1) (equivalent to 400mg of fresh beetroot powder)
- Turmeric powder (95% Curcumin)
- Burdock root extract (5:1) (equivalent to 200mg of fresh burdock root)
- Fennel seed extract (4:1) (equivalent to 120mg of fresh fennel seed powder)
- Dandelion root extract (4:1) (equivalent to 100mg of fresh dandelion root powder)
- Liquorice root extract (5:1) (equivalent to 100mg of fresh liquorice)
- N-acetyl L-cysteine
- Alpha lipoic acid
- Garlic (black aged garlic) extract (100:1) (equivalent to 500mg of fresh garlic powder)
- Ginger root powder
- Cayenne (Capicum Frutescens) extract (8:1) (equivalent to 30mg of fresh cayenne powder)

Another herbal formula called COLFORM. This is a fast-acting, herbal colon cleanser and bowel support formula with 10 active herbal ingredients, including glucomannan.

COLFORM is a well-known herbal colon cleanser and bowel support combination, based on a formula by American master herbalist, Dr. John R. Christopher.

Beneficial for...

- Constipation
- Sluggish bowels
- Haemorrhoids
- Clearing bowel 'pockets'
- Diverticula
- Internal cleansing and detoxification
- Stool softening
- Prior to, following or between colonic hydrotherapy treatments

You should take one capsule x 3 times daily. Each capsule contains:

- Rhubarb powder
- Barberry powder
- Burdock root powder
- Cayenne powder
- Ginger root powder
- Rhubarb root extract (30:1)
- Fennel seed powder
- Aloe vera extract (200:1)
- Clove bud powder
- Dandelion root extract (4:1)

Another herbal remedy called CONSTFORM, based on one of Dr. John R. Christopher's formulas, is good to add when there has been a history of constipation.

It is a fast-acting colon cleanser, designed for the chronically constipated in need of strong treatment for a blocked bowel.

Beneficial for...

- Chronic constipation
- Internal cleansing
- Lower bowel function
- Bowel regularity
- Laxative abuse
- Use by colonic hydrotherapists before, during and after treatments

You can take one capsule x 3 times daily. Each capsule contains:

- Rhubarb powder
- Barberry powder
- Glucomannan 90%
- Alfalfa powder
- Cayenne powder
- Garlic powder
- Aloe vera extract (200:1)
- Dandelion root extract (4:1)
- Ginger root extract (20:1)
- Nettle leaf extract (4:1)

Another herbal formula that I recommend to my patients during the 15-day detox is called PARAFORM PLUS ONE. This one is designed to eliminate parasites from the intestine; we pick these up from food and water all the time, so a couple of times per year it is good to detox from these too.

The ingredients have been hand-picked for their anti-parasitic, anti-bacterial, anti-microbial, anti-fungal and anti-viral activities.

Beneficial for...

- Internal parasites, flukes and worms
- Candida albicans overgrowth
- Irritable Bowel Syndrome (IBS)
- Diarrhoea
- Constipation
- Fungal infections
- Mouth sores and herpes
- Certain skin conditions, such as acne and eczema
- Colon cleansing
- Travel abroad to locations where food hygiene and/or water quality may be less then ideal

Each capsule contains:

- Magnesium caprylate – **175mg**
- Cinnamon powder – **100mg**
- Cloves powder – **100mg**
- Shiitake mushroom powder – **100mg**
- Garlic powder extract (10000mg/g) – **75mg**
- Glucomannan (95%) – **50mg**

- Pumpkin seed P E 4:1 (40%) (equivalent to 200 mg pumpkin seed powder) – **50mg**
- Chicory root P.E 4:1 (equivalent to 120mg chicory root powder) – **30mg**
- Grapefruit seed P.E 5:1 (equivalent to 100mg grapefruit seed powder) – **20mg**
- Cayenne extract 7:1 (equivalent to 100mg cayenne powder) – **14.3mg**
- Fenugreek seed P.E 4:1 (equivalent to 48mg fenugreek seed powder) – **12mg**
- Olive leaf extract 15:1, 6% Oleurpein (equivalent to 50mg olive leaf powder) – **3.35mg**

Yet another supplement that I recommend during the detox that gives the body a good energy boost is called SUPER GREENS PLUS. This is a 100% organic (Soil Association registered) superfoods powder, that can be used as a plant protein powder, light meal shakes or daily nutrient booster. In fact, it is one of the most nutrient-dense organic superfood combinations per serving you will find.

It provides a broad range of vitamins, minerals, antioxidants and powerful phyto-nutrients through its multiple organic superfood, superfruit and herbal ingredients.

High in vegetable-source proteins, this full-spectrum blend also contains over 20 natural enzymes and 70 beneficial nutrients.

A great all-round supplement to support energy levels, cleanse, detox, and alkalise the body – daily organic nourishment made easy!
For every 300 g of powder, it contains:

*Activated Pre-Sprouted Barley
*Apple
*Linseed / Flaxseed
*Wheatgrass
*Quinoa
*Barley Grass
*Alfalfa
*Kelp (Ascophyllum)
*Spirulina
*Acai Berry
*Carrot
*Turmeric
*Bilberry Fruit
*Spinach Leaf
*Lemon Peel

Stay with the detoxification process, and allow yourself time to rest, particularly during the first few days. It is best starting on a Friday, given that you will have the weekend at home to get organized and rest when you need to.

I do not recommend vigorous exercise during this initial period, but a 20-30-minute walk with a friend or loved one in an open-air park is fine. You need to conserve your energy levels for the detoxification process. Under normal circumstances, the body uses 80% of its energy for detoxification, which is a substantial amount, and this will increase during the 15 days of this intensive detox programme.

The Good News!

The good news is that after the initial healing crisis you WILL FEEL A LOT BETTER. This is literally a guarantee that I can give you personally, as I have witnessed it hundreds of times with my patients, as well as myself.

I personally detoxify twice a year for 15 days, and another 7 days in the summer when fruit and juices are plentiful here in Cyprus.

I KNOW how it feels when your body begins to get rid of the toxins and you are over the healing crisis – a clarity of mind that is crystal clear, increased concentration, increased energy levels, better sleep, calmer, more reflective state of being, increased awareness of your environment, better digestion, your constipation improves, body pains dwindle or melt away, arthritis improves, chests and throats clear, skin colour and tone greatly improves and I have had many clients who cut down or actually stopped smoking, as the body rebels harder during a detox programme.

These are all benefits that you will experience, so STICK WITH THE PROGRAMME and achieve OPTIMUM HEALTH. Once you experience this state of optimum health you will wonder what the hell you were doing when you had moderate health, just like most people walking the planet today.

The Alkaline Detox Diet is one of the most positive steps you can take and should be treated and enjoyed that way – treat yourself for 15 days, eat as much as you like, whenever you like, of the foods that you are allowed during the detox.

Before Starting the Detox Programme

There are a few indications which would exclude some people from starting the detox programme and you should not do so if any of the following apply:

- You are pregnant – the toxins released during the detoxification process can harm the embryo because the embryo's capacity to detoxify is limited due to its poor organ functionality at such early stages of development.

- You are breastfeeding – toxins released into the mother's blood will travel to the milk, so the baby will get a dose of toxic milk that will not help them in any way. Wait until after the baby is weaned off the breast and meanwhile you could start eating healthily.

- You are presently being treated for an illness or condition such as diabetes or heart problems without medical supervision. It is important for your doctor or health practitioner to know what you are doing. With diabetics, for example, it is possible that you might go into a hypoglycemic episode where your blood sugar levels fall below normal, due to the increased insulin production by the pancreas.

  I have seen this several times – as the pancreas begins to clear of toxic overloads, it begins to function better, so it can begin to produce MORE insulin than before, resulting in a sudden decrease of blood sugar levels. This is fine if a health practitioner is aware of what is going on and can adjust the dosage of drugs to suit.

- You are recovering from a serious illness without expert medical supervision – if you are recovering from cancer, any type of operation, an accident or other serious disease, then you should be extremely careful of detoxifying by yourself. The toxins released in the body could upset the healing process and period of convalescence. Seek guidance from an experienced health practitioner who has experience in detoxifying. It is pointless asking a doctor who has no idea of detoxifying, as you are more than likely going to get a negative report, just from pure ignorance. Seek the help of an experienced person in these matters and take note that not many medical doctors are knowledgeable of the detoxification process, nor have experience in these matters. Only very few do, so do not take it for granted that all are knowledgeable because they are doctors.

- You are taking any prescribed or non-prescribed medication – again, the toxins mixed with the drugs could exacerbate further the healing crisis and cause more symptoms than are necessary.

- You are not ready at this moment in time to begin – the detox programme does require a little discipline and organization so would not be suited to a person who is travelling continuously, or eating out continuously with business associates, or who is under a lot of stress from marital or domestic problems. We need to prepare ourselves psychologically and emotionally before we begin. If you feel that this is not the right time for you, then postpone it for another time when you are ready.

Preparing for the Detox

Preparing for the detox is not difficult, nor is it costly, but should be done some time BEFORE you decide to begin. There are several things that you need to gather before you start. A checklist of essentials is outlined below:

- A large stock of fresh vegetables and fruit in season – kept in the fridge for freshness. If you have access to ORGANIC FRUIT and VEGETABLES, then this should be your obvious first choice. Organic produce is free from the pesticides and chemical fertilizers that are harmful to the body but are also richer in nutrients due to the organic fertilizers that are used. One famous doctor, Dr. Gerson, said, *"The soil is our second metabolism."* What he meant by this profound statement was that the nutrient quantity and quality of the soil is going to determine the quality of our bodily functioning. Organic produce has been 'fed' the right ingredients of minerals, trace elements and vitamins that our bodies require to function optimally. I sincerely wish I had a steady supply of organic produce at my disposal here in Cyprus where I work and live, but unfortunately, we are not that health conscious as a nation to begin organic farming yet.

- A good thermos flask – you can use this for transporting freshly squeezed fruit or vegetable juices to and from work. It is important to remember, however, that the live enzymes and vital energy in freshly squeezed juices have a life-span of ONLY THREE HOURS. So, it is crucial that you drink the juice within these 3 hours and try to keep the juice as cool as possible – heat can destroy these very vulnerable enzymes. You may also use the flask to transport herbal teas, either hot or cold (with ice cubes) if you wish.

- A good quality juicer – there are many different types of juicers on the market, and it is a true science to choose the right one. Most of the juicers on the market for domestic use are centrifugal juicers. If you are buying one, try to find the best that money will buy as this is going to be a sound health investment that will see you through many years of life. There are cheaper ones at half the price that will probably only last a year or less, so choose carefully. You could pick up a good one for less than $100, but if you can pay to buy the Rolls Royce of juicers, go for something like a Champion juicer (about $300), which will extract 25% more nutrients from vegetables and juices than the centrifugal juicer. The Champion juicer is a masticating juicer – it grinds the fruit or vegetable into a paste before spinning at high speed, to squeeze the juice through a screen set into the juicer bottom. The ultimate in juicers is the Health Stream Press which can extract up to 50% more juice than a centrifugal juicer but can cost from $500 to over $2,000 for the automated press.

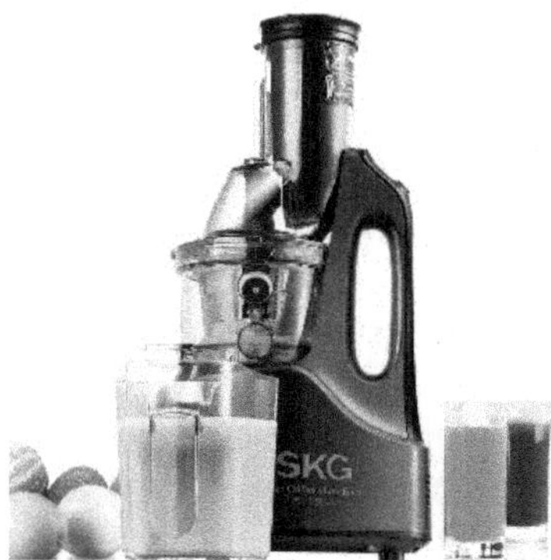

- A steamer – metal (stainless steel) or bamboo – the type you place over or in the pan of hot water to steam vegetables. Steaming is far more preferable to boiling because when you boil vegetables in water, they lose minerals such as potassium, which is crucial to health. Steaming vegetables decreases the losses of these important minerals.

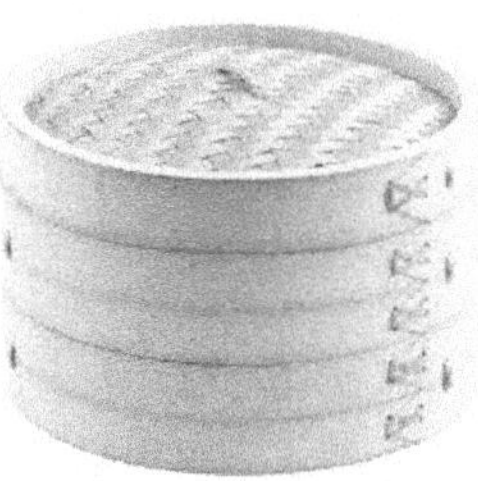
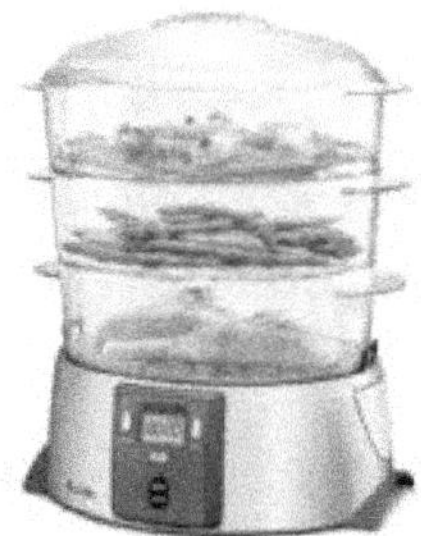

- Extra virgin olive oil – this is extracted using a cold press method from whole, ripe, undamaged olives. It is made without heat and is unrefined, as compared with olive oil that is not virgin or extra virgin. It still contains many of the natural factors unique to olives, which are normally lost through degumming, refining, bleaching and deodorizing. Virgin olive oils do not suffer nutrient losses and molecular changes that negatively affect human health. Choose this oil over ones that do not have the word 'virgin' or 'extra virgin' on the label.

- Fresh garlic – have plenty of fresh garlic at hand - it would be wise to eat one clove a day as this contains more than 200 chemical compounds, most of them having therapeutic qualities. Eating fresh parsley and lemon juice or sucking on a whole clove can help to neutralize garlic odour on the breath. Garlic can inhibit and kill bacteria, fungi and parasites; lower blood pressure, blood cholesterol and blood sugar; prevent blood clotting; protect the liver and contains anti-tumour properties. It can also boost the immune system to fight off potential disease and maintain health.

Regarding detoxification, which particularly interests us here, garlic can stimulate the lymphatic system, which expedites the removal of waste from the body. It can nourish most of the organs such as the heart, stomach, circulation and lungs, as well as protect the cells from damage by nasty free radicals (molecules that harm the body). The sulphur elements in garlic also help to stimulate certain enzyme systems that are beneficial for detoxifying, such as the liver's glutathione pathways, which help to remove toxins from the body; there are going to be plenty of these passing through the liver in the next 15 days.

So, now you understand why garlic is so important. It is one of the true wonders of nature, and I cannot understand why people dismiss it because of its odour, yet we accept so many other disgusting smells such as smokers smelling like ashtrays!

- A brush made of natural fibre – this is going to be used for SKIN BRUSHING (see details below).

- Water – you will need a large supply of either mineral or distilled water throughout the detoxification process. I suggest that you drink at least 10 glasses daily – this may mean having a glass next to you at home and the workplace and keeping it topped up. You will be surprised how many glasses you can drink in a day if you do this systematically. It really is a matter of habit, but what I have found is that if you don't have the water to hand, you will not remember to drink it.

Water is crucial to detoxification. It is part of the flushing process, which gets the toxins that are released by the cells out of the body. After a lot of research regarding water filters, I have personally settled for the reverse osmosis unit with a vortex energizer – there are many companies now that can fit the unit under your sink and add a separate small tap specifically for the drinking water. This is connected to your tap water, but the reverse osmosis filter will eliminate literally everything from chlorine, fluoride, heavy metals, pesticide residues as well as micro-organisms – it is squeaky clean water that you can drink and cook with.

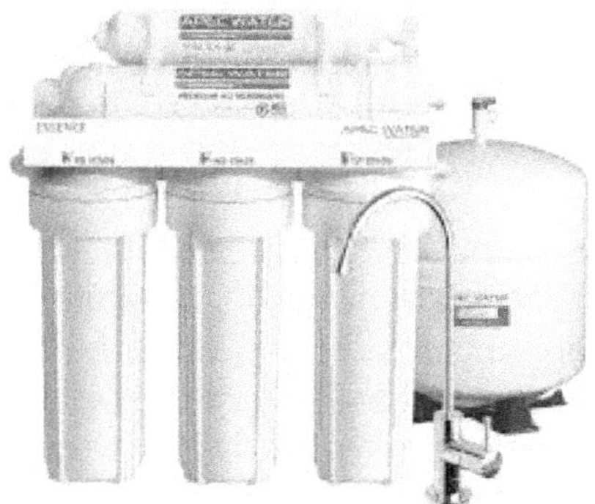

- Fresh lemons or cider vinegar – what you use is really a matter of taste, but both are excellent and healthy condiments. Cider vinegar made from apples is very rich in potassium, a mineral that is required by all cells during metabolism. In his book, *'Cider Vinegar'*, Cyril Scott talks about how cider vinegar can help overweight people, citing several case histories. He recommends two teaspoons of cider vinegar in a tumbler of water, to be taken on rising in the morning. Exactly how it works is an enigma, but even if it does not work for weight loss, it will certainly help to alkalize the blood and help clean it.

- Herbal teas – there are several herbal teas that you could drink every day throughout the detox programme. Green tea is excellent. Apart from being rich in vitamin A, E, C, calcium and iron, it contains healthy phytonutrients called Epigallocatechin Gallate (EGCG), which inhibit the growth of cancer and lowers cholesterol levels. Dandelion 'coffee' is also excellent, as this herb purifies the blood, detoxifies and stimulates the function of the liver. It's also a natural diuretic. It's good to drink teas that help to drain the detoxification organs and get rid of the toxins. Another good one is stinging nettle tea, which helps to drive excess fluid out of the tissues and helps with metabolism by increasing the elimination through the kidneys. Other goodies are chamomile, peppermint, rosehip, blackcurrant, elder flower, strawberry and Melissa. Most of these can be found in good health food shops – either in tea bags, or loose.

The Theory of Autointoxication

The compelling suspicion that a stagnant bowel filled with putrefying matter can leak out and become a source of infection for the rest of the body was first suggested by the ancient Egyptians. In the 19th century, this became known as 'The theory of autointoxication – self poisoning from one's own retained wastes.'

This idea has been enthusiastically embraced by every subsequent generation. One of the main causes is constipation.

Constipation

Constipation has done more to provide the health profession with an obvious solution to un-diagnosable ailments than any other simple complaint. It is defined as 'The difficult or infrequent passage of faeces' and it is associated with the presence of dry, hardened stools.

Constipation is a national pastime and slow bowels are more common today than years previous. For one thing, people not only ate better 100 years ago, they were more active and got out doors more.

When the bowels slow down, toxins are not eliminated but are reabsorbed and carried back to the liver for recycling and elimination. Reabsorbed bile salts have been linked to increased cholesterol levels. Therefore, high cholesterol is a major precursor of constipation. Also, when the bowels get slow and toxin levels increase, the pathogenic microorganisms grow to out-number the normal flora, causing dysbiosis.

Although friendly bowel flora such as Acidophilus (small intestine) and Bifidobacteria (colon) are needed to correct this, it is the clogged bowels that are the major problem. When the bowels move again, everything else will fall into order.
Our endocrine glands (which control metabolism), are also involved since it is our thyroid that controls metabolism and metabolism affects how our bowels function. In this way, constipation can be seen as a symptom of hypothyroidism. Low body temperatures (a symptom of hypothyroidism) are very common today –although they are not 'normal' – as many authors have reported.

Intestinal toxaemia (a form of blood poisoning), is caused by the absorption of bacteria and their toxins through the intestinal wall. The large intestine (colon) is the most prolific source of bacterial contamination in the entire body. Thirty-six toxic substances have been isolated from the human colon, including such compounds as indole, skatole, phenol and cresol.

When these kinds of toxins are passing through the intestinal wall, they can enter the lymphatic or portal system and be directly transported to the liver. Temporary increases in the toxic load of the liver occur during periods of stagnation in the colon. Any prolongation of this state will impede the detoxification and bacteria-killing function of the liver. The importance of this function cannot be overlooked when one realizes that blood from the intestinal tract enters the liver before it is delivered to the tissues of the body.

An overburdened liver, which cannot handle the toxic load from the intestine, transfers the task of detoxification onto another organ - the kidney. Unfortunately, the kidney is not able to reduce the amount and kind of toxins that enter the liver, nor can it detoxify them as efficiently as the liver. The toxins that the kidneys do not remove from the blood increase circulating body-toxin levels.

The Oxford Dictionary defines constipation as, *'Irregular and difficult defecation.'* The question is, *'What is a regular bowel movement when there is no norm?'* Regularity becomes a meaningless expression when some people have a bowel movement regularly every Sunday morning, while others regularly empty their bowels after every meal.

Defecation is a reflex action, stimulated by distension of the rectum with faeces. It is under voluntary control in adults and normally takes place only when time and circumstances are suitable. The presence of food in the stomach stimulates a reflex action called peristalsis, which moves food residue into and along the colon. Mass peristalsis gives us the feeling that we need to empty our bowels. This reflex action usually occurs after the first meal of the day but can also be stimulated by only drinking some liquid on rising.

If the call to defecate is persistently neglected, the reflex mechanism becomes less sensitive and constipation can result. This is likely to happen when there are time constraints causing hurry and stress (stress ceases peristaltic action in the colon). Some healthy people don't defecate every day and do not have any discomfort. Many others open their bowels every day with excruciating agony – passing dark, rock hard, compacted stools. Both cases would be considered constipated.

Ideally, one should defecate as many times as we have a proper meal, usually 3 times per day. Although the main rule is that we should have a bowel movement at least once a day. The stool should be fibrous, light in colour, float in the water, break up easily and cause no pain or discomfort to pass – in fact no toilet paper should be needed. Pain or discomfort whilst passing hard or dry stool at less than daily intervals can be considered as constipation. Many people have suffered heart attacks as a result of vigorous efforts to have a bowel movement as continuous efforts to evacuate material from the rectum increases the heart rate, blood pressure and respiration.

Referred to essentially as a Western disease, constipation is virtually unheard of among third world people adhering to traditional fibre-rich diets. Constipation is implicated in many Western diseases such as diverticulosis, obesity, varicose veins, cancer of the colon and rectum, appendicitis and haemorrhoids. These are all very rare in undeveloped countries.

Whatever the causes of constipation, it is important that you should try to use some gentle herbal formulas and supplements in order to help the transit time of the gut.

At the Da Vinci Center, I use the following formulations to help my patients. They can all be combined if required and the dosages can vary depending on the condition and the patient:

1. CONSTFORM
2. COLFORM
3. OXYGUT

Nature Needs Some Help and Urgently

- In the U.S., approximately 80 million people suffer from bowel problems.
- 100-120,000 a year lose their lives – usually from bowel cancer.
- Colon cancer is the second leading killer in the Western World.
- Behind these statistics are also those saved by colostomies (surgical removal of the large intestine), which in the US only approximately 250.000 people a year receive.
- In UK and the rest of Europe, the numbers are more or less the same.

Bowel experts all over the world now agree that poor bowel management is the root of most health problems. The faulty Western commercialized diet is the focal point of the problem. A diet high in meat, white sugar, white flour, fat, and low in dietary fibre and water is believed to be connected with constipation.

The root of the problem is clearly indicated by laxative sales, estimated at *600–800 million dollars a year.*

Laxatives aggravate the problem of constipation by interfering with the colon's ability to eliminate normally on its own. The chemicals within laxatives irritate and stimulate the colon to abnormally contract, to expel the irritating substances. In addition, the oral route of administration is the least optimal method for evacuation of the colon because crucial digestive processes occurring in the stomach and small intestine are interfered with. Most laxatives and purgatives precipitate dehydration.

Hippocrates took the view of not disturbing and messing up the entire peptic system with harsh laxatives, as the problem lies at the extreme end of this same system. Standard enemas, even highly recommended as first aid, only cleanse the rectum and last portion of the colon, missing out most of the large intestine.

Colon Hydrotherapy is an extended and more complete form of an enema. This method extends beyond the rectum to cleanse the entire colon and offers greater therapeutic benefits. It addresses the cause or source of the constipation problem. Other methods treat only the symptoms and provide temporary relief of the problem.

Why constipated? The biggest reasons? Dietary (lack of natural dietary fibre and consumption of devitalized foods, especially white sugar, white flour and all their by-products); neglecting the urge to eliminate; dehydration (too little water); stress; too little exercise (sitting for long hours); abuse of stimulants and drugs; irregular hours (work – rest, wake – asleep) and pathological conditions.

The most common signs and symptoms due to an impacted, constipated colon are:

- Infrequent or difficult bowel movements; hard compacted stools and low stool weight
- Tiredness, fatigue, lethargy, lack of energy, poor concentration and irritability
- Bloating and flatulence
- Headaches, mental depression or dullness
- Irritable Bowel Syndrome, diverticulosis, colitis, leaky gut, cancer of the bowel, Crohn's Disease, appendicitis, hiatus hernia
- Malabsorption, bad breath and a coated tongue
- Haemorrhoids, varicose veins, obesity and cellulite

Colon Hydrotherapy

Colon Hydrotherapy is one of the most powerful and effective ways of cleansing and detoxifying our entire system. The mucous membrane of the large intestine is the first and most important defence system against toxic substances (followed by the liver, the lymph system, lungs and the skin), thus a very important part of the body's immune system.

As I outlined above, nearly all doctors and practitioners of natural medicine take the view that most disease originates in an unhealthy colon.

Exogenous toxins such as poor nutrition, sterilized and denatured foods, environmental toxins and poisons, abuse of medicines and narcotics as well endogenous toxins from emotional conflicts and stress, clog detoxifying channels on an on-going basis.

Having three bowel movements a day does not negate the fact that after years of dietary indiscretion, a gradual build-up of mucus and undigested foods begin to form in the lining of the colon.

Dehydration and stagnation occur. Our bodies are being poisoned by these toxic substances which can cause inflammation, damage the intestinal wall and cells, and intoxicate the nerves and glands. These toxins can also be absorbed through the walls of the colon into the blood and lymph; ultimately to into the cells and tissues. The resulting toxaemia can become a chronic condition, but for most of us it creates erratic conditions in the body that we call *disease.*

Heavy Metal Detoxification

We will discuss this in a separate chapter on toxicity, but we can briefly mention that heavy metals such as arsenic, aluminum, antimony, cadmium, lead, mercury and uranium are insidious in today's world. There is probably not a person on this planet that does not have some of these in their system, leading to heavy metal toxicity, which is the cause of many illnesses.

The early signs of heavy metal poisoning are vague or often attributed to other diseases. These include headaches, fatigue, muscle pain, indigestion, tremors, constipation, anemia, indigestion and tremors. Mild toxicity symptoms include impaired memory and distorted thinking ability. Severe toxicity can lead to death.

Hair mineral analysis is a convenient but often unreliable screening test. The most accurate measurement is by blood analysis of actual toxin levels within the red blood cells. Many toxic metals tend to accumulate inside the cell, where most of the damage is done.

One of the safest and most effective ways to remove heavy metal toxicity is to use a natural heavy metal chelating therapy named HMD ULTIMATE DETOX PACK[97]. The main formulation that mobilizes the metals is called HMD™ – you will need to take 45 drops, three times a day shortly before meals, in some water or juice.

In addition, there are two other drainage remedies that can be taken along with the HMD™, and are part of the HMD Ultimate Detox:

Chlorella (500mg) for absorbing the stray heavy metals that may get reabsorbed from the gut. Recommended adult dosage: 2 tabs three times per day.

[97] www.detoxmetals.com

'Organic Lavage' combines several organic herbs that help to clean the blood and help the kidneys, liver and lymphatic system to open up and drain the toxins out of the body. Recommended adult dosage: 25 drops x 3 daily for 3-6 months, along with the HMD™ and chlorella.

Killing Uninvited Guests

Schmidt and Roberts in their 1989 *'Foundations of parasitology'*[98] book noted that 25%–30% of people living in the south-eastern US (mainly children) were infected with whip worm (the trichuris species)[99].

Meanwhile, the Centers of Disease Control also stress that parasitic infections affect persons living in developed countries, including America. Zoonotic diseases, i.e. those transmitted from animals, are often caused by parasites, and infected people can even experience symptoms so severe they become life-threatening.

Food can become contaminated if livestock (i.e. cows and pigs), are infected with parasites such as cryptosporidium and trichinella. People can acquire trichinellosis by ingesting trichinella-infected, undercooked meats. Cryptosporidiosis can be passed to humans if orchards or water sources near cow pastures become contaminated by infected bovine faeces; or if tainted fruit is consumed without being washed adequately beforehand.

In addition, pets too can act as parasite hosts and pass them on to humans. Young animals, such as puppies and kittens, are more likely to be infected with Ascaris and hookworms. According to official CDC data:

> *"Trichomonas is the most common parasitic infection in the USA, accounting for an estimated 7.4 million cases per year. Giardia and cryptosporidium are estimated to cause two million and 300,000 infections respectively in the US annually. Cryptosporidiosis is the most frequent cause of recreational water-related disease outbreaks in the US, causing multiple outbreaks each year. There are an estimated 1.5 million new toxoplasma infections and 400 to 4,000 cases of congenital toxoplasmosis in the US each year; 1.26 million persons in this country [US] have ocular involvement due to toxoplasmosis;*

---

[98] Schmidt, GD and Roberts, LS., Foundations of Parasitology (4th ed). USA: Times Mirror/Mosby College Publishers, 1989.

[99] For a brief history of human parasitology, visit the site: http://cmr.asm.org/cgi/content/full/15/4/595. Further information can also be found at: http://www.alternative-doctor.com/allergies/parasites.htm

and toxoplasmosis is the third leading cause of deaths due to food-borne illnesses (375+ deaths).[100]"

In the EU, the European Food Safety Authority (EFSA) was set up in January 2002 following a series of food crises, which have hardly subsided since then; mad cow/sheep/goat disease, foot-and-mouth disease, bird flu and so on. In its latest report, the EFSA says the most commonly reported zoonotic infections in humans in the EU are, by far:

> *"... those caused by bacterial zoonotic agents that can be shed by asymptomatic farm animals: the 2004 data indicates salmonellosis (192,703 reported cases) and campylobacterosis (183.961) – followed by yersiniosis (10,381), human listeriosis (1,267), parasitic zoonoses is 2,349 (trichinellosis, toxoplasmosis and echinococcosis put together). Compared to the main bacterial food-borne infections mentioned above (395,455 put together), reported human cases of 'classic' zoonoses are relatively low: brucellosis (1,337), tuberculosis due to M. bovis (86) and rabies (two imported)."*

But perhaps even harder to accept is that the parasites within you are infected by their own parasites in turn – parasites within parasites! The story is endless. For an enlightening exposition on the nature of symbiotic, as well as parasitic endobiotic relationships (microorganisms living within other organisms), Dr. Peter Schneider's article, *'Prof. Enderlein's research in today's view. Can his research results be confirmed with modern techniques?'*[101] is enlightening.

Parasites are everywhere. In their most pathogenic states cause havoc in body, mind and spirit. Doctors respond with a range of treatments intended to suppress the symptoms, while failing to attack their source – the parasites themselves.

So, what can we do about these parasites we carry? Dr. Hulda Clark, Ph.D., N.D., a naturopathic physician, has brought the issue of parasitically-caused diseases and other types of toxicity back into the spotlight in recent years, dealing with this subject at length in her book, '*The cure for all diseases.*'[102] Clark describes various methodologies and procedures to cleanse the body from these nasty creatures. This is not the only herbal parasite cleanse that is used at the Da Vinci Centre. Sometimes other therapies are combined using Sanum remedies, homeopathics, other herbal formulas and bioresonance therapy.

---

[100] The CDC's A-Z index listing of Parasitic diseases can be accessed at: http://www.cdc.gov/ncidod/dpd/parasites/index.htm

[101] Schneider, P. Prof. Enderlein's Research in Today's View: Can his research results be confirmed with modern techniques? First published in the German language in the *SANUM-Post magazine* (56/2001) Semmelweis-Institut, Germany, 2001.

[102] Clark, HR. The Cure for All Diseases. San Diego, CA: New Century Press, 1995.

At the Da Vinci Holistic Health Center, we use Bioresonance diagnostics to identify the specific parasites in question and can therefore design bespoke anti-parasite programmes. However, generally we use the PARAFORM PLUS ONE (one capsule x 3 times daily, away from food) mentioned above, along with a PARAFORM TINCTURE (2 teaspoons in the morning, in a little water away from food). Both can be taken together.

The Liver and Gallbladder Flush

The liver is the gateway to the body and in this 'chemical age' its detoxification systems are easily overloaded. Thousands of chemicals are added to food and over 700 have been identified in drinking water.

Plants are sprayed with toxic chemicals, animals are injected with potent hormones and antibiotics, and a significant amount of our food is genetically engineered, processed, refined, frozen or cooked. All this can lead to destruction of delicate vitamins and minerals, which are needed for the detoxification pathways in the liver. The liver must try to cope with every toxic chemical in our environment, as well as damaged fats that are present in processed and fried foods.

This is why it is crucially important to cleanse your liver, much like you clean your house, bedroom, car and external self. Cleansing at least once per year is a good thing. When the liver gets overloaded it cannot metabolize fats and cholesterol easily, and this is when your cholesterol level start increasing and gall stones form.

As well as this, the liver itself becomes 'fatty.' Fatty livers are usually found in about 50% of people over the age of 50 – this is often seen by radiologists over time when examining patients routinely. Any imbalances in the liver will have a direct effect on the gallbladder, since it's the liver that produces the bile and gallstones.

Let's look at the gallbladder and how this organ can be easily cleansed, with amazing health benefits.

The gallbladder is a pear-shaped organ that stores about 50ml of bile until the body needs it for digestion. Bile is a bitter, yellow/green alkaline fluid secreted by hepatoacytes (special cells) in the liver. The human liver can produce close to one litre of bile per day. The bile stored in the gallbladder is between 5-10 times more concentrated and potent that the bile secreted directly by the liver. This bile is discharged into the duodenum (the first part of the small intestine) mainly for the emulsification (breakdown) of fats during digestion. This is why people who have had their gallbladder removed are likely to have a tough time digesting fatty food.

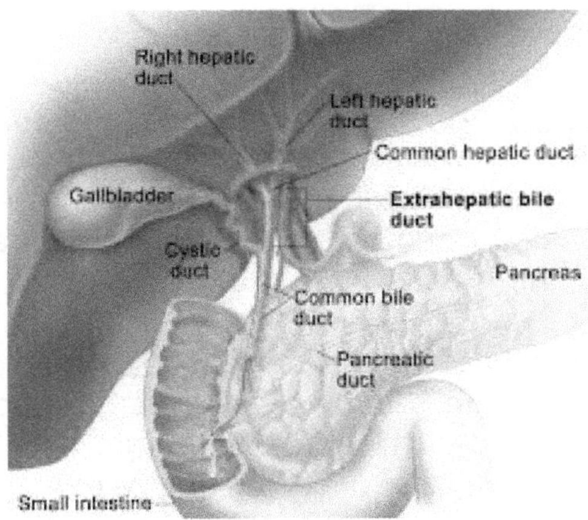

Gallstones

If the ducts or tubing of the gallbladder is filled with gallstones, then this can cause several health problems including allergies or hives. However, some people have no symptoms. These stones cannot be seen by ultrasound scan or X-rays as they are not actually in the gallbladder, but in the ducts. They may also not be calcified stones. There are many types of gallstones, most of which have cholesterol crystals in them. They can be black, red, white, green or tan coloured.

As the stones grow and become more numerous, the back-pressure on the liver causes it to make less bile. This is also thought to slow the flow of lymphatic fluid. Imagine if your garden hose had small stones in it; the result would be that much less water would flow. When there are gallstones present, much less cholesterol leaves the body, resulting in elevated cholesterol levels.

Moreover, gallstones are porous so can pick up all the bacteria, cysts, viruses and parasites that are passing through the liver. These masses or 'nests' of infectious material hang around the liver and supply the blood flowing through it with lots of fresh bugs daily. This is one way that parasites are circulated and reproduce. These parasites and infectious nests must be removed, and the simplest way of doing that is to remove the gallstones.

The Pathogenesis of Gallstones

The stones consist mainly of cholesterol, bilirubin and calcium salts, with smaller amounts of protein and other materials. In Western countries, essentially all gallstones, whether cholesterol or pigmented, arise in the gallbladder. In Asia, a significant fraction of pigmented stones originate in the bile ducts. In Western countries cholesterol is the principal constituent of more than three quarters of gallstones.

In the simplest sense, cholesterol gallstones form when the cholesterol concentration in bile exceeds the ability of bile to hold cholesterol in solution. Non-cholesterol stones are categorized as black or brown pigment stones, consisting of calcium salts of bilirubin.

Most of the stones are made of cholesterol (75-80%), with bilirubin stones being rarer and consisting of calcium bilirubinate, with large amounts of mucoprotein. Brown pigment stones are usually the hardest and smallest of the stones and these are usually made of calcium salts of unconjugated bilirubin, with variable amounts of protein and cholesterol.

Gallstones Effect Many Millions of People

It is estimated that 20% of the world's population will develop gallstones in the gall bladder at some stage in their lives. This figure does not take account the numerous stones that accumulate in the liver and its ducts.

In the United States, over 10% of the total population has gallstones. Each year 1,000,000 new patients are diagnosed. Performance of 500,000 cholecystectomies (gallbladder removal) leads to an annual expense of more than $5 billion in direct costs.

Gallstone prevalence varies with age, sex and ethnic group. Ultrasound surveys show a female: male ratio of 2:1 in the younger population and an increasing prevalence in both sexes with age. After the age of 60, 10-15% of men and 20-40% of women will have gallstones. Childbearing, oestrogen-replacement therapy and oral contraceptives increase the risk of developing gallstones.

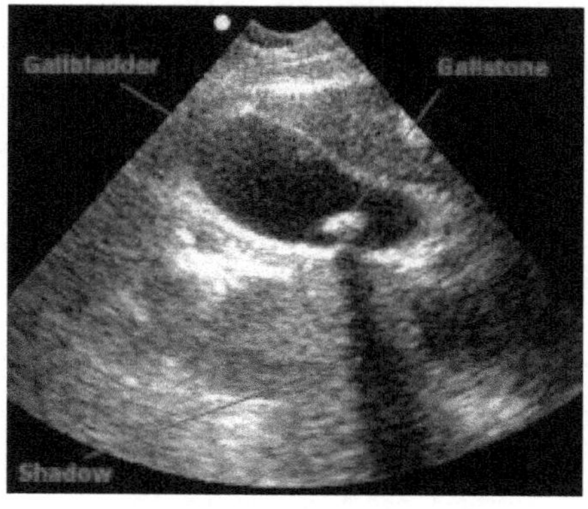

Ultrasound scan of gallstones

How do we remove gallstones without resorting to surgery?

Cleansing the liver of gallstones dramatically improves digestion, which is the basis of your whole health. You can expect your allergies to disappear, too, with each cleanse you do! Incredibly, it also eliminates shoulder, upper arm, and upper back pain. You'll also have more energy and an increased sense of well-being.

I have personally witnessed the removal of gallstones from hundreds of patients. Some of them with gallbladder symptoms expelled many stones that did not even appear on an ultrasound, probably because they were trapped in the liver and gallbladder ducts and were not sitting in the gallbladder where the radiologists usually look.

Most, however, did not have any symptoms at all, yet would flush out literally hundreds of stones – no exaggeration! One woman in her 50's had three scans and the radiologists found nothing. She had pains in the gall-bladder region for 20 years. When she did the gall bladder flush she removed 280 stones the first time around, and about 200 the second time! Here's her first flush with the gallstones – the coins are there to indicate size ratios and are Cypriot.

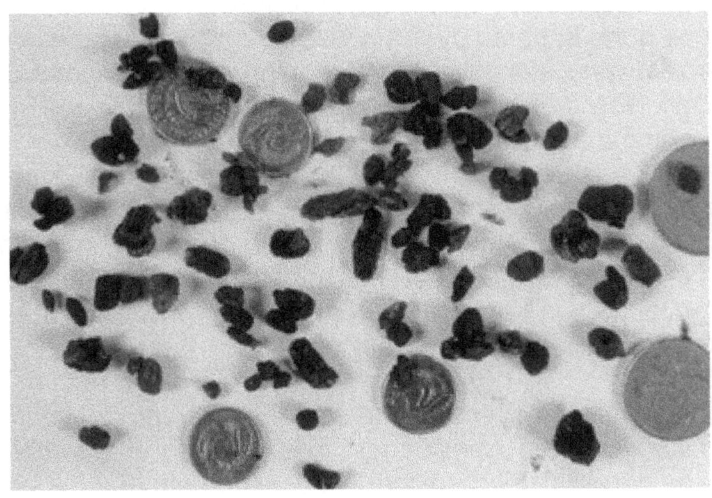

Gallbladder stones flushed naturally

About a week before I did my first gall bladder flush (on myself), I went to see a friend who is an ultrasound specialist. He checked my gall bladder and found it as clean as a whistle. When I flushed a week later I removed 5 LARGE stones (about the size of a walnut), and about 150 smaller stones, including gravel – here is a photo of some of them:

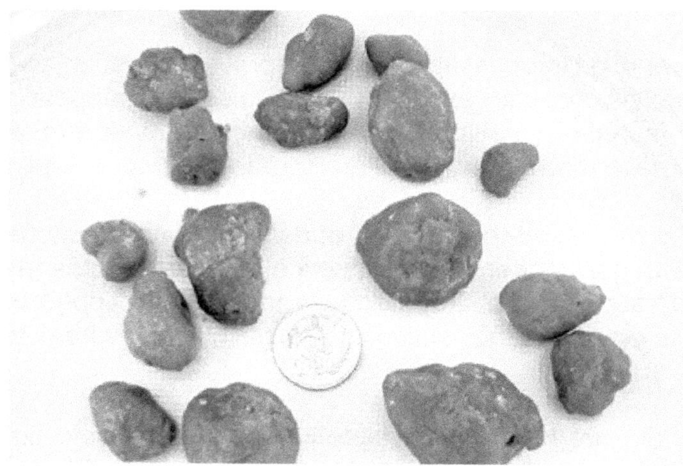

My stones on the first gallbladder flush

It is believed by many naturopathic doctors that EVERYONE has gallstones, even children, with all the junk food that they eat these days (some less than others), and I have validated this many time in clinical practice.
The cleanse that I recommend below takes place within a period of less than 14 hours and can be done at home over the weekend. It is a harmless, pain-free and natural way of removing stones, without requiring invasive procedures such as surgery, laser, etc. Now *that* is a statement that will not be believed by most general surgeons performing their gallbladder removals!

I had a personal experience of a 78-year old nun from a local convent here in Cyprus who was under my care for various health problems, including gallstones. She collected her stones in a jam- jar after her flush and took them to the surgeon at the local hospital here in Larnaca. His first reaction was, *'But that's impossible; you can only remove gallstones surgically or with a laser!'*

The nun looked at him in amazement and said*, 'But Doctor, do you think I am lying to you?'* whilst holding her rosary beads. The surgeon adamantly persisted his point of view. The nun said, *'OK Doctor, you scanned me about 3 weeks ago, and you found stones and said that I require an operation. Is it possible that these stones disappeared by themselves?'* He replied, *'No, this is not possible, once they are in the gallbladder they will stay there until they are removed, and yours were quite large, too.'*

The nun wisely replied, *'OK Doctor, if this is the case, then why don't you scan me again and let's see if they are in the gallbladder or in the jam jar?'* So off they went to the ultrasound room, where he performed another scan. They emerged 30 minutes later after a thorough examination.

There were absolutely NO STONES in the gallbladder at all and now the surgeon looked really surprised. After a short silence, he perked up and said, *'I cannot see any stones now, so this may have been a wrong diagnosis, but you certainly have quite a lot of sludge, so the operation should proceed.'* The nun was flabbergasted and did not know what to say, but before leaving, they agreed to have the stones analyzed in the hospital lab – the results came back: 'GALLBLADDER STONES!'

The moral of this interesting story is: do not try to persuade your doctors and surgeons. There is a mindset akin to brainwashing where it is difficult for them to accept new concepts and treatments, particularly when they are based on the principles of Nature, who they are not too friendly with! Just keep the information to yourself. It is your health that you are trying to optimize, so why go through all the hassle of creating enemies with your doctor? Who you may need on other occasions.

Remember that many years ago, people and scientists were convinced that the world was flat, and it's ironic that there are still these believers in the 21st Century!

Preparations for the Gallbladder Flush

OK, enough of the stories, let's proceed with the details of the gallbladder flush, beginning with the ingredients that you should first collect:

Apple juice (which is high in Malic acid and pectin); it acts as a solvent in the bile to weaken adhesions between solid globules, while softening the stones. This is crucial to the success of the procedure as it enables them to pass HARMLESSLY through the gall ducts.

The apple juice should be coarse, unfiltered and free of additives and preservatives – you will need to drink close to ONE LITRE (3-4 GLASSES) DAILY FOR 14 DAYS PRIOR TO THE FLUSH. In the worst-case scenario, if you cannot find fresh apples to juice, then you can use packaged apple juice, which should still contain these ingredients, but see if you can pick up some organic ones. An alternative to apple juice, which is just as effective, is taking Malic Acid in capsule form (magnesium malate). You will need to take one capsule, three times daily for 14 days before attempting the flush).

Four tablespoons of **Epsom salts** (magnesium sulphate). This allows magnesium to be absorbed into the bloodstream, therefore relaxing smooth muscles that surround the gallbladder ducts. This enables larger stones that may otherwise create spasms to pass through a relaxed bile duct. This is a very crucial part of the therapy and you CANNOT do the flush without taking these salts, which are freely available in most pharmacies. Ask for the B.P. variety for internal use, not those used for soaking in the bath – you will require about 70 grams per flush.

Half a cup of **Extra Virgin Olive Oil**, which stimulates the gall bladder and bile duct to contract powerfully, thus expelling the stones into the duodenum or small intestine. Once you drink the cup of olive oil and citrus fruits it enters the gut and the gallbladder which, detecting huge quantities of fat or oil, begins to go into spasm, expelling all the waste rubbish that has been stored for years.

At least a couple of large **grapefruits** (oranges will do if there are no grapefruits) mixed together with the juice of two fresh **lemons or limes**. The more acidic the juice, the faster the transit of the olive oil through the stomach and into the duodenum, which helps prevent or minimize nausea.

I have supervised hundreds of such cleanses using exactly this protocol that I am recommending here, without one patient suffering any harm whatsoever. But please follow the instructions carefully, and it must be said that you have ultimate responsibility, given that none of you are actual patients of mine.

On the day of the gallbladder flush there are some rules to follow:

1. Take no medications, vitamins or pills that you can do without on the day of the flush. They could prevent success.
2. Eat a NO-FAT breakfast and lunch such as cooked cereal with fruit, fruit juice, brown bread with a little honey (no butter, milk or margarine), baked potato or other vegetables with salt only.
3. 2:00 PM – Do NOT drink or eat anything after 2:00 PM – only mineral water is fine, non-fizzy.
4. 6:00 PM – Drink one serving (3/4 cup) of ice-cold Epsom salts. Mix one tablespoon Epsom salts into 3/4 cup cold water and stir well. You may add 1/8 teaspoon of vitamin C powder to improve the taste. You may drink a little water afterwards or rinse your mouth out. Epsom salts can also be mixed in with apple juice to make it taste nicer, or a few drops of lemon or lime can be added; or a little orange juice.
5. 8:00 PM – Repeat the Epsom salt drink as above.
6. 9:45 PM – Pour 1/2 mug (a large 10 oz. mug) of olive oil and squeeze 1/2 cup of orange or grapefruit juice into this, with the juice of two whole fresh lemons. Shake or stir hard until the oil and fruit juice mix thoroughly. Visit the bathroom now, shower, brush your teeth, go to the toilet etc. so that you are ready to lie down as soon as you have taken the olive oil mixture.

7. 10:00 PM – Drink the olive oil and juice you have mixed. Drinking through a plastic straw helps it go down easier. Drink it standing up, not sitting or lying. You may use a little honey between sips to help it down. Try to drink it as quickly as you can, within 5 minutes.

TIPS: If you find it difficult drinking the olive oil mixture by itself, it is possible to mix it with prune juice or grape juice with a tablespoon of honey and put it in a blender for a minute or so.

If you can obtain ozonated olive oil – maybe your naturopath has an ozonator and can make some ozonated olive oil for you – it may be better to use this as it will kill off any bacteria, parasites or other micro-organisms that may be lingering in the bile when it enters the intestine.

LIE DOWN IMMEDIATELY, ON YOUR RIGHT SIDE! You may fail to get stones out if you don't. The sooner you lie down, the more stones you will get out. Try to keep perfectly still for 20 minutes as the more you move the less stones your gallbladder will expel. You may feel a train of stones travelling along the bile ducts like marbles. There is no pain because the bile duct valves are open, thanks to the Epsom salts. GO TO SLEEP.

NEXT MORNING – upon awakening take another dose of Epsom salt. Drink 3/4 cup of the mixture. You may go back to bed. Don't drink this before 6:00 a.m.

2 HOURS LATER – take your 4th and last dose of Epsom salts. Drink 3/4 cup. You may again go back to bed and rest if you wish. Between the first and this dosage of Epsom salts, expect to frequent the toilet more often with diarrhea.
AFTER 2 MORE HOURS – you may begin to eat. Start with fruit juice or a carrot juice. Half an hour later eat some fruit. One hour later you may eat regular food but keep it light – salads, steamed vegetables, fruit, juices, etc. It's probably a good idea to drink some prune juice too as this will help to clear the gut.

BY SUPPER you should feel well. There are occasions when you may feel a little unwell for a couple of days, particularly if you have not done a liver flush before the gallbladder flush. Parasites in the liver can also cause symptoms to linger. Other times this may be due to stones and debris remaining in the colon and causing irritation and inflammation. Colon hydrotherapy or a good, deep enema can help this problem.

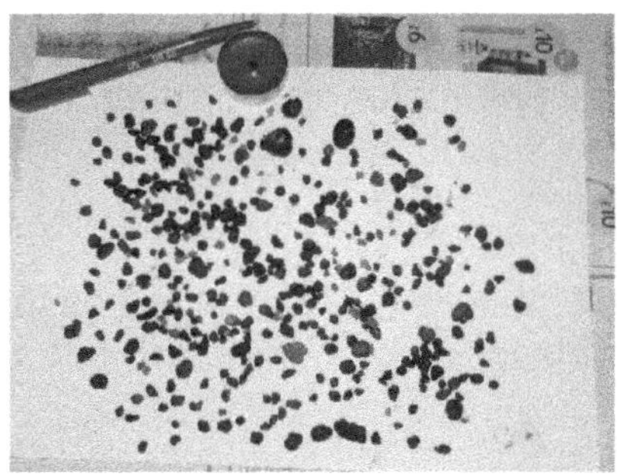

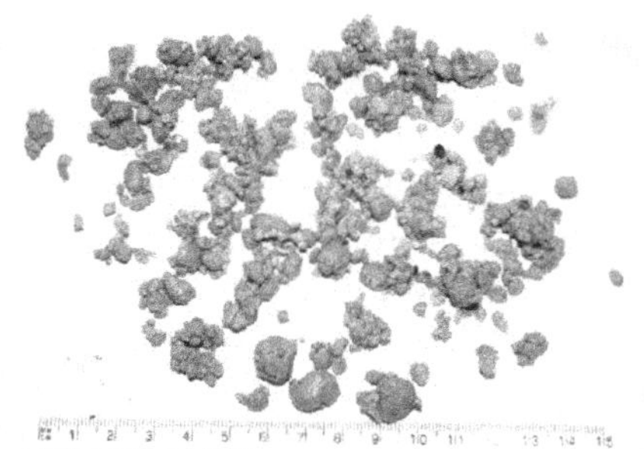

IN THE MORNING expect diarrhea. Try to catch the gallstones in a sieve placed on the toilet pan so that you can see them. If any of you have a digital camera, please take photos and send me a copy for my clinical archives – admin@docgeorge.com.

Most of the stones will be SOFT and green, breaking easily, or even dissolving. All these green stones are as soft as putty thanks to the malic acid in the apple juice and are mostly made of cholesterol. Some stones may be dark, near black in colour because of the bilirubin they contain. Other stones may be small and hard, made of calcium and oxalates (see image below). You may see all these types in one flush, but most of them will be the soft green ones made of cholesterol, as about 80% of the stones in the gallbladder are made of these.

A few days after the flush (maybe 10-15 days) stones from the rear of the liver will have travelled 'forward' towards the main bile ducts leaving the liver and fill the gall bladder again! Therefore, it is sometimes necessary to do up to 6 cleanses (perhaps one each month) in order to get rid of all the stones. If a cleanse produces no more stones, your liver can be in excellent condition!

Helpful Tips

On rare occasions, some people may feel nauseous. This is related to the toxic bile leaving the gallbladder, causing discomfort and the feeling of wanting to vomit. There are a few things that may help in such cases:

- Taking one hydrochloric acid tablet at bedtime will help reduce any nausea during the night – these are sold in health food stores.
- If you tend to get nauseated from the oil, take 2 tablespoons of Aloe Vera juice after your doses of oil and citrus juice.
- Placing a hot water bottle over the liver area (under the right ribcage) during the night also helps relieve nausea.

Many people complete this procedure with minimal discomfort, and nearly everyone feels much better after completing it. Flushing the liver and gall bladder in the manner described (if the gall bladder is present) stimulates and cleanses these organs like no other process does.

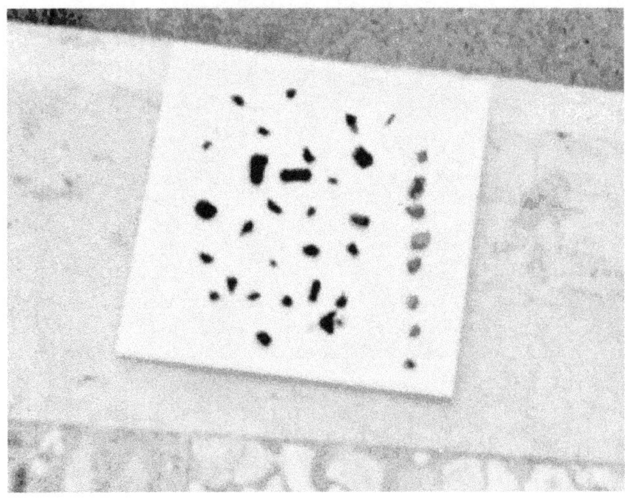

Small hard stones on the right of image

Oftentimes, people suffering for years from gallstones, lack of appetite, biliousness, backaches, nausea, and a host of other complaints, will find gallstone-type objects in the stool the day following the flush. These objects are light to dark green in colour, very irregular in shape, gelatinous in texture, and of sizes varying from 'grape seed' size to 'cherry' size. If there seems to be many these objects in the stool, the flush should be repeated in 2-4 weeks.

In the next chapter we will look at how food intolerances can lead to chronic inflammation and then on to chronic diseases.

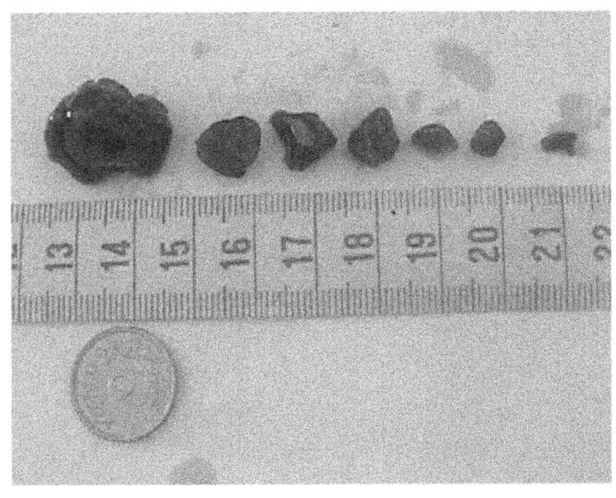

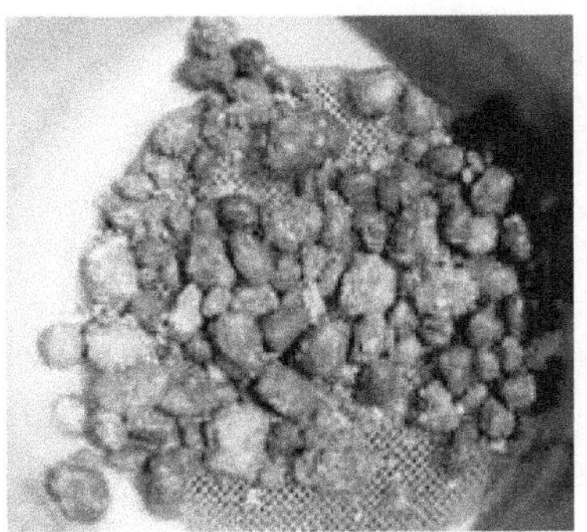

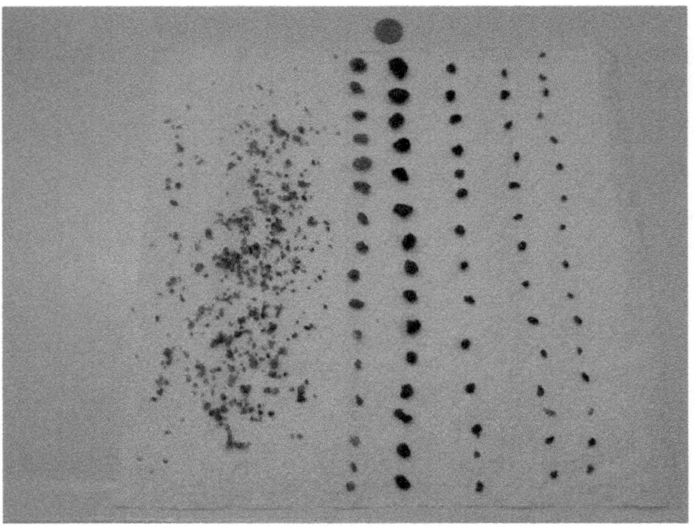

Chapter 5

Food Intolerances, Inflammation and Disease

"One man's food is another man's poison" is a centuries-old saying that implies that different people can have different reactions to exactly the same food. This has been known for eons, but modern medicine is still in the dark regarding this very important cause of many health issues and symptoms. One of the greatest enigmas in modern medicine is food intolerances.

Food intolerances are important to avoid for diabetics too as they will exacerbate the diabetes, as well as all other chronic diseases.

The reason that food is extremely important to health is that the body can react to certain foods in a negative way, causing the body to have an inflammatory reaction.

There are basically two levels of reactions. One is the life-threatening FOOD ALLERGIES, which can cause anaphylactic shock and difficulty breathing which requires immediate medical attention.

The other is FOOD INTOLERANCES, that still cause a reaction, but it is much slower and more prolonged. The symptoms are not so life-threatening, even though they can cause chronic diseases over time.

We will not spend much time discussing food allergies per se, as these only involve about 1% of the population. This chapter is more devoted to food *intolerances*, that involve far more people. According to research by the charity Allergy UK, up to 45% of the population suffer from food intolerances, otherwise known as *Food Hypersensitivity*.

Before we leave the topic of food allergies and concentrate on food intolerances, let's look at the difference between FOOD ALLERGIES and FOOD INTOLERANCES/HYPERSENSITIVITIES.

Food Allergies

Over 140 different foods have been identified as causes of allergic reactions. According to a recent report by the U.S. Centers for Disease Control, 90% of food allergies are associated with only 8 food types:

- Cow's milk
- Hen's eggs
- Peanuts
- Soy foods
- Wheat
- Fish
- Crustacean shellfish (such as shrimp, prawns, lobster, and crab)
- Tree nuts (such as almonds, cashews, walnuts, pecans, pistachios, Brazil nuts, hazelnuts, and chestnuts)

When people with these food allergies consumed the food, can go into anaphylaxis and can die within minutes if they ingest even one molecule of their allergic food. This is a serious issue requiring immediate medical attention.

Should such a reaction occur, taking **Sodium Cromoglycate,** a non-steroidal anti-inflammatory commonly used with asthmatic patients, or the natural bioflavonoid **Quercetin,** are both effective agents in blocking mast cell degranulation and slowing down the adverse reaction until medical help arrives. Under no circumstances, however, should you try treating such food allergic reactions at home, even if you are a practitioner. Immediate medical intervention will most likely be required.

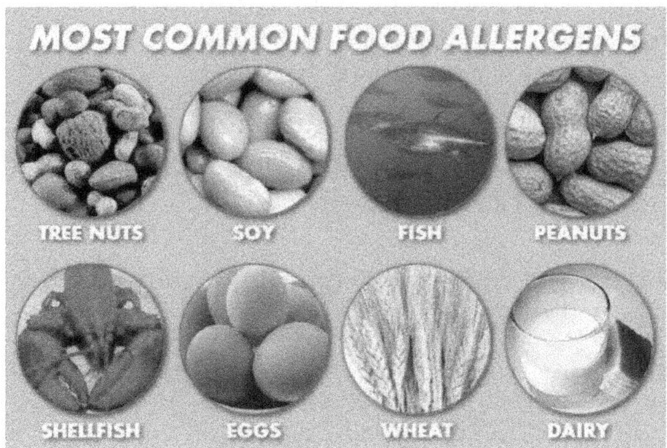

So, what happens in the body when we ingest a food that we are allergic to? During an allergic response, the body reacts to the allergen by producing several antibodies. In the case of food allergies, it is called Immunoglobulin E (IgE). This is a Type 1 allergic reaction.

Diagram 1 demonstrates how the allergen or food is detected by a white blood cell called a **B-lymphocyte cell (Plasma cell).** This plasma cell will produce an IgE antibody.

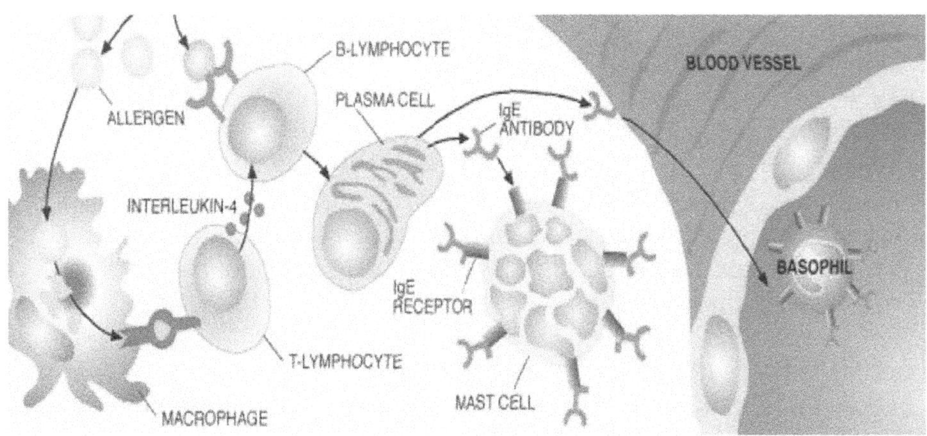

Diagram 1. Classic allergy response

This IgE antibody will then attach itself onto a **mast cell** (another type of white blood cell), which releases potent inflammatory chemicals. This action signals the mast cells and the Basophil cells to begin disintegrating, thereby releasing **histamine** and other chemicals such as proteoglycans (e.g. heparin and chondroitin), and proteolytic enzymes (e.g. elastase and lysophospholipase).

They also secrete lipid mediators like leukotrienes, and several cytokines that contribute to inflammation.

Immediate reaction to foods may involve the **skin, respiratory tract, GI mucosal and cardiovascular system.** Usually the throat or pharynx that begins to constrict and the person has difficulty breathing.

Table 2 shows a comparison between food intolerances and food allergies:

Food Intolerances

Food intolerances do not involve an immediate response. There is a delay in symptoms that can take from 45 minutes to several days for them to become apparent.

The delayed onset of symptoms and complex physiological mechanisms involved in food intolerances make them an especially difficult puzzle to try to solve either on your own or with most laboratory tests. In fact, food sensitivities often go undiagnosed or misdiagnosed.

The medical name for FOOD INTOLERANCES is “Non-IgE mediated food hypersensitivity”, which is sometimes loosely referred to as “food hypersensitivity”. This is also known as a “Type III Allergy” and is IgG-mediated, characterised by the production of IgG antibodies and the gradual formation of antigen/antibody complexes which are deposited in tissues, which cause chronic inflammation.

The best example of food intolerance is lactose intolerance. This condition is characterized by bloating, loose stools, diarrhoea and gas. Lactose intolerance is caused by an inability of the body to produce enough of the enzyme *lactase*, which breaks down lactose, the primary sugar found in milk. Avoiding milk products or supplementing the diet with lactase enzyme is the best way for a person with lactose intolerance to overcome the problem.

Signs and Symptoms

Food intolerance is more chronic, less obvious in its presentation, and often more difficult to diagnose than a food allergy. Symptoms of food intolerance vary greatly and can be mistaken for the symptoms of a food allergy. While true food allergies are associated with fast-acting immunoglobulin IgE responses, it can be difficult to determine the offending food causing a food intolerance because the response generally takes place over a prolonged period.

Food intolerance symptoms usually begin about half an hour after eating or drinking the food in question, but sometimes symptoms may be delayed by up to 48 hours. Diagram 2 shows some of the symptoms that are commonly encountered in cases of food intolerances.

The most common symptoms include: irritable bowel (Jones, VA, 1982; Nanda, R et al, 1983), headaches, migraines, fatigue, behavioural problems (Pelsser, LMJ et al, 2008; McCann D et al, 2007; Bateman, B et al 2004; Breakey, J. 1997; Swain, A et al, 1985) or urticaria (Di Lorenzo, G et al, 2005). Asthma symptoms can also be triggered in some patients and, occasionally, anaphylactoid reactions occur.

Withdrawal, super-sensitivity, tachyphylaxis and tolerance are often observed (Loblay, RJ, 1982). Food chemicals implicated include artificial food colours, preservatives, flavour enhancers, glutamates, vasoactive amines and salicylates (Loblay, RH, 1986; David, TJ, 2000; Perry, CA et al, 1996). It is common for patients with food intolerance to react to several chemicals – all of which can be found in a wide range of foods. A family history of symptoms and specific chemical intolerances is common (Loblay, RH et al, 1986).

Item Compared	FOOD INTOLERANCES	FOOD ALLERGIES
Body Organs Involved	Any organ system in the body can be affected	Usually limited to airways, skin, gastrointestinal tract
Rate of Response	From 45 min up to 3 days after ingestion	From seconds to 1 hour after ingestion
Severity	Not life-threatening	Can be fatal
Are symptoms acute or chronic?	Usually chronic, sometimes acute	Usually acute, rarely chronic
Percentage of Population Affected	30 - 45%	1-2%
Permanence	Can last a lifetime	Can be reversed or reduced after eliminating problem foods
Immunologic Mechanisms	White blood cells – rapid release of histamine IgG antibodies	Gradual formation of Antigen/Antibody complexes IgE antibodies
Non-Immunologic Mechanisms	Toxic, pharmacologic	None
How much food is needed to trigger the allergy?	From small amount to large amount; often dosage dependent	1 molecule of allergic food needed to trigger reaction
Half-life of Immunoglobulins	IgG – 21 days – 3 months	IgE – 1 – 14 days

Table 2. Food intolerances vs food allergies

Food intolerances can present with symptoms affecting the skin, respiratory tract, and gastrointestinal tract (GIT), either individually or in combination. Skin problems may include rashes, urticaria, angioedema, dermatitis and eczema.

Respiratory tract symptoms can include nasal congestion, sinusitis, pharyngeal irritations, asthma and an unproductive cough. GIT symptoms include mouth ulcers, abdominal cramp, nausea, gas, intermittent diarrhoea, constipation, irritable bowel syndrome and anaphylaxis.

Food intolerance has been found to be associated with Irritable Bowel Syndrome and inflammatory bowel diseases such as Crohn's disease.

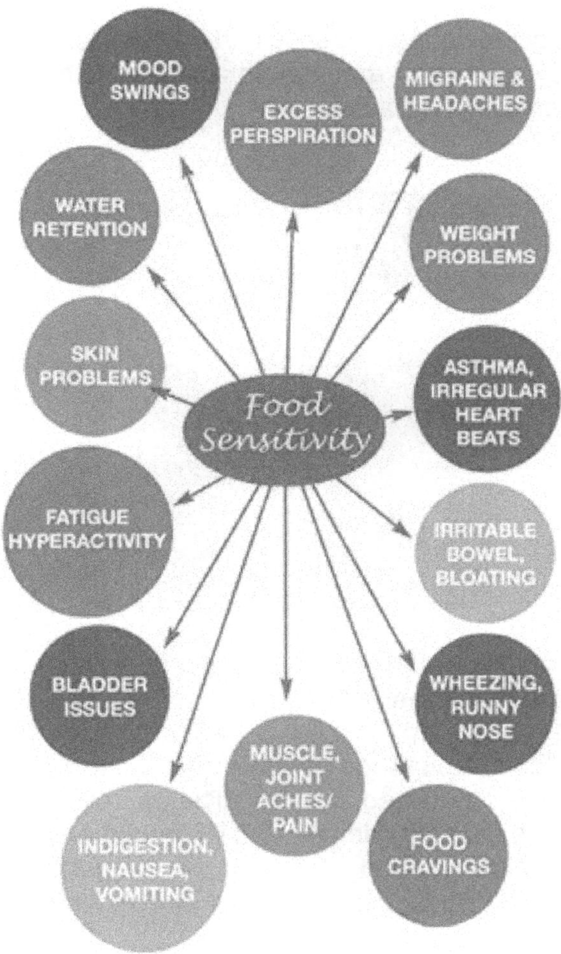

Diagram 2. Symptoms of Food Intolerances

Other general symptoms include chronic constipation, chronic hepatitis C infection, eczema, NSAID intolerance, respiratory complaints, asthma, rhinitis, headaches, functional dyspepsia, eosinophilic esophagitis and ENT illnesses, as well as a myriad of other symptoms. Therefore, it is very difficult to find a correlation between these symptoms and foods that we eat.

Apart from these symptoms, food intolerances may also cause commonly encountered symptoms that most people feel are "normal," given that so many people have them. These include symptoms such as fatigue, gas, bloating, mood swings, nervousness, migraines and eating disorders.

Clinical research is accumulating evidence that food intolerances can also increase the severity of the symptoms of rheumatoid arthritis, asthma and other diseases normally not considered food related.

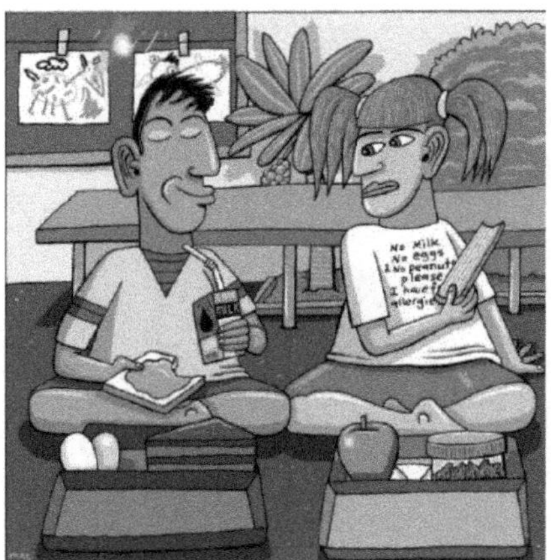

Mechanisms of Food Intolerances

The mechanism of food intolerance involves the production of antigen/antibody complexes which are deposited in the tissues, triggering the release of inflammatory chemicals causing damage and inflammation in that particular tissue. This could be in any part of the body, for example, the gut, causing IBS symptoms or Crohn's; in the joints, producing symptoms of arthritis; in the head producing migraines and so forth.

The sequence of events is as follows (diagram 2 shows this diagrammatically):

- Partially digested foods pass between gut cells into the blood.
- These proteins are recognised as 'foreign' and food specific IgG are produced in response.
- Antigen/antibody complexes form between the partially digested foods and the IgG antibodies. The symptoms of food intolerance tend to be delayed because this formation of complexes is a gradual process – it does not happen immediately.
- The complexes are deposited in tissues (could be anywhere in body such as gut, head, skin etc.).

- Complement is activated which causes respiratory burst in neutrophils, release of proteolytic enzymes, mast cell mediators and vasoactive peptides, and aggregation of platelets.
- Complement and macrophages stimulate inflammation, although complement helps to prevent smaller complexes going on to form larger complexes.
- C2 and C5 (part of the enzyme cascade) can release histamine too.
- Macrophages release inflammatory mediators such as interleukin-1, tumour necrosis factor, reactive oxygen species and nitric oxide (N.B. The complement system is an enzyme cascade that helps defend against infection).

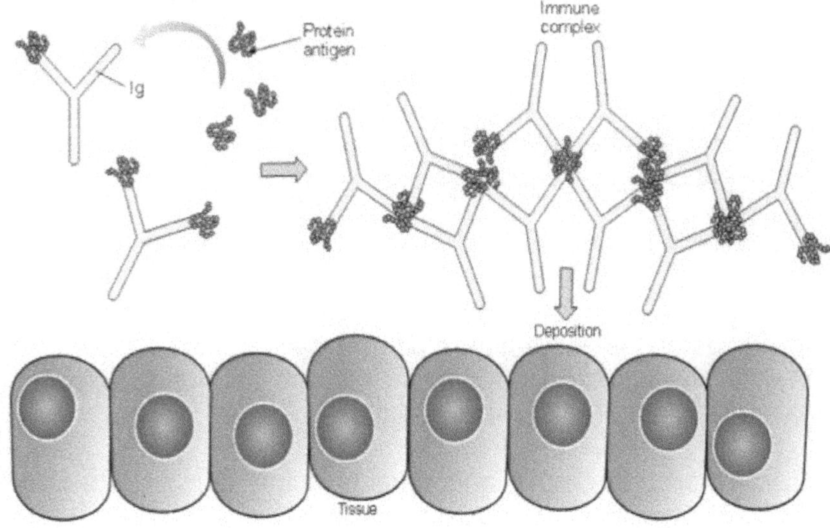

Diagram 2. showing IgG Response

Tests for Determining Food Intolerances

In clinical practice, I use Bioresonance testing to determine what foods the patient may be intolerant to. I have been doing this for over 20 years now; it is possible to test for over 100 foods in less than 15 minutes, and the accuracy is around 85% which is akin to the IgG tests already discussed. It is a quick, easy, efficient and cost-effective way of testing for this critical health parameter that is important to identify and eradicate.

I have always said to my friends that if I were ever stranded on a remote island somewhere in the Pacific and had to work as a therapist, the only piece of equipment I would take with me would be my Bioresonance device and some testing ampoules. I personally use the German VEGA Bioresonance device, as well as the Russian Deta Elis PROFESSIONAL. This has its roots in the work of

Dr. Reinhold Voll, MD, who ingeniously merged and transformed traditional Chinese acupuncture into a modern form of electromedicine called EAV (Volls' so-called Electro Acupuncture).

In the early 1950s, Reinhold Voll[103], a German medical doctor, developed an electronic testing device for finding acupuncture points electrically. He was successful in demonstrating that specific acupuncture points, known to Chinese acupuncturists for millennia, had a different resistance to a tiny electrical current passing through the body, compared to the adjacent tissues[104]. Many other researchers have also verified that electrical conductance at the acupuncture points is significantly greater than the surrounding tissue.

Voll then began a lifelong search to identify correlations between disease states and changes in the electrical resistance of the various acupuncture points. He thought that if he could identify electrical changes in certain acupuncture points associated with certain diseases, then he might be able to identify those diseases more easily, or earlier, when treatment intervention was likely to be more effective.

Voll was successful in identifying many acupuncture points related to specific conditions and published a great deal of information about using acupuncture points diagnostically[105]. He found, for example, that patients with lung cancer had abnormal readings on the acupuncture points referred to as 'lung points'. Changes also occurred in the electrical conductance of the acupuncture points supplying musculoskeletal structures that were inflamed.

Voll also discovered that certain acupuncture points showed abnormal readings when subjects were reacting allergically[106]. He made several serendipitous discoveries related to "allergy" testing. He noted some unusual readings on certain acupuncture points when a patient had a bottle of medicine in his pocket. He could remove the bottle and consistently get different readings when the bottle was in his pocket compared to when it was not.

At first, he was baffled as to how a closed bottle of medicine outside the body could affect the acupuncture readings. It was even more baffling when he discovered that the glass bottle of medicine could change the readings when it was in contact anywhere along the closed electric circuit involved with the testing procedure[107].

---

103 Voll, R. 1980. The phenomenon of medicine testing in electro-acupuncture according to Voll. American Journal of Acupuncture 8:97-104.

104 Voll R.: Topographic Positions of the Measurement Points in Electroacupuncture. (Illustrated Vol. I). Med. Liter. Verlagsgesellschaft, Uelzen, 1977.

105 Voll, R: Twenty Years of Electroacupuncture Therapy Using Low Frequency Current Pulses. *Amer. J. Acupuncture*, 3(4): 291-314, 1975.

106 http://www.youtube.com/watch?v=Jltzy072hxY

107 Kenyon JN. 21st century medicine: a layman's guide to the medicine of the future. Wellingborough, Northants: Thorsons, 1986.

Personally, I have spent more than 20 years working with the VEGA[108] machine and I can say that I truly resonate with it. The analogy that I give to illustrate this is that the VEGA is akin to a musical instrument. We often see a maestro playing a guitar so beautifully that we are in awe - how beautiful those notes seem to flow and with such ease the maestro plays. Of course, if we take the same instrument that the maestro is playing in to our own hands, without devoting a lot of time and arduous effort in really learning to play it, then our attempts to perform like the maestro will be in vain.

This is really what happens with the VEGA machine, or any other Bioresonance testing device using VRT testing. In the wrong hands it can make more wrong predictions than pure guesswork – in the maestro's hands it can be as accurate as any medical scanning device at determining anything that you ask of it. It will accurately determine what food intolerances a person has; as well as whether they have viruses or residual particles of viruses in their tissues that may have been left from an old infection or vaccination.

It can identify bacteria, parasites, fungi and moulds and tell what drugs or remedies a person is adversely reacting to. It can also identify organ weaknesses and prioritise them; it can identify whether the person has electromagnetic stress, X-ray stress, mobile phone stress, geopathic stress and the like; as well as being able to identify the specific potency of any remedy that a person needs to take.

All these tests can be done quickly and in less than an hour. It is not difficult to scan all the organs of the body; test for food intolerances[109]; identify the weak organs; identify the specific potency required to make a homeopathic sarcode in order to strengthen a weak organ; as well as scan for vaccination stress, viruses, bacteria, fungi, Candida and parasites.

The Bioresonance device helps the practitioner to take the guesswork out of working out the pathogenesis of disease, as well as guessing which dosage or homeopathic potency the patient is resonating with. It is my belief that when there is a paradigm shift in thinking from mechanistic to *holistic*, then most health practitioners of all disciplines will be proud owners of a Bioresonance testing device.

In the early days when I began using the VEGA, I was astounded by its accuracy as I was testing the organ systems of an athlete who wanted to optimize his health and sports performance. I really did not find much as this athlete was fairly healthy

---

108 Fehrenbach J, Noll H, Nolte HG, et al. Short manual of the Vegatest-method. Schiltach: BER, 1986.
109 Krop J, Swiertzek J, Wood A. Comparison of ecological testing with the Vega test method in identifying sensitivities to chemicals, foods and inhalants. *Am J Acupuncture* 13 253-259, 1985.

and was on an optimal diet and supplement programme. But one thing that came up on the VEGA was the reproductive system – it was showing weaknesses in the testes, epididymis and prostate.

It turned out that he was indeed sterile but did not mention this in his history as he was ashamed and embarrassed; this was a real blow to his vision of having a family with his wife. Further testing showed that he was afflicted with systemic Candidiasis and certain protozoa, along with vaccination stress. When these issues had been addressed with a 90-day protocol, his wife became pregnant a couple of months later. This was a professional athlete who had consulted at least 5 doctors about his sterility problem, but no amount of medical testing could determine what the VEGA had helped me to diagnose in less than 30 minutes.

I also use other Bioresonance testing devices which I have found to be just as good, but more cost effective as they have over 20,000 digitized ampoules already programmed into the device. One such device is called the DETA PROFESSIONAL from the Russian company Deta Elis. This has the capabilities of treating using Bioresonance and other treatment modalities – see www.deta-elis-uk.com.

The Link with Chronic Disease

Food intolerance (as defined by elevated levels of IgG food antibodies), is being increasingly associated with the low-grade inflammation which characterises most chronic conditions such as Crohn's, Irritable Bowel Syndrome, atopic allergies, obesity and arthritis.

Research supports this with studies showing how testing for IgG antibodies has helped in improving conditions like obesity, migraines, arthritis and IBS.

The mechanisms behind this link are thought to include the following:

1. Formation of antigen/antibody immune complexes. The immune system may occasionally react to substances, including foods that adversely affect it. Under normal conditions, the formation of antigen/antibody complexes are dealt with and eliminated by the immune system.

However, if the immune system is overwhelmed or over-worked, then these complexes can accumulate in places such as joints or the digestive tract resulting in the production of inflammatory cytokines, which lead to the manifestation of symptoms of food intolerance.

2. Increased intestinal permeability. This is linked to the promotion of low grade inflammation as a result of lipolysaccharides moving across the

disturbed gut mucosa. Disturbance of the tight junction proteins which maintain the gut membrane also allows the migration of large peptides into the circulation which would otherwise be blocked.

These peptides can induce an adverse immune response. Studies have found increased intestinal permeability in patients with food intolerances (Dupont et al 1989, Schrander et al 1990).

The "Leaky Gut"

One major theory as to how delayed food sensitivities develop revolves around the concept of a "leaky gut."

Ordinarily, the digestive tract will efficiently break down and absorb consumed food as small molecules, amino acids, simple carbohydrates, etc., which are, in general, non-antigenic.

The efficiency of the digestive system today with all the additional stressors that it has to deal with results in digestion becoming less efficient and the intestinal lining becoming more permeable to large molecules. It is assumed that this "leaky gut" condition allows macro-molecular food fragments into the circulation, where they can stimulate a typical immune response where IgG is the primary antibody produced to defend the body against perceived non-self-invaders.

Inadequate digestion of food products due to hypochlorhydria (insufficient secretion of hydrochloric acid by the stomach) and pancreatic enzyme deficiency is also thought to be a significant cause of food allergies.

Insufficient brush border enzymes such as lactase and sucrase also affect the body's ability to breakdown food to an elemental form.

When proteins are not digested to amino acids, dipeptides, or short chain polypeptides, they retain their antigenic properties. These antigenic molecules may then be absorbed through a damaged mucosal barrier or "leaky gut" and become exposed to the immune system.

This in turn can create a state of chronic immune hypersensitivity and inflammation.

In general, foods with a higher protein content (>20%) are more likely to be allergenic.

The following factors can all put stress on a person's health and can lead to increased gut permeability or leaky gut:

- **Low levels of secretory IgA**. Secretory IgA is an immune marker and is the first line of defence in the gut against bacteria, food residue, fungus, parasites and viruses (Walker & Bloch 1983).
- **Stress** can deplete the body of secretory IgA and hence reduce the body's defence system against foreign bodies. Also, stress depletes the gut of good bacteria, and therefore allows an overgrowth of bad bacteria and yeast such as Candida.
- **Imbalanced gut flora**. An overgrowth of bad gut bacteria (dysbiosis) can exacerbate intestinal permeability through inhibition of genes which regulate tight junction proteins protecting the gut mucosal barrier (Kennedy et al 2002).
- **Mucosal injury** due to infection or certain medical drugs. Non-steroidal anti-Inflammatory Drugs (NSAIDS) e.g. Aspirin, damage the intestinal wall causing inflammation resulting with an increase in permeability (Bjarnson et al 1987).
- **Parasites** also damage the intestinal wall causing inflammation, eventually resulting in an increase in permeability.
- **Low stomach acid** can arise due to lack of digestive enzymes caused by nutritional deficiencies or as a result of H. Pylori infection. Low stomach acid results in incomplete breakdown of protein leading to large peptides in the small intestine which can potentially cross the gut wall if there is increased intestinal permeability, pass into the bloodstream, stimulate antibody response and cause further inflammation (Gardner ML 1984).
- **Low pancreatic enzymes**. When the intestinal lining is damaged, the microvilli are also damaged thus reducing absorption of nutrients vital for the manufacture of digestive enzymes. Consequently, foods are not fully digested, pass into blood stream and stimulate antibody response.
- **Poor nutrient status**. Damage to the intestinal lining reduces nutrient absorption with the consequence of impaired gut repair, and therefore further impaired digestion and absorption.
- **A high fat diet** has been closely linked with increased intestinal permeability and the formation of chylomicrons, which transport inflammatory lipopolysaccharides across the gut wall and into the circulation. This results in systemic inflammation in tissues. It is possible they also promote intestinal absorption and systemic dissemination of dietary antigens (Wang et al 2010).

Leaky gut can be healed by taking supplements such as L-GLUTAMINE and BUTYRIC ACID to heal the mucosa of the gut, along with VITAMIN D3.

Have GMOs Contributed to the Rise in Allergies?

There is some discussion about the role that genetically modified (GM or GMO) food might play in the escalating incidence of food allergy, food intolerance, and digestive illnesses. Genetically modified food is the result of scientists inserting DNA from another species into the plant - typically corn, soybeans, canola, cotton (the source of cottonseed oil), and sugar beets - to make the plant resistant to insect damage, viral infections, and certain herbicides.

The FDA says that the GMO foods that have been evaluated through its voluntary consultation process are not more likely to cause an allergic or toxic reaction than foods from traditionally bred plants. When new genetic traits are introduced into plants, the developer evaluates whether any new material could be allergenic or toxic.

Yet some consumer groups are questioning whether there's a link between the dramatic rise in allergies in the past two decades and the introduction of GMO soybeans into the U.S. food supply in 1996.

GMO soy is now ubiquitous in many processed foods. While the timing does not prove any causal link between GMO food and allergies, these groups say it merits research. However, there is currently a lack of long-term independent scientific studies published in peer-reviewed journals that examine how ingesting GMO foods affects humans.

How Do These Foods Damage My Body?

It has been reported that while individuals may sometimes have adverse reactions to foods, these reactions are not always consistent. This is because the response to food involves not only the immune system or a sensitivity to some of the molecules in foods but is also the health of the entire digestive tract and whether it is providing a good barrier for your body.

Therefore, when the health of your digestive system is compromised you may have a sensitivity to foods which otherwise would not affect you adversely, like in times of extreme stress. Thus, it is very important when dealing with any inflammatory disease of the bowel to make certain that all stressors that may be playing a role are eradicated concomitantly within a holistic model. This is the only way of succeeding.

The role of your gastrointestinal tract, which includes your oesophageal area, stomach, and your upper and lower intestinal tracts, is to take in the food you eat, break it down to molecule-size pieces, and allow it to be absorbed into your body in a controlled way.

Your gastrointestinal tract provides a protective barrier between the food you eat and the inside of your body. When it is healthy and functioning efficiently, it lets in specific food molecules in specific places at specific times. Many things can affect this barrier and, when it is compromised in any way, it can let in food molecules that are not properly digested. This can cause a reaction to a certain food, not because you are sensitive to it, but because it is in the wrong place at the wrong time.

Food Sensitivities, Oesophageal Reflux and Your Stomach

The beginning of food digestion occurs in the stomach at the upper end of the gastrointestinal (GI) tract. The stomach has a protective mucosal layer called the stomach lining which protects it from the strong acid that is produced by specialized stomach cells called parietal cells. The acid in the stomach is a vital component in breaking down food particles.

As already mentioned, the stomach lining contains specialized cells for producing hydrochloric acid called PARIETAL CELLS (Diagram 4) along with CHIEF CELLS that produce Pepsinogen. The pepsinogen is activated once it reaches the stomach, so it doesn't harm the cells that produce it.

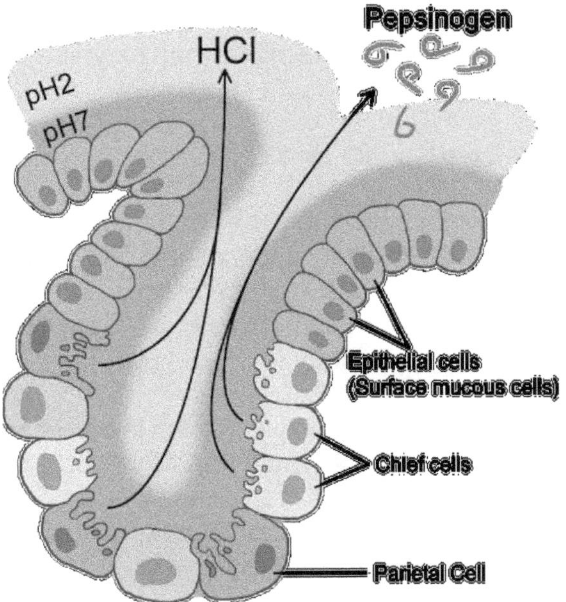

Diagram 4: Parietal and Chief Cells of Stomach

An allergic response in the stomach can produce inflammation in the stomach wall. This can cause lesions or sores as well as potentially destroy the parietal cells.

The reduced number of parietal cells results in less acid production, ultimately inhibiting the proper breakdown of food in the stomach.

When food is improperly broken down in the stomach, large undigested particles are transported to the intestines where they cause additional inflammation and allergic responses as well as increasing the severity of symptoms that are already being experienced.

Along with toxic foods, alcohol consumption and non-steroidal anti-inflammatories (NSAIDs) can also destroy the stomach lining causing stomach inflammation and inadequate digestion of food. Medications that decrease stomach acid production also decrease the ability to digest food properly.

One specific type of food allergy in the stomach is called, allergic eosinophilic gastroenteritis. This condition is characterized by symptoms of acid reflux, severe abdominal pain after eating, vomiting, and diarrhoea. With allergic eosinophilic gastroenteritis, the oesophageal area, stomach and upper intestinal tract can become inflamed, compromising proper function.

Oftentimes, people who have serious acid reflux problems that are not responsive to medications have this condition. Although this condition is caused by an allergic reaction to food, food allergy tests reveal positive results in only about half of all cases. If left untreated, the inflammation in the stomach can result in ulceration and degeneration of the stomach lining, leading to additional problems.

Gentle foods that can support healing of an inflamed stomach include:

- Rice
- Lamb
- Vegetables such as cabbage in juices

These foods can be used with an Allergy Avoidance Diet to support healing of the stomach. Also, avoiding alcohol and the most commonly allergenic foods would also prove to be beneficial. These foods are:

- Cow's Milk
- Tomato
- Wheat
- Chocolate
- Peanuts
- Shellfish

Food Sensitivities and Systemic Responses

The travel of toxic food particles via the bloodstream to other parts of the body can account for a rash on your arms or legs as a result of an allergic response. Many scientists and clinicians have looked at the role of food allergy in a number of systemic (whole body) diseases and conditions.

Most notably, conditions associated with inflammation, such as red, inflamed patches of skin called dermatitis, asthma and joint pain all have been related to toxic food responses. Several studies have been published on the beneficial effects of using allergy-avoidance (elimination) diets to help decrease the symptoms of rheumatoid arthritis. It has also been observed that the symptoms of asthma become worse in some individuals after consuming certain foods.

Avoidance of these foods has helped decrease the number and severity of symptoms in these individuals.

Food Sensitivities and Processed Foods

Reports suggest the incidence of conditions such as asthma, allergic rhinitis, and atopic dermatitis has increased during the past decade. While the increase in damaging pollutants - particularly in large cities - is most often attributed for this increase, many scientists believe the consumption of processed foods and the increased level of stress in our daily lives are also major contributors to the rise in the frequency of these conditions.

As mentioned above, processed foods contain higher levels of additives such as preservatives (benzoate-containing substances like sodium benzoate, sulphites, hydroxytoluene-containing substances like BHT), flavouring agents (salicylates), and dyes. Processed, non-organically grown foods may also contain pesticides which can also promote toxic responses in the body. Candies like chocolates, also contain many colourings, additives and preservatives as well as simple sugars.

Processed foods can also contain small amounts of residue of foods that are not listed on the label. Most manufacturing plants produce several types of food products and although regulations exist to assure these companies manufacture products under clean conditions, they do not require sterile conditions that would prevent any cross-contamination from the production of other food products.

For example, a manufacturer may use the same equipment to produce wheat and non-wheat bread. It is possible that a small amount of wheat residue could inadvertently end up in a non-wheat product. However, these residues would not be listed as an ingredient on its label.

This is of concern with peanut residue which can cause a severe allergic reaction from amounts so small that they are undetectable by all tests used to determine the cleanliness of equipment. Government agencies are responding by requiring manufacturers that use the same equipment to produce peanut products and non-peanut products to label their non-peanut products as 'possibly containing peanut residue'.

Processed foods also add colours and flavourings which raise additional concerns. Colours, and particularly flavourings, are usually produced with "carrier" ingredients. In the past, manufacturers have been required to only list the main ingredients in the products, so carrier ingredients were not included on this list.

This practice has recently come under scrutiny by the FDA and other food industry organizations as reports of food intolerance or allergic reactions from allergens that were present in foods but were not listed on the labels continue to grow. The FDA is starting to require labels that list all ingredients, including carrier ingredients. However, it may be many years before all the processed food on our grocery shelves will have all the ingredients clearly labelled.

Whole, organically grown foods do not contain colourings, flavourings, preservatives or other hidden ingredients which may cause food sensitive reactions. This is a particularly important consideration for individuals with any type of food sensitivity.

Why Do I Crave Foods to Which I am Sensitive?

It is not clear why we often crave foods to which we are sensitive, but several theories have been proposed to help explain why this may occur.

Some researchers suggest that our bodies can become addicted to the chemical messengers, such as histamine or cortisol, which are secreted by immune cells in response to allergens in the body. It is hypothesized that while eating foods to which you are allergic can cause a rash or sneezing, the body also may experience a soothing response from the presence of the chemical messengers, increasing the desire to eat more of that food.

Another theory proposed by a well-known immunologist is based on the science of how antibodies and antigens connect (bind) to each other. Antibodies can bind to more than one site on an allergen in the food. Therefore, when there is very little antigen but many antibodies present, the antibodies will become cross-linked and make large complexes.

It is theorized that these large complexes can cause an increase in symptoms. In this theory, symptoms are related to the number of antibodies in relation to antigens, rather than being caused by the number of antigens themselves. In fact, it is suggested that if you eat more of the antigen, you can decrease the number of antibody complexes by allowing each antibody to bind to an antigen rather than forming the large complexes, thereby *reducing* the number of symptoms.

Normal metabolism works to remove the food antigens and as the ratio of antibodies to antigens begins to rise, symptoms will begin to increase. Cravings and addiction to food may be the result of the body's attempt to increase the number of antigens present in order to prevent the formation of the large antibody complexes that are associated with an increased number of symptoms (Diagram 5).

The Cycle of Addiction

Eating more of the toxic food introduces more antigens into the body. These antigens bind to the antibodies and dilute the complexes, leading to reduced symptoms. However, the antibodies are still present in the body.

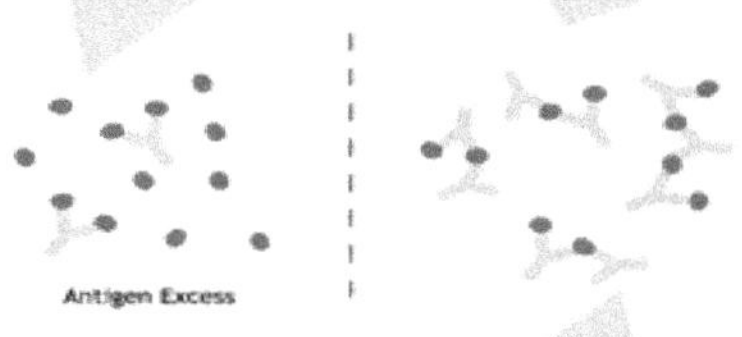

The antigen is removed by metabolism over time and the antibodies start forming lager complexes with the reduced amount of antigen. The complexes lead to more symptoms. So, the body is signaled to eat more of the toxic food to reduce the symptoms again, and cycle continues.

The Way Out of the Cycle: the Elimination Diet (Allergy Avoidance Diet)

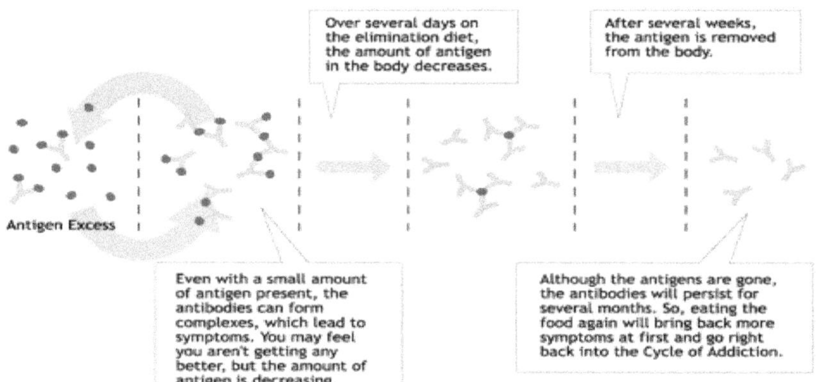

Diagram 5. Antigen excess and antibody excess Marinkovich model

Succumbing to food cravings to help alleviate symptoms is the beginning of a cycle of short-term relief from symptoms, then craving the food as symptoms increase again. This yo-yo effect is believed by some allergy specialists to be the reason why people who stop eating the foods to which they are allergic (go on elimination or avoidance diets) first go through several days when they feel worse before they start feeling much better.

An allergy avoidance diet (also called the Elimination Diet) is instrumental in avoiding allergic reactions to food and is the way to break the cycle of addiction. An allergy avoidance diet allows the body to completely remove the antigen, providing no reason for the formation of antibodies which will then also disappear. Clinicians suggest that this is the reason why some people can go back to eating a food to which they were once allergic after a year or two of avoiding the food.

In my clinical experience, however, having tested many thousands of patients over the years for food intolerances, I have found that patients who have food intolerances will always have them, unless they are treated using Bioresonance therapy. It appears that there is an *immune memory* that never forgets the food molecules that it reacts to, however many years go by.

Occasionally, a person will experience more symptoms for the first several days to a week when beginning an allergy avoidance diet. While some clinicians believe this is caused by the cross-linking of antibodies as explained in the model above, others believe it is because the body is starting to mobilize toxins that have been stored in fat tissue and other storage sites in the body. Whatever the reason, it is important to remain on the allergy avoidance diet, even though symptoms may appear to be worsening. After staying on the diet for several weeks, you should begin to feel relief from symptoms and generally feel much better.

Other Treatments of Food Intolerances

Perhaps one of the simplest and most effective ways of treating food intolerances (not allergies) is to use Bioresonance therapy. At the Da Vinci Holistic Health Center (www.naturaltherapycenter.com) where I work, we use the BICOM device for treating food intolerances.

It generally requires 3 treatments per food group. It is a simple procedure where the patient lies on a couch and holds an electrode in each hand. The foods being tested are placed into the INPUT pot of the device.

The patient's body signals are conducted from the right hand into the input of the device using a BICOM electrode. In the BICOM device the disharmonious frequencies are filtered out and inverted. These inverted therapeutic oscillations are now given back to the patient via the left hand using another electrode.

BRT has been tested and approved throughout Europe and Canada, and it is in use in 85 countries worldwide. In Germany, where it was developed by Regumed, BRT has been in use for over 25 years.

Developing a Healthy Diet

1. *Avoid foods which you are intolerant and/or allergic to.* First and foremost, you must know your own body and what foods are toxic to you. Food sensitivities are very individual. You can be sensitive to a food that no one else in your family or groups of friends finds problematic. It's part of why we are all individuals, and you should determine for yourself what foods may be causing damage to your body. Many healthcare practitioners are knowledgeable about food sensitivities and, especially if you are experiencing significant symptoms, you should consider talking with your healthcare practitioner about your diet and suspected food sensitivities.

2. *Eat organically-grown foods whenever possible.* Especially if you suspect food sensitivities, you should avoid foods with pesticides, artificial colourings and preservatives. These synthetic food additives can cause food sensitivities and may intensify other symptoms you are experiencing. Avoiding these artificial additives is essential in determining the foods to which you are sensitive and in developing a diet that promotes your optimal health.

3. *Support healthy digestion.* One way you can support healthy digestion is to ensure you have adequate amounts of digestive factors. After chewing, the food's next stop is the stomach, where an adequate amount of stomach acid (hydrochloric acid) is the next necessity. Stomach acid is required for adequate breakdown of proteins, and without proper breakdown, all proteins are potential antigens and toxic food molecules.

Low stomach acid (hypochlorhydria) is common, especially in older people since as we age, we make less stomach acid. Research suggests that as many as half of people over 60 years old have hypochlorhydria. A variety of factors can inhibit enough stomach acid production, including the pathogenic bacteria, *Helicobacter pylori*, and frequent use of antacids.

Hypochlorhydria is also associated with many diseases, such as asthma, celiac disease, hepatitis, rheumatoid arthritis, osteoporosis, and diabetes mellitus. Signs of hypochlorhydria include a sense of fullness after eating, bloating, excessive belching, indigestion, multiple food allergies, undigested food in the stool, and peeling and cracked fingernails.

In addition to hydrochloric acid, the production of pancreatic enzymes and bicarbonate is also compromised in some people. If necessary, these digestive factors can be replaced with appropriate supplementation.

Digestive enzyme support can also be obtained from fresh pineapple or papaya, both of which contain the enzyme bromelain, as well as other fresh vegetables and herbs. Processed foods like canned pineapple contain little enzyme activity since digestive enzymes are proteins, which are destroyed by heating which occurs in the sterilization process.

4. *Support the gastrointestinal barrier.* The gastrointestinal cell wall is the barrier between potentially toxic food molecules and the inside of your body. Therefore, the integrity of this barrier is vital to your health. Support for the mucus that covers the cells in the gastrointestinal tract is very important, especially in the stomach.

The mucus layer is one way the stomach and upper small intestine protect themselves against the damaging effects of stomach acid. Alcohol, over-the-counter anti-inflammatory drugs called NSAIDS (e.g., aspirin), and the pathogenic bacteria, *Helicobacter pylori* can all reduce the mucous layer, leading to lesions in the stomach and small intestinal tract walls.

Choline provides nutritional support for a healthy mucous layer and is found in vegetables such as cauliflower and lettuce. Choline can be obtained from lecithin (phosphatidylcholine) as well, which is high in eggs and soybeans. Some foods also help combat or protect against the damage of *Helicobacter pylori*; these include catechins found in green tea, some spices such as cinnamon, carotenoids found in vegetables, and vitamin C, found in many fruits and vegetables.

Given that many food intolerances are acquired, the best advice to anyone is to ROTATE foods and never eat foods continuously, day-in, day-out. This is most certainly the best way to acquire food intolerances. It is very important that we DO NOT eat the same foods every day, even though our fast pace of life often entraps us into modes of convenience that are often difficult to break.

In the next chapter we will examine why Candida is another important underlying cause of many diseases and what we can do about it.

References

Ahmed T, Fuchs GJ. Gastrointestinal allergy to food: A review. *J Diarrhoeal Dis Res.* 1997;15(4):211-223.

Amre DK, D'Souza S, Morgan K, Seidman G, Lambrette P, Grimard G, Israel D, Mack D, Ghadirian P, Deslandres C, Chotard V, Budai B, Law L, Levy E, Seidman EG: Imbalances in dietary consumption of fatty acids, vegetables, and fruits are associated with risk for Crohn's disease in children. Am J Gastroenterol 2007; 102: 2016–2025.

Andre F, Andre C, Feknous M, Colin L, Cavagna S. Digestive permeability to different-sized molecules and to sodium cromoglycate in food allergy. *Allergy Proc.* 1991;12(5):293-298.

Bateman B, Warner JO, Hutchinson E, et al. The effects of a double-blind, placebo controlled artificial food colourings and benzoate preservative challenge on hyperactivity in a general population sample of preschool children. Arch Dis Child 2004; 89:506–11.

Breakey J. The role of diet and behaviour in childhood. J Paediatr Child Health1997; 33:190–4.

Cooney R, Jewell D: The genetic basis of inflammatory bowel disease. Dig Dis 2009; 27: 428–442.

David TJ. Adverse reactions and intolerance to foods. Br Med Bull 2000; 56:34–50.

Di Lorenzo G, Pacor ML, Mansueto P, et al. Food-additive-induced urticaria: A survey of 838 patients with recurrent chronic idiopathic urticaria. Int Arch Allergy Immunol 2005; 138:235–42.

Dominus S. *The Allergy Prison*. New York Times. June 10, 2001.

Edwards CRW. Lessons from licorice. N Engl J Med 1991, 325: 1242-3

Farrell RJ, Kelly CP. Celiac Sprue.*N Eng J Med.* 2002;346(3):180-188.

Fuglsang G, Madsen C, Halken S, et al. Adverse reactions to food additives in children with atopic symptoms. Allergy 1994; 49:31–7.

Gitzelman R, Steinmann B, Van den Berghe G Disorders of fructose metabolism. In: Scnver CR, Beaudet AL, Sly WS, Valle D (Eds) The Metabolic and Molecular Bases of Inherited Disease, 7th edtn New York: McGraw-Hill, 1995; 905-34

Hafstrom I, Ringertz B, Spangberg A, et al. A vegan diet free of gluten improves signs and symptoms of rheumatoid arthritis: the effects of arthritis correlate with a reduction in antibodies to food antigens. *Rheumatology.* 2001; 40:1175-1179.

Halmos, EP, Power VA, Shepherd SJ, et al. A Diet Low in FODMAPs Reduces Symptoms of Irritable Bowel Syndrome. Gastroenterology 2014; 146(1)67-75

Helm RM, Burks AW. Mechanisms of food allergy. *Current Opin Immunol.* 2000; 12:647-653.

Henderson WK, Raskin NH. 'Hog-dog' headache: individual susceptibility to nitnte. Lancet 972; u. 1162-3

Johnson JD, Kretchmer N, Simoons FJ Lactose malabsorpnon. its biology and history. Adv Pedtatr 1974; 21: 197-237

Jones VA, McLaughlan P, Shorthouse, Workman E, Hunter JO. Food intolerance: A major factor in the pathogenesis of irritable bowel syndrome. Lancet 1982; 8308:1115–7.

Kweon M-N, Takahashi I, Kiyono H. New insights into mechanism of inflammatory and allergic diseases in mucosal tissues. *Digestion.* 2001;63 (Suppl 1):1-11.

Lebenthal E, Rossi TM. Lactose malabsorpnon and intolerance. In Lebenthal E (Ed) Textbook of Gastroenterology and Nutrition in Infancy New York Raven, 1981; 673-88

Lichtenstein LM. Allergy and the immune system. *Sci Am.* 1993;269(3):117-124.
Loblay RH, Swain AR. Food intolerance. Rec Adv Clin Nutr 1986; 2:169–77.

Malone MH, Metcalfe DD. Histamine in foods: its possible role in non-allergic adverse reactions to ingestants. N E R Allergy Proc 1986; 7: 241-5

McCann D, Barrett A, Cooper A, et al. Food additives and hyperactive behaviour in 3-year-old and 8/9-year-old children in the community: A randomized, double-blinded, placebo-controlled trial. Lancet 2007; 370:1560–7.

Moneret-Vautrin DA, Einhorn C, Tisserand J. Le role du nitnte de sodium dans les urticaires histaminiques d'ongine ahmentaire. Ann Nutr Alim 1980; 34: 1125-32

Nanda R, James R, Smith H, et al. Food intolerance and irritable bowel syndrome. Gut 1983; 30:1099–104.

Nossal GJV. Life, death and the immune system. *Sci Am.* 1993;269(3):53-62.

Nsouli TM, Nsouli SM, Linde RE, O'Mara F, Scanlon RT, Bellanti JA. Role of food allergy in serous otitis media. *Annals Allergy.* 1994; 73:215-219.

Ong DK, Mitchell SB, Barrett JS, Shepherd SJ, Irving PI, Biesiekierski JR, Smith S, Gibson PR, Muir JG. Manipulation of dietary short chain carbohydrates alters the pattern of hydrogen and methane gas production and genesis of symptoms in patients with irritable bowel syndrome. J Gastroenterol. Hepatol. 2010 Aug ;25(8):1366-73

Paul G, Khare V, Gasche C: Inflamed gut mucosa: downstream of interleukin-10. Eur J Clin Invest 2012; 42: 95–109.

Pelsser LMJ, Frankena K, Toorman J, et al. A randomized controlled trial into the effects of food and ADHD. Eur Child Adolesc Psychiatry 2008; DOI 10.1007/s00787–008–0695–7.

Perry CA, Dwyer BA, Gelfand JA, et al. Health effects of salicylates in foods and drugs. Nutr Rev 1996; 54:225–40.

Perry CA, Dwyer J, Gelfand JA, Couris RR, McCloskey WW. Health effects of salicylates in foods adnd drugs. *Nutr Rev.* 1996;54(8):225-240.

Prenner BM, Stevens JJ. Anaphylaxis after ingestion of sodium bisulfite. Case report. Ann Allergy 1976; 37:180–2.

Sakamoto N, Kono S, Wakai K, Fukuda Y, Satomi M, Shimoyama T, Inaba Y, Miyake Y, Sasaki S, Okamoto K, Kobashi G, Washio M, Yokoyama T, Date C, Tanaka H: Dietary risk factors for inflammatory bowel disease: a multicenter case-control study in Japan. Inflamm Bowel Dis 2005; 11: 154–163.

Samartin S, Marcos A, Chandra RK. Food hypersensitivity. *Nutr Res.* 2001; 21:473-497.

Sampson HA. Food anaphylaxis. *Br Med Bull.* 2000;56(4):925-935.
Sampson HA. Food hypersensitivity: Manifestations, diagnosis, and natural history. *Food Tech.* 1992; May:141-144.

Sensenig J, Marrongelle J, Johnson M, Staverosky T. Treatment of migraine with targeted nutrition focused on improved assimilation and elimination. *Alt Med Rev.* 2001;6(5):488-494.

Shepherd SJ, Parker FJ, Muir JG and Gibson, PR Dietary triggers of abdominal symptoms in patients with irritable bowel syndrome- randomised placebo-controlled evidence Clin. Gastroenterol. Hepatol. 2008;6(7):765-771

Sicherer SH, Sampson HA. Food hypersensitivity and atopic dermatitis: Pathophysiology, epidemiology, diagnosis and management. *J Allergy Clin Immunol.* 1999; 104: S114-S122.

Sicherer SH. Manifestations of food allergy: evaluation and management. *Am Fam Phys.* 1999;59(2):415-24, 429-430.

Sinclair S. Migraine Headaches: nutritional, botanical and other alternative approaches. *Alt Med Rev.* 1999;4(2):86-95.

Soderholm JD, Perdue MH. Stress and the gastrointestinal tract II. Stress and intestinal barrier function. *Am J Physiol Gastrointest Liver Physiol*. 2001; G7-G13.

Swain A, Soutter V, Loblay R, Truswell AS. Salicylates, oligoantigenic diets and behaviour. Lancet 1985; 2:41–2.

Taylor SL, Hefle SL. Food allergies and other food sensitivities: A publication of the Institute of Food Technologists' Expert Panel on Food Safety and Nutrition. *Food Tech*. 2001; 55(9):68-83.

Taylor SL, Leatherwood M, Lieber ER. A survey of histamine levels in sausages. / Food Protect 1978; 41 634-7

Walker WA, Sanderson IR. Epithelial barrier function to antigens. *Neuro-Immuno-Physiology Gastrointestinal Mucosa*. 1992; 664:10-17.

Walker-Smith J. Food sensitivity enteropathy: Overview and update. *Acta Paediatrica Japonica*. 1994; 36:545-549.

Wuthrich B. Adverse reactions to food additives. Ann Allergy 1993; 71:379–84.

Xavier RJ, Podolsky DK: Unravelling the pathogenesis of inflammatory bowel disease. Nature 2007; 448: 427–434.

Chapter 6

Candida: A Universal Cause of Many Diseases

One of the health challenges that I was facing many years ago was Candida. This is also known as Systemic Candidiasis; 'systemic' means "all body."

It took me over 11 years to finally rid myself of Candida after pursuing many different therapies from experts who had written books on the subject.

I will share with you the secrets that I discovered while formulating the Da Vinci Candida Protocol that has now been published in peer-reviewed journals[110, 111]. The protocol has been implemented with over *5,000* patients at the Da Vinci Holistic Health Centre that I founded and direct in Larnaca, Cyprus, with astounding success.

It was not until I began investigating the issue myself after completing a number of degree and diploma courses in natural medicine that I eventually managed to heal myself of Candida. Through trial and error, I found that many practitioners that I had seen and read about where trying to kill off the pathogenic, mycelial form of Candida using natural substances, without converting the pleomorphic, pathogenic Candida back to the normal, budding type; this really is the key to success that I will share with you in this book.

Another important element of success is to change the internal milieu using the detoxification protocols that I will talk about later below. Cleaning and adjusting the pH of the body are critical elements of success.

Let's look at the topic of Candida in more detail. With the abuse of antibiotics and sugar-laden products, I find Candida in probably 30% – 35% of all patients that I see. This percentage exceeds 70% when the patient is suffering from chronic disease. I have never seen a cancer patient who does not have Candida, particularly if they have had chemotherapy and radiation treatments.

---

110 Georgiou, G.J. (2008) British Naturopathic Journal, Vol. 25.,No. 1 & 2.
111 Georgiou, G.J. (2005) Explore! Volume 14, No. 6.

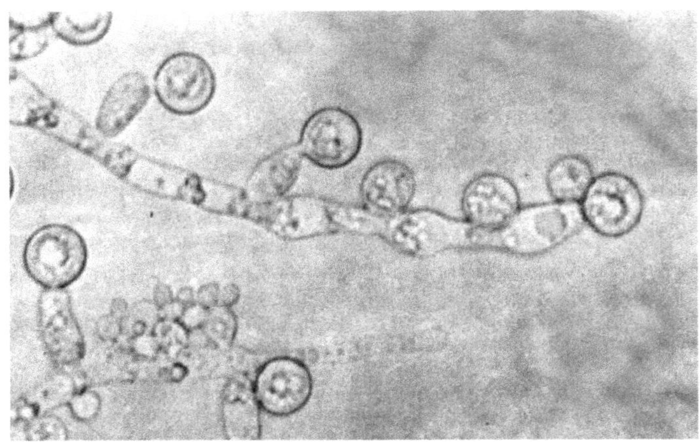

Pathogenic, Mycelial Candida albicans: Credit Wikipedia

There have been several books written on Systemic Candidiasis that are considered classics, which you may want to read.[112,113,114,115]

According to various surveys, Candida may be present in up to 62% of healthy people. This was shown by more than 40 surveys published between 1960 and 1986. Indeed, as long ago as 1924, candida was found in the mouths of 54% of many infants aged 2–6 weeks; in 46% of those up to 1 year old; and in 39% of those aged 1–6 years (Al-Doory, 1969).

In 1938, experimental vulvitis was produced by applying glucose to healthy vaginal surfaces which carried candida; while controls, free from the yeast but treated similarly, produced no signs of the disorder (Hesseltine, 1938).

This organism is responsible for buccal (oral) thrush, a disease which has been recognized for over 2,000 years. The renowned Greek physician, Hippocrates

---

112 Trowbridge JP and Walker M The Yeast Syndrome Bantam Books, New York, New York 1986.

113 Truss C: The Missing Diagnosis Birmingham Alabama (The author) 1983.

114 Crook, WG. The Yeast Connection and the Woman. Professional Books, Jackson TN 1987.

[115]115 Crook WG: The Yeast Connection, A Medical Breakthrough 2nd Addition Professional Books, Jackson, TN, 1984.

Odds FC. 1988. Candida and Candidosis, 2nd edn. Bailli`ere Tindall: London.

Al-Doory Y. 1969. The mycology of the freeliving baboon (Papio sp.). Mycopathologia et Mycologia Applicata 38: 7–15.

Hesseltine HC, Campbell LK. 1938. Diabetic or mycotic vulvovaginitis. American Journal of Obstetrics and Gynecology 35:
272–283.

(460–~370 BC), mentions oral thrush: aphthae in the mouth. Thrush usually refers to an infection by Candida within the mucous membranes of the mouth (particularly of babies), the throat or the vagina.

Many people have non-clinical infections of Candida, but its pathogenic effects are often experienced after treatment with antibiotics, which eliminates competing bacteria.

Those with an immune system which is suppressed (using immune suppressants, or from infection such as AIDS), are also particularly subject to the pathogenic effects of Candida and other yeasts.

Modern Medicine Negates its Existence

Many researchers have spent decades studying Candida and its virulent properties, yet modern medicine still negates its existence and does not believe that "normal" people can be carriers of this virulent, disease-causing, pathogenic form.

Modern medicine believes that it exists, but only in seriously ill patients whose immune system has literally become destroyed, like AIDS patients, or those who have been given drugs to suppress their immune system. Modern medicine believes that this is the best way of dealing with auto-immune diseases such as Crohn's, Lupus, Ulcerative colitis and the like.

Given that fungal candida is associated with so many symptoms, conditions, and diseases, one would think that a medical doctor would be aware of well-documented, evidence-based, scientifically-backed research that demonstrates time and time again a common causative agent. Scientists have published more than 54,000 studies on Candida, just go to https://www.ncbi.nlm.nih.gov/pubmed/?term=candida where they are listed.

Ideally, medical doctors SHOULD be aware of the possible consequences that their prescription medication could have on the patient. Giving antibiotics time and time again, without also giving prebiotics in parallel, is a sure way for patients, even young children, to develop systemic Candidiasis.

I personally have gotten into debates with various medical doctors who simply did not want to understand the relationship between Candida and the internal milieu. It appeared that they could not understand that destroying the complex and highly sensitive microbiome of the patient would not have any dire consequences.

This ignorance needs to be transcended by medical doctors to serve their patients better. There is simply no justification for it. Hopefully this book will provide enough knowledge for all to be aware of the side effects of powerful drugs, one of which is the development of systemic Candidiasis.

The widespread use of antibiotics, which induce neutropenia (an abnormally low number of neutrophils or white blood cells) and immune system suppression, is commonly attributed by science to be the most consistent cause of systemic Candida – the scientific papers on this are too many to mention here.

Corticosteroids can also suppress the immune system, and this too can lead to pathogenic candidiasis. Intestinal homeostasis is critical for human health and we should nurture it, not destroy it with powerful drugs.

The science of candida and how it affects the body goes far beyond what is written here. The ability of antibiotics to create systemic fungal candida is documented in thousands of studies dating back to the introduction of antibiotics in the 1940s. This gap between science and the practice of modern medicine is a major cause of sickness and illness today.

The consequences are often *dire* to many people's health. Only recently (July 2016) the National Geographic magazine published headlines such as: *"New and Deadly Drug-Resistant Yeast Emerges Globally."* The article goes on to say:

> *"One highly resistant form of yeast, called Candida auris, has been found in several hundred cases in nine countries since 2009: on the Pacific Rim, in South Asia, in the Middle East, in the United Kingdom, and in South America. The Centers for Disease Control and Prevention (CDC) is so concerned that it recently sent an alert to U.S. hospitals, even though only one possible case of the resistant fungus has been identified in the United States so far."*

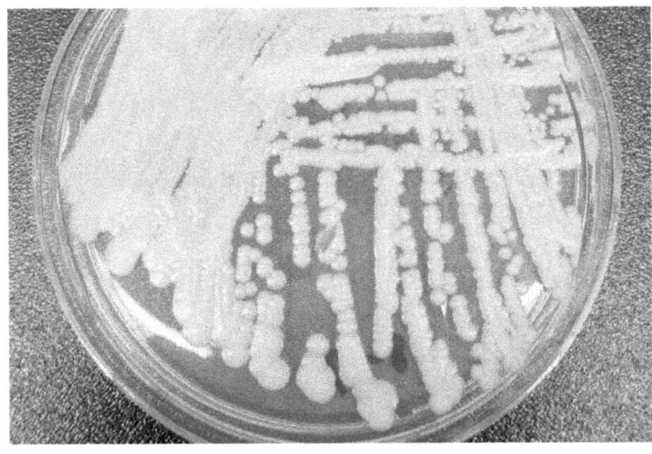

Fatal Candida auris yeast. Credit: National Geographic

They continue:

> *"By themselves, fungal infections - even ones that invade the bloodstream or bones - aren't a new problem. Yeasts exist throughout our environment and move from there to our guts, where their growth is held in check by the complex interactions of all the bacteria that live there. But when some of those bacteria are killed off by antibiotics - especially the long courses of drugs given in intensive-care units - or when illness or infection disrupt the immune system, yeasts can surge out of control and cause a whole-body infection. These invasive infections can be deadly, killing maybe a third of patients who develop them."*

Again, in June 2016, the Daily Mail reports:

> *"Thirteen cases of a sometimes deadly and often drug-resistant fungal infection, Candida auris, have been reported in the United States for the first time, health officials have confirmed.*
>
> *The infection, which often spreads in hospitals and other health care settings, was identified by the US Centers for Disease Control and Prevention in June 2016 as an emerging global threat.*
>
> *Four of the patients diagnosed with the infection have died, although the precise causes remain unclear, the CDC said."*

Indeed, Candida overgrowth can be fatal under varying circumstances, particularly anti-fungal resistant forms that are now appearing and spreading around the world.

This simply cannot be referred to as a gap in knowledge - it is a wide chasm that millions of people fall into while under modern medical care.

As modern medicine continues its decline, patients will search for the truths that lead them back to a state of health and a life of vitality. This is the premise of this book and I see hundreds of patients from all over the world who are on this search to be healed of their Candida and other related problems.

So, let's delve into this topic so that you can really understand what Candida is, how do you get it, and more importantly, how do you treat it.

What is Candida?

Every person lives in a virtual sea of microorganisms (bacteria, viruses, parasites, stealth organisms and fungi). These microbes can reside in the throat, mouth, nose, intestinal tract, almost anywhere; they are as much a part of our bodies as the food we eat. Usually, these microorganisms do not cause illness, unless our resistance becomes lowered.

Candida albicans is yeast that lives in the mouth, throat, intestines and genitourinary tract of most humans and is usually considered to be a normal part of the bowel flora (the organisms that coexist with us in our lower digestive tract). It is a member of a broader classification of organisms known as fungi.

Candida are unicellular yeasts, somewhat larger than bacteria, that divide mostly asexually, can switch between a yeast and a pseudohyphal or hyphal form and, like other yeasts, flourish in habitats where there is an abundance of sugar.

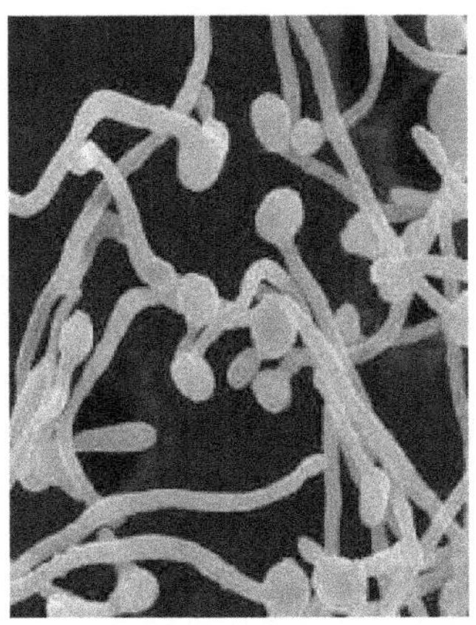

Pathogenic, mycelial Candida

Candida are normal human commensals, particularly in the mouth, skin, vagina and intestine. Candida can be cultured from faeces in up to 80% of healthy adults[116]. Candida numbers increase significantly following antibacterial therapy[117], but the numbers seem to be unaffected by a refined carbohydrate diet[118]. It seems

116 Bernhardt H, Knoke M. Mycological aspects of gastrointestinal microflora. Scand J Gastroenterol 1997; 32(suppl 222) :102–106.
117 Seelig MS. Mechanisms by which antibiotics increase the incidence and severity of candidiasis and alter the immunological defences. Bacteriol Rev 1 1966; 30 :4442–4459.
118 Weig M, Werner E, Frosh M, Kasper H. Limited effect of refined carbohydrate dietary supplementation on colonization of the gastrointestinal tract of healthy subjects by Candida albicans. Am J Clin Nutr 1999; 69 :1170–1173.

likely that intestinal Candida numbers are regulated in a similar way to intestinal bacteria[119].

C. Albicans and C. glabrata are the two most common Candida species that cause Systemic Candidiasis. There are 81 different types of Candida species such as C. glabrata, krusei, lusitaniae, parapsilosis, tropicalis and more, but only half a dozen are commonly found in humans, with C. albicans dominating. More than 70% of Candida species found in humans are Candida albicans.

How Does Candida Behave?

Some strains of Candida produce gliotoxin which may impair neutrophil function[120]. However, it is a polyantigenic organism containing up to 178 different antigens[121], which might explain the number of cross-reactions to yeasts (Malassezia, bread/brewer's yeast) and moulds[122] and even human tissue[123].

It was shown recently that there is a potential cross reactivity with gluten. Such a mechanism might lead to wheat intolerance with its accompanying symptoms and even trigger celiac disease in genetically susceptible people[124]. Furthermore, a placebo-controlled crossover study revealed that dietary yeast may affect the activity of Crohn's disease[125].

Candida produces alcohol and contains glycoproteins which have the potential to stimulate mast cells to release histamine and prostaglandin (PGE2), inflammatory substances which could cause IBS-like symptoms[126,127].

119 Fitzsimmons N, Berry DR. Inhibition of Candida albicans by Lactobacillus acidophilus: evidence for the involvement of a peroxidase system. Microbios 1994; 80 :125–133.

120 Shah DT, Jackman S, Engle J, Larsen B. Effect of gliotoxin on human polymorphonuclear neutrophils. Inf Dis Obster Gynecol 1998; 6 :168–175.

121 Poulain D, Hopwood V, Vernes A. Antigenic variability of candida albicans. CRC Crit Rev Microbiol 1985; 12:223-70.

122 Koivikko A, et al.. Allergenic cross-reactivity of yeasts. Allergy 1988; 43:192-200.

123 Vojdani A, Rahimian P, Kalhor H and Mordechai E. Immunological cross reactivity between candida albicans and human tissue. J Clin Lab Immunol 1996; 48:1-15.

124 Nieuwenhuizen WF, Pieters RH, Knippels LM, Jansen MC, Koppelman GJ. Is Candida albicans a trigger for the onset of coeliac disease? Lancet 2003; 361 :2152–2154.

125 Barclay GR, McKenzie H, Pennington J, Parratt D, Pennington CR. The effect of dietary yeast on the activity of stable chronic Crohn's disease. Scand J Gastroenterol 1992; 27 :196–200.

[126] Romani L, Bistoni F, Puccetti P. Initiation of T-helper cell immunity to Candida albicans by IL-12: the role of neutrophils. Chem Immunol. 1997; 68:110-35.

127 Kanda N, Tani K, Enomoto U, Nakai K & Watanabe S. The skin fungus-induced Th1- and Th2-related cytokine, chemokine and prostaglandin E 2 production in peripheral blood

Secretory immunoglobulin A (SIgA) is front-line in the defence of mucous membranes, especially in the intestine where it is active against infectious agents and certain antigens[128]. At least three different Candida species are able to produce proteases[129]. This protease can induce inflammation. An infection of the intestinal mucosa with Candida might lead to inflammation in patients with IBS symptoms.

Candida is sensitive to several antifungal agents, such as nystatin, which is not absorbed from the gastrointestinal tract after oral administration.

Candida is a diploid organism which has eight sets of chromosome pairs. Interestingly, Candida is one of the few microorganisms that have a diploid gene controlling the same protein – this means that it is capable of pleomorphic activity, being able to mutate forms from the budding form to the mycelial, pathogenic form.

When Does Candida Become a Problem?

The problem begins when the normal, budding Candida species that we have in our gut, which 90% of babies are born with, changes form to the mycelial or hyphae form, which is pathogenic or disease-causing. This only happens when the internal milieu of the gut and other tissues becomes more acidic, either through taking a variety of drugs such as antibiotics that wipes out the friendly flora of the gut, or through eating very acidic foods such as sugar and other refined products.

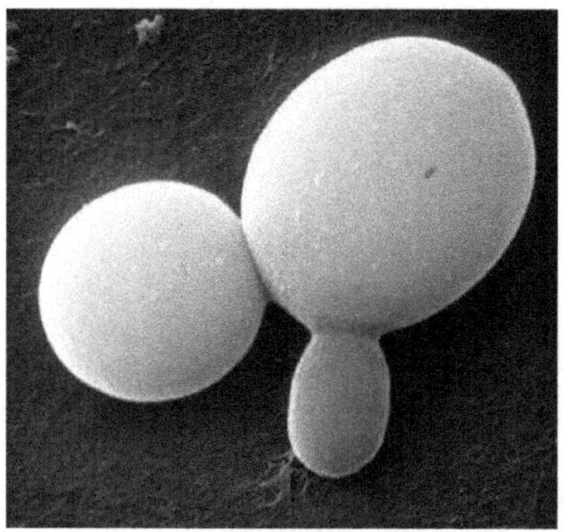

Normal, budding Candida

mononuclear cells from patients with atopic dermatitis and psoriasis vulgaris. Clinical & Experimental Allergy; 32(8):1243-50.

[128] Brandtzaeg P. The mucosal B cell and its functions. In: Brostoff J, Challacombe S (eds): Food Allergy and Intolerance. London: Saunders; 2002:127-171.

[129] Reinholdt J, Krogh P, Holmstrup P. Degradation of IgA1, IgA2, and S-IgA by candida and torulopsis species. Acta Path Microbiol Immunol Scand, Sect C 1987; 95:65-74.

It appears that this change in pH can trigger genes in the Candida to begin a pleomorphic change into a stealth organism that is very virulent. If fed with sugar, it can increase itself from 1 to 100 cells in 24 hours. These 100 cells can then produce 100 each in the next 24 hours, and so on, so by the 4th day we will have 100 million Candida cells – this is exponential, explosive growth!
Research has shown that it does not take longer than 1-2 days for this pathogenic form to get deep into the body tissues, inflaming them and damaging them in the process.

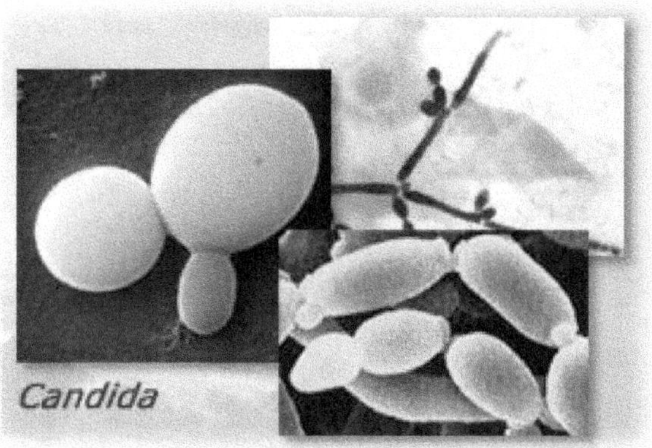

Normal, budding Candida on left; pathogenic on right

Fungus has many faces

A distinctive characteristic of Candida is its ability to grow with three distinct morphologies:

1. Yeast
2. Pseudohyphae
3. True hyphae

See Fig 1 below that illustrates the difference between these 3 forms. This is the same fungus, but it can change forms when given the right circumstances. This is typically known as PLEOMORPHISM, which is the Greek word for "many shapes or morphologies".

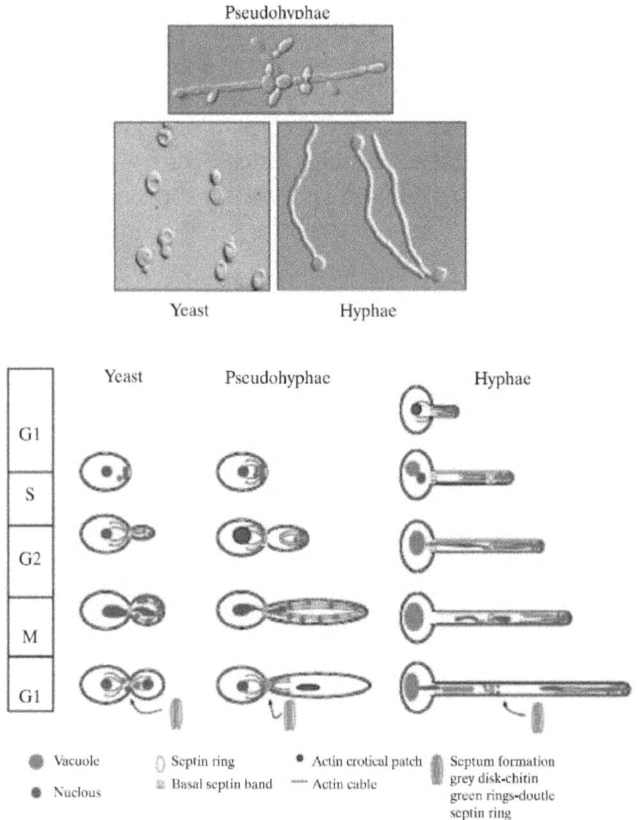

Fig 1. Different growth morphologies of Candida (reproduced from Sudbery et al., 2004).

Of all these forms, the Hyphal form is the worst. It can be aggressive and destroy tissues, causing disease. In other words, it is virulent or disease causing.

This form of virulent fungus is created when environmental conditions are conducive; 37°C growth temperature, the presence of serum, neutral pH, high CO2, growth in embedded conditions, and the presence of N-acetylglucosamine.

Figure 3 shows this aggressive, hyphal form of Candida aggressively infiltrating the human small intestine.

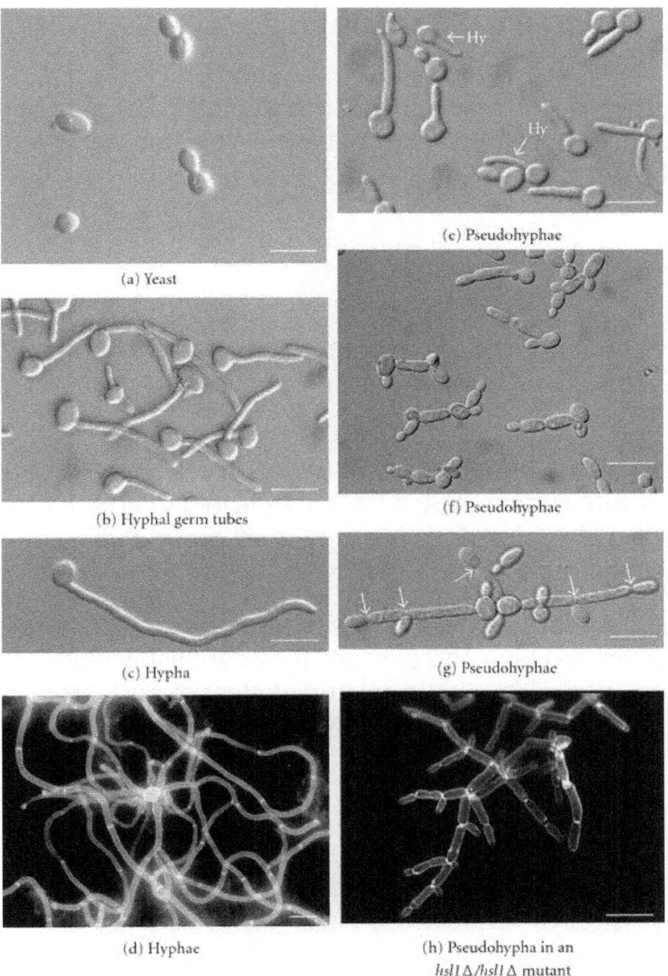

Figure 2: Yeast, hyphal and pseudohyphal morphologies

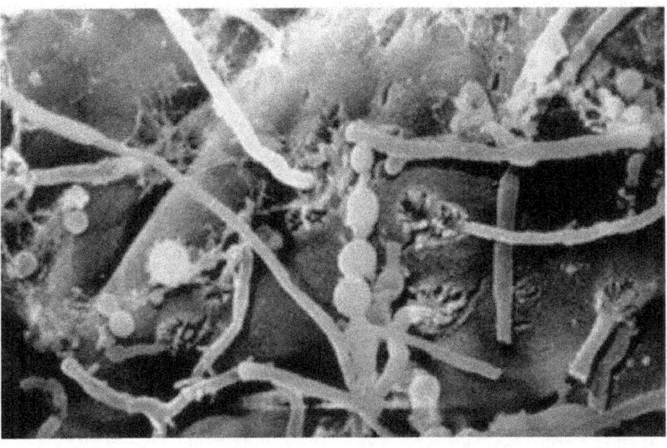

Fig 3. Candida albicans on human small intestine mucosa

The less virulent, yeast form of Candida favours a 30°C growth temperature and acidic pH (pH 4.0).

Pseudohyphal growth is an intermediate, transitional stage between the yeast form (less virulent) to the most virulent, hyphal form. This can occur in temperatures of 35°C or a pH of 5.5.

Biofilms

Have you ever picked up a rock from a nearby stream and wondered why it's slimy on the surface? That slimy layer is a group of microorganisms, collectively called a biofilm.

A biofilm is a community of bacteria that attach to a surface by excreting a sticky, sugary substance that encompasses the bacteria in a matrix. This might be the first time you've heard the term biofilm, but they're all around us, in streams, in drains, in fish tanks, even on our teeth.

A biofilm can be composed of a single species or a conglomerate of species. In many cases, biofilms are only bacteria, but they can also include other living things such as fungi and algae, creating a microbial stew of sorts. Biofilms are complex systems that are sometimes compared to multicellular organisms.

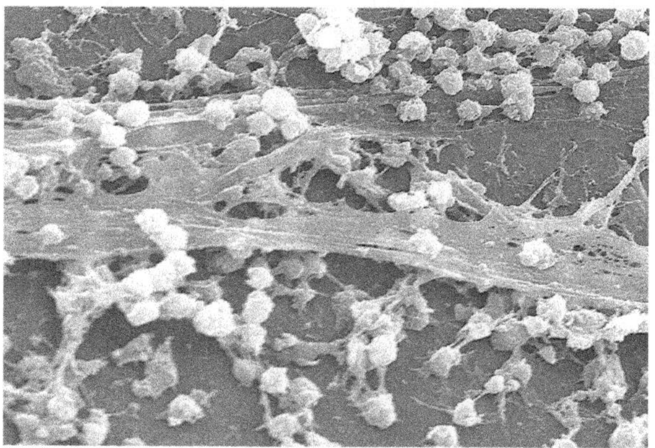

Biofilm of Candida

Candida can form a biofilm that basically protects it from being attacked by the immune system of the host (Blankenship and Mitchell, 2006; Nobile and Mitchell, 2006).

This biofilm of Candida is composed of protein polypeptides, polysaccharide carbohydrates, fibrinogen or fibrin and polynucleotides that contain RNA and DNA material. This structure is bound together with ligands that have stickiness properties.

As we will see later, the Enlyse™ enzymes present in one of the remedies used for treating Candida – CANDA PLUS - can eradicate this biofilm, hence allowing the immune system to do its work.

How Does Candida Attack the Body?

When candida attacks the body, it does it in various stages. First is interaction with the host cells by adhesion. Candida acts bit like glue, binding to extracellular matrix proteins of mucosal or endothelial cells (Calderone, et al, 2001; Grubb et al, 2008).

The close association with cell surfaces stimulates the formation of biofilms that we have already mentioned above (Kumato et al, 2005). The biofilm surrounds the yeast cells like a protective cocoon and keeps out attacks from the environment, including the immune system.

These biofilms can also make the Candida more resistant to anti-fungal drugs by pushing out these drugs from the cells. It also reduces production of ergosterol in the cell membrane, which makes the yeast cells less sensitive to anti-fungals by a factor of 30 to 2000 (Douglas, L.J., 2003).

Candida is also able to rapidly change its cell surface structure, making it more difficult for the immune system to recognize it. This is known as "phenotypic switching" (Soll, D.R., 2002; Morita, E 1999; Pappas et al, 2004; Reinel et al, 2008).

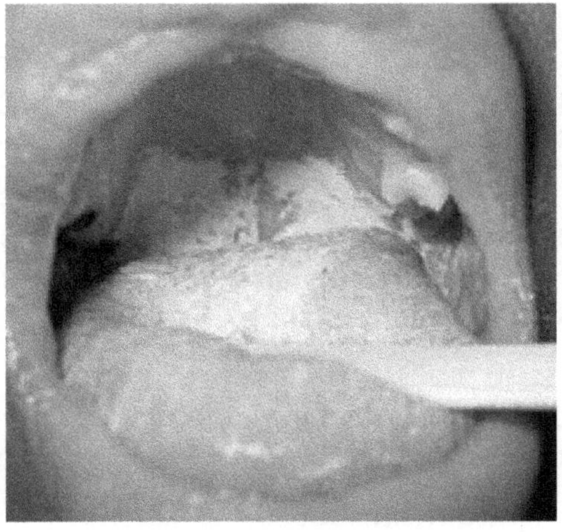

Candida attacking the mouth

As a consequence, the immune system can no longer recognize the fungi or initiate an immune reaction (Bastidas et al, 2009; Romani et al, 2003; Berman, J, 2006).

Some Candida strains avoid the attacks of the immune system by concealing themselves in host cells. They can survive unharmed in epithelial cells (Filler et al, 2006) or in non-activated white blood cells called macrophages (Raska et al, 2007; Dalkilic et al, 1991) and even replicate there.

In summary

Traditionally, fungi are considered plants, but they contain no chlorophyll and cannot make their own food. Fungi tend to inhabit cool to tropical climates.

The problem begins when the normal, budding yeast cell Candida that we have in our gut, which 90% of babies are born with, change forms to the mycelial or hyphae form which causes disease. This only happens when the internal milieu of the gut and other tissues changes, either through taking a variety of drugs such as antibiotics that wipes out the friendly flora of the gut, or through eating acidic foods. Repressing the immune system certainly does not help matters either.

How is Candida Diagnosed?

Dr. Crook, an American trained medical doctor and lecturer, after repeated observations of his patients became interested in chronic health complaints related to yeast overgrowth and to nutritional and environmental factors.

Dr Crook was one of the modern-day pioneers who published, *The Yeast Connection* and brought the concept of yeast infections to the public eye, while also trying to teach his colleagues, which was not easy at the best of times. In his book, he developed a comprehensive questionnaire of many of the symptoms that are related to systemic Candidiasis.

Dr. Crook's Candida questionnaire (see Appendix) is very helpful because it enables the patient to score their symptoms and arrive at a number. Anything above 180 for women, and 140 for men is highly significant and represents most symptoms that relate to Candida infestation.

There are also other testing procedures for picking up the Candida; the Vegetative Reflex Testing (VRT) biodermal screening, a form of Bioresonance testing initially invented by Dr Voll and later adapted by Dr Schimmel, is one.

The VRT testing can highlight the causes of illnesses by using homoeopathic biosonodes, this is usually a small portion of diseased tissue from a diseased organ that is ground up and made into a homoeopathic remedy.

When a particular biosonode that is placed on the honeycomb on the Bioresonance testing device induces a resonance reaction in the acupoint, then this infers a relationship between the diseased organ being tested and the related organ of the patient.

Even bacteria, viruses, fungi, stealth organisms and more can be tested for resonance with the patient and identified much quicker than any other type of biological testing.

In the case of identifying the pathological, hyphal form of Candida, as long as the practitioner has an ampoule of this form, then it is very easy to test whether the patient is resonating to it. In the hands of an experienced practitioner, this is an accurate and efficient way of testing, given that there are no real clinical tests for pathological Candida that have been developed yet.

There are several Bioresonance testing devices including the VEGA, the BICOM, the DETA PROFESSIONAL and more. The most cost-effective device is the DETA PROFESSIONAL (http://www.deta-elis-uk.com).

I run 5-day intensive clinical workshops 3-4 times per year training practitioners to use VRT Bioresonance testing and treatment in Larnaca, Cyprus. There is also an online course to help practitioners understand the theory entitled, *Energy Medicine and Bioresonance* (http://www.collegenaturalmedicine.com).

Another method of testing for Candida is to use a form of kinesiological muscle testing called Autonomic Response Testing (ART), invented by a German neurologist, Dr. Dietrich Klinghardt, M.D. Ph.D. ART grew out of the importance of detecting and correct problems of the autonomic nervous system (ANS).

ART allows the practitioner to correct the problems of the ANS and to help restore the self-regulating mechanism of the body, allowing the patient to return to a state of health naturally.

To date, there is no conclusive blood or clinical test for diagnosing pathogenic Systemic Candidiasis. There are expensive genetic tests that can determine the genome of the mycelial, hyphal, pathogenic Candida, but these are not generally available on the open market yet and are more used for research purposes. The other way is to examine tissue taken during a biopsy, as I have already mentioned above.

Conclusive laboratory tests have not yet been developed, even though there are several tests that can help in the diagnosis.

Other Factors Creating Pathogenesis

When other health conditions become involved, Candida becomes known as Candida-related complex (CRC). CRC, an excess of Candida in your system can cause a host of uncomfortable signs and symptoms which are syndromes within themselves, such as chronic fatigue syndrome, hypoglycemia, leaky gut syndrome, fibromyalgia, allergy or sensitivity, hormonal, thyroid, and adrenal dysfunction.

This syndrome isn't caused by Candida itself, but by the number of metabolites yeast colonies release inside the human colon when they exceed tolerable amounts.

Patients with CRC often have widespread symptoms affecting multiple organs systems such as:

- Gastrointestinal symptoms and haemorrhoids
- Chronic allergies
- Unexplained fatigue; always tired
- CNS fog, mood swings, depression
- Skin rashes, fungal infections
- Cravings for sugar, bread, beer

Toxicity in the colon affects the health of the whole body, particularly if one's elimination is slowed as in the case of constipation due to an imbalance in intestinal flora.

The delicate hormonal and chemical balance that orchestrates our emotional health can also be affected causing symptoms of mental illness.

Everyone can be Affected with Candida!

Anyone can be infected with Candida today! Women can be infected because of antibiotics, steroids, anti-inflammatory medications, hormones and birth-control pills. Men are also being infected with Candida from antibiotics, steroids, anti-inflammatory drugs, pain medications, and sexual relations with an infected partner (even though this often results in a topical infection, not a systemic spread).

Teenagers can get Candida from routine treatment with tetracycline or other antibiotics for acne. Babies have Candida from the birth canal or breast milk of the infected mother. That is why babies often have thrush (a white- coated tongue), which is a yeast infection.

Millions of people all over the world are infected with Candida. It is estimated that at least one out of three people in the Western world are affected. Because so many of the population can be infected and because so many factors can cause the condition, Candida is an enormous health problem today.

Candida coexists in our bodies with many species of bacteria in a competitive balance. Other bacteria act in part to keep Candida growth in check in our body ecology, when health is present, the immune system keeps Candida proliferation under control. But when the immune response is weakened, Candida growth can proceed unchecked.

What is the role of Candida?

Candida has two parasitic functions:

1. Gobble up any putrefied food matter in our digestive system (mostly caused by improper digestion due to low stomach acid).
2. After we die, Candida acts to decompose the body, feeding off our corpse and returning us to Mother Earth!

When conditions are right, they transform their yeast form into the hyphal, mycelial state, where filament-like roots invade deep into the mucosa in search of nourishment. The mycelia release enzymes such as phospholipase that attacks cell membranes of the mucosa, splitting fatty acids, generating free radicals, and causing inflammation in the intestine and other tissues.

Wherever the yeast colonizes they cause symptoms, whether an itchy anus or vagina, diarrhea, heartburn or sore throat. The mycelial forms release 79 different toxic by-products that damage specific tissues and organs and will determine which symptoms will occur.

These toxins, such as aldehyde, can also compete with hormone receptor sites and cause hypothyroidism, hypoestrogenism as well as binding cortisone, progesterone and other hormones for its own use and causing endocrine deficiency states.

How do you get it?

Candida albicans prefers people. Candida enters newborn infants during or shortly after birth. Usually, the growth of the yeast is kept in check by the infant's immune system and thus produces no overt symptoms. But, should the immune response weaken, the condition known as oral thrush can occur. By six months of age, 90% of all babies test positive for Candida and by adulthood, virtually all humans play host to Candida albicans and are thus engaged in a life-long relationship.

Unfortunately, there are many factors in our modern society that can upset the ecological balance of the body, weaken the immune system and allow the yeast to overgrow. The major risk factors, which may predispose one to the proliferation of Candida, are:

- **STEROID HORMONES, IMMUNOSUPPRESSANT DRUGS** such as cortisone, which treat severe allergic problems by paralyzing the immune system's ability to react.

- **PREGNANCY, MULTIPLE PREGNANCIES or BIRTH CONTROL PILLS** which upset the body's hormonal balance.

- **DIETS HIGH IN CARBOHYDRATE AND SUGAR INTAKE, YEAST AND YEAST PRODUCTS, AS WELL AS MOULDS AND FERMENTED FOODS.**

- **PROLONGED EXPOSURE TO ENVIRONMENTAL MOULDS.**

- **ANTIBIOTICS and SULPHA DRUGS** - probably the chief culprit of all. Antibiotics kill all bacteria. They do not distinguish good bacteria from bad. Antibiotics kill the "good" flora which normally keeps the Candida under control. This allows for the unchecked growth of Candida in the intestinal tract.

In the Kaiser Health News report in June 2016, this was what was said against antibiotics and the lethal fungus that can be created (a Candida species known as C. auris):

> *Hospitalized patients are at especially high risk from the fungus because many have had antibiotics, which can kill off healthy bacteria that help protect us from disease, said Peter Hotez, dean of the National School of Tropical Medicine at Baylor College of Medicine in Houston.*
>
> *It's a warning or wake-up against the indiscriminate use of antibiotics, especially in hospital settings," Hotez said.*
>
> *Hospitals have been testing for the fungus more frequently due to outbreaks in Asia and the United Kingdom, said Amesh Adalja, senior associate at the UPMC Center for Health Security in Baltimore.*
>
> *In earlier outbreaks, the fungus has killed 59 percent of patients, including 68 percent of patients whose infection spread to the bloodstream, said Adalja, who published a brief report on the infection Friday. Previous patients have had a median age of 54, Adalja said. The most common underlying medical problem was diabetes, and half of the patients had undergone surgery within 90 days. Nearly 80 percent of patients had a catheter placed in a major vein in the chest and 61 percent had a urinary catheter.*

"Candida auris is a major threat that carries a high mortality," Adalja said. "Candida fungal species are ubiquitous. ... As we learn more about this species, it will be essential to understand how it spreads in health care facilities and what the best infection control and treatment strategies are."

Antibiotic Abuse and Inappropriate Prescribing

The prevalence today of Candida may be most directly related to the widespread societal exposure to antibiotics - from prescriptions for colds, infections, acne, and from additional consumption of antibiotic-treated foods such as meats, dairy, poultry and eggs.

Notably, antibiotics do not kill viruses; they destroy bacteria. Yet, they are universally prescribed for all colds, flus and other viral problems. Such indiscriminate and extensive use of antibiotics is not only considered a primary cause of Candida overgrowth but is recently being found to be responsible for the unbridled development of "killer bacteria."

The rapid and direct proliferation of the yeast following antibiotic use strongly suggests that the problem of Candida is one which stems from an inner state of imbalance, rather than from an outside attack by a microbe or disease. This is a very important point to understand if one wishes to get rid of an overgrowth problem, suggesting that Candida is not so much a problem as is the body's own failure to control it!

- Incorrectly prescribed antibiotics also contribute to the promotion of resistant bacteria (Center for Disease Control and Prevention).
- Studies have shown that treatment indication, choice of agent, or duration of antibiotic therapy is incorrect in 30% to 50% of cases (Luyt, C.E, 2014).
- One U.S. study reported that a pathogen was defined in only 7.6% of 17,435 patients hospitalized with community-acquired pneumonia (CAP) (Barlett, J.G., 2013).
- In comparison, investigators at the Karolinska Institute in Sweden were able to identify the probable pathogen in 89% of patients with CAP through use of molecular diagnostic techniques (polymerase chain reaction [PCR] and semiquantitative PCR), therefore prescribing the correct antibiotics for this particular health problem, as opposed to experimenting with many different types, to the detriment of the patient.
- In addition, 30% to 60% of the antibiotics prescribed in intensive care units (ICUs) have been found to be unnecessary, inappropriate, or suboptimal (Luyt, C.E., 2014).

- Incorrectly prescribed antibiotics have questionable therapeutic benefit and expose patients to potential complications of antibiotic therapy (Lushniak, B.D., 2014).
- Sub-inhibitory and sub-therapeutic antibiotic concentrations can promote the development of antibiotic resistance by supporting genetic alterations, such as changes in gene expression, HGT, and mutagenesis (Viswanathan, V.K.,2014).
- Changes in antibiotic-induced gene expression can increase virulence, while increased mutagenesis and HGT promote antibiotic resistance and spread.
- Low levels of antibiotics have been shown to contribute to strain diversification in organisms such as *Pseudomonas aeruginosa*. Sub-inhibitory concentrations of piperacillin and/or tazobactam have also been shown to induce broad proteomic alterations in *Bacteroides fragilis.*

Symptoms Related to Candida

There are many symptoms that can be caused by Candida – the following list is Dr. Jeff McComb's, D.C., a chiropractor working in the U.S. who has also created a Candida Library with hundreds of research papers on Candida – see http://www.candidalibrary.org/cand_lib/.

This is a list of 100 Common Candida Symptoms associated with systemic fungal candida from his website:

ADD	ADHD	Acid reflux	Acne	Allergies
Anxiety	Arthritis	Asthma	Athlete's foot	Autism
Autoimmune conditions	Bladder infections	Blisters in mouth	Bloating	Blood sugar imbalances
Body odour	BPH	Brain fog	Bronchitis	Burping
Cancer	Chemical sensitivities	Chronic Fatigue Syndrome	Colitis	Concentratio n difficulty
Confusion	Congestion	Constipation	Crohn's Disease	Cough
Cystitis	Depression	Dermatitis	Diabetes	Diarrhoea

Eczema	Endometriosis	Excess mucous	Fibromyalgia	Flatulence
Fluid retention	Food allergies	Food cravings	Frequent colds	Frequent infections
Fungal infections	Gas	Gastritis	Genital rashes	Headaches
Haemorrhoids	Hormonal imbalances	Hypoglycaemia	Hypothyroidism	Irritability
Inflammatory Bowel Disease	Immune system dysfunction	Impotence	Indigestion	Infertility
Irregular menstruation	Itchy skin	Joint pain	Lack of mental clarity	Leaky gut
Lethargy	Lupus	Migraines	Memory problems	Mood swings
Muscle pain	Nail fungus	Osteoarthritis	Penile itching	PMS
Poor concentration	Poor memory	Prostatitis	Prostate enlargement	Psoriasis
Rashes	Rectal itching	Rheumatoid arthritis	Rhinitis	Scleroderma
Sexual dysfunction	Sinus problems	Sores	Sore throat	Sugar cravings
Swollen joints	Thrush	Urethritis	Vaginitis	
Weakness	Weight gain	White coating on tongue		

Why is it a serious problem?

Once begun, if not recognized and treated appropriately, Candida overgrowth can result in a self-perpetuating, negative cycle. Large numbers of yeast germs can weaken the immune system, which normally protects the body from harmful invaders. Even though Candida is part of the ecological balance in the body since birth, it is still recognized by the immune system as a foreign body that needs to be controlled.

So, when overgrowth occurs, a chronic stimulation to the immune system results - every second, every minute, every hour, every day, every month, every year - in an attempt by the immune system to regain control. In time, it is believed that this can exhaust the immune system, predisposing one to more serious degenerative processes. Many believe chronic drains on the immune system such as Candida and parasites can play a direct role in the development of cancer and AIDS. Seen in this light, Candida overgrowth should not be taken lightly.

Candida produces its effects by two routes. Firstly, there is a direct route initially by invasion of the gut and the vagina; Candida can spread along the entire length of the gut – from mouth to anus. The presence of chronic vaginitis can often indicate wide-spread Candidiasis. Secondly, there can be indirect effects caused by spread of mycotoxins through the bloodstream to other sites.

In the gut, Candida can alter its form from a simple yeast organism to a "mycelial fungal form" with a network of root-like fibres called rhizoids. These can penetrate and damage the gut lining, allowing foreign food proteins to be absorbed into the bloodstream and to challenge the immune system so that multiple food allergies or intolerances may result.

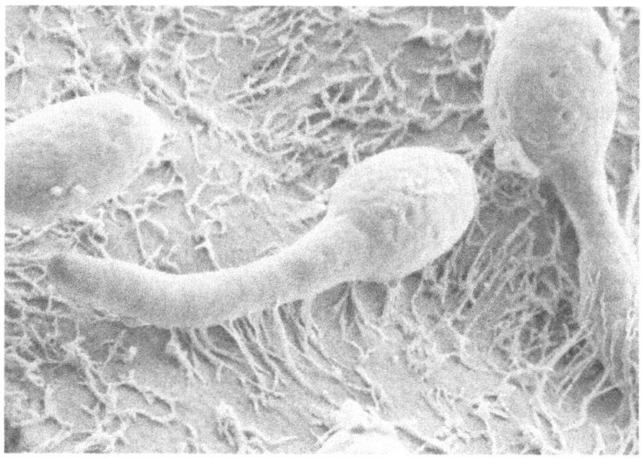

Electron micrograph of Candida

Toxic waste from Candida infestations can also be absorbed into the bloodstream causing "Yeast Toxin Hypersensitivity" leading to many symptoms such as anxiety, depression and impaired intellectual functioning. The main toxin implicated here is acetaldehyde, which is a normal by-product of metabolism, produced in small amounts and rendered harmless by the liver.

If, however, there is excess production of this by Candida, particularly in low-oxygen environments, and a lack of the appropriate liver enzymes which tend to be deficient in 5% of the general population, the acetaldehyde will bind strongly to human tissue. This may cause impaired neuro-transmission in the brain, resulting in anxiety, depression, defective memory and cloudy thinking.

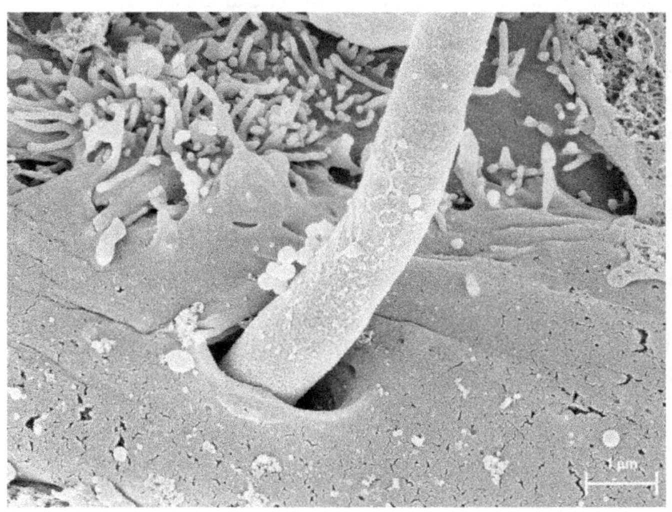

Electron micrograph of Rhizoid penetrating tissue

Acetaldehyde, one of the mycotoxins secreted by Candida, mediates a good part of the cellular damage that occurs. Acetaldehyde in the intestinal wall and liver will disrupt intestinal absorptive processes, as well as impairing the function of lymphocytes and red blood cells. Acetaldehyde is damaging to host cells by free radical and peroxidative mechanisms. When yeast cells are limited in oxygen, they are also more resistant to immune defenses. Patient hypoxia is a major contributing factor to yeast susceptibility, for these two reasons.

Adequate amounts of glutamine, selenium, niacin, folic acid, B6, B12, iron, and molybdenum will allow the aldehydes to be metabolized into acetic acid, which can be excreted, or converted further into acetyl coenzyme A. Certainly, patients exhibiting toxic syndrome while treating Candida are highly recommended to take these food supplements for their own protection.

Effects on Immunity

Some 40 to 60% of all the immune cells in our body are in the gut. The immune system may concurrently be adversely affected by poor nutrition, heavy exposure to moulds in the air, as well as an increasing number of chemicals in our food, water and air, including petrochemicals, formaldehyde, perfumes, cleaning fluids, insecticides, tobacco and other indoor and outdoor pollutants.

Over 10,000 chemicals have been added to our food supplies alone that were not there just 100 years ago! We do not have the genetic recognition of these substances as foods or as useful additions to our bodies.

Specifically, yeast tend to secrete a toxin called Gliotoxin[130], which can disrupt the immune system by inactivating enzyme systems, producing free radicals, interfering with the DNA of leukocytes and being cytotoxic.

Resulting lowered resistance may not only cause an overall sense of ill health, but also may allow for the development of respiratory, digestive and other systemic symptoms. One may also become predisposed to developing sensitivities to foods and chemicals in the environment. Such "allergies" may in turn cause the membranes of the nose, throat, ear, bladder and intestinal tract to swell and develop infection.

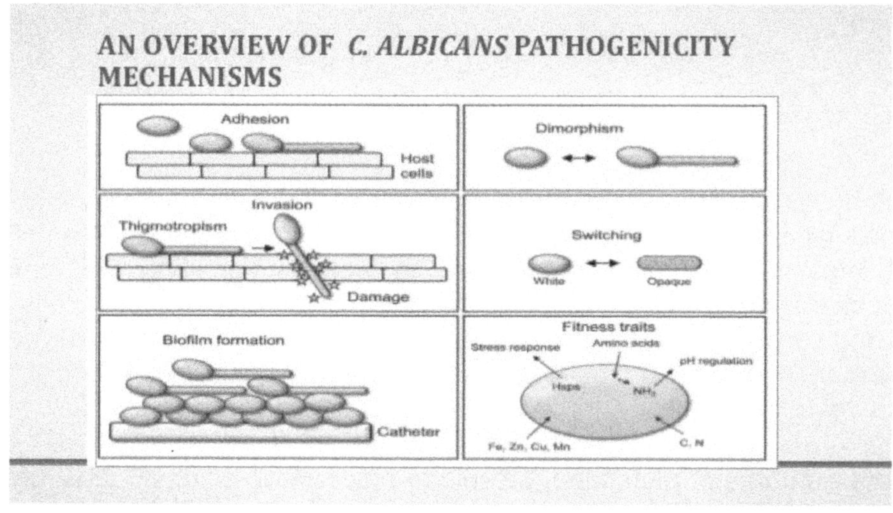

Such conditions may lead the physician to prescribe a "broad spectrum" antibiotic which may then further promote the overgrowth of Candida and strengthen the existing negative chain of events, leading to further stress on the immune system and increased Candida-related problems.

---

[130] Iwata, K.; Yamamoto, Y "Glycoprotein Toxins Produced by Candida albicans." Proceedings of the Fourth International Conference on the Mycoses, PAHO Scientific Publication #356, June 1977.

I have seen this happen in clinical practice many times. If only physicians could think laterally for a minute, many hundreds of thousands of superfluous antibiotic prescriptions could be done away with to the benefit of the patient as opposed to the pharmaceutical industry. Physicians talk about evidence-based medicine, but often drugs such as antibiotics are prescribed for the wrong infections because testing was not done in the first place.

Candida overgrowth results in production of the highly toxic canditoxin and ethanol which are known to cause fatigue, toxicity, and depressive symptoms. Another study found such impairment of neutrophils decreases the body's ability to combat viruses such as those that cause heart damage, resulting in more inflammatory damage.

The diagram below (Fig 5) clearly shows how Candida is known to impair immune functioning by directly and negatively impacting the helper-suppresser ratio of T lymphocytes.

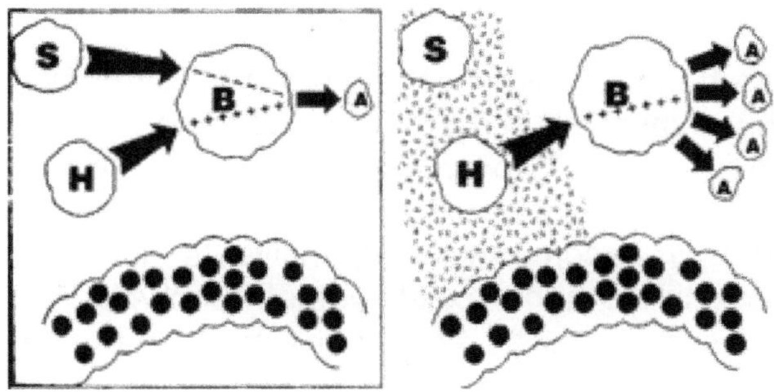

Fig 5: How Yeast Toxins Injure the Immune System

S=Suppressor cell; H=Helper cell; B=B-cell; A=Antibodies

First diagram: Yeast and intestinal lactobacilli bacteria in balance = normal immune function. A balance between intestinal lactobacilli bacteria and yeast allow for normal immune lymphocyte function. Helper cells stimulate the B-cells to make antibodies, whereas suppressor cells appropriately oppose B-cell antibody production. Antibody production is in balance.

Second diagram: Overgrowth of intestinal yeast, release of toxins into the bloodstream, and altered immune function. Intestinal yeast overgrowth and yeast toxins released into the bloodstream inhibit suppressor cell function. Stimulation of antibody production by helper cells is now unopposed, and inappropriate antibody production occurs. Here we have a heightened state of allergy, as well as an increased susceptibility to autoimmune conditions.

The main components of the immune system are:

1. B-lymphocytes; these produce proteins called immunoglobulins, which bind antigenic substances and render them harmless. An antigen is a substance which the body recognizes as being alien and therefore potentially harmful. An immunoglobulin is a particular kind of protein which coats the antigen; by being made harmless the antigens can then be digested by other cells.

2. T-lymphocytes; there are three types:

   a. The killer cells; this attack and destroy substances with enzymes and hormones.

   b. The helper cells; these help B cells to make the immunoglobulins.

   c. The suppressor cells; these protect the body from the excesses of the body's defense system.

T-cell efficiency can be influenced to a useful extent by nutrition. It is largely the suppressors which are involved in fighting the Candida challenge, partly because Candida's adaptability allows it to produce disguising antigens which deter the immune system from recognizing it as foreign and harmful. In this way, the immune system may eventually become non-responsive to the presence of Candida albicans. Candida toxins will then circulate virtually unchallenged, and Candida will grow in a range of tissues either as a yeast or a mycelial fungus.

This apparent tolerance of Candida by the immune system can only be reversed in the long term by ending exposure of the body to yeast antigens and toxins. A high percentage of serum from symptomless people has been found to contain yeast toxin immunoglobulins. This indicates that the B-cell immune defenses must be constantly counteracting Candida toxin.

When alive, yeasts can invade the immune system to a certain degree. When they are killed, proteins making up the yeast cell wall are absorbed through the lining of the intestine and can cause heightened allergy reactions, resulting in a phenomenon called 'Die off' or the 'Herxheimer reaction'. This may in fact signal a good response to treatment.

What are the signs of Candida infection?

Basically, the characteristics of Candida overgrowth fall under three categories, those affecting:

1. The gastrointestinal and genitourinary tracts
2. Allergic responses
3. Mental/emotional manifestations

Initially, the signs will show near the sights of the original yeast colonies. Most often the first signs are seen in conditions such as nasal congestion and discharge, nasal itching, blisters in the mouth, sore or dry throat, abdominal pain, belching, bloating, heartburn, constipation, diarrhea, rectal burning or itching, vaginal discharge, vaginal itching or burning, increasingly worsening symptoms of PMS, prostatitis, impotence, frequent urination, burning on urination, and bladder infections.

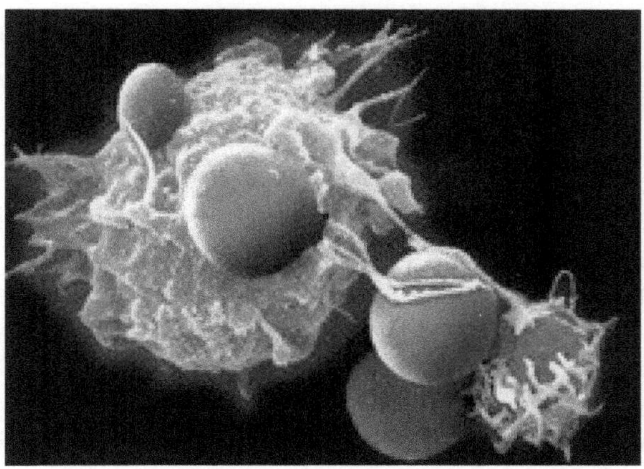

White blood cell killing Candida

But, if the immune system remains weak for long enough, Candida can spread to all parts of the body causing an additional plethora of problems such as fatigue, drowsiness, incoordination, lack of concentration, mood swings, dizziness, headaches, bad breath, coughing, wheezing, joint swelling, arthritis, failing vision, spots in front of the eyes, ear pain, deafness, burning or tearing eyes, muscle aches, depression, irritability, sweet cravings, increasing food and chemical sensitivities, numbness and tingling, cold hands and feet, asthma, hay fever, multiple allergies, hives and rashes, eczema, psoriasis, chronic fungal infections like athlete's foot, ringworm and fingernail/toenail infections.

In addition, *79 different toxic products* are released by Candida, which places a considerable burden on the immune system. These get into the bloodstream and travel to all parts of the body where they may give rise to a host of adverse symptoms. Yeasts in the body produce a by-product called acetaldehyde, a toxic substance resulting in several health consequences. In fact, acetaldehyde is the compound that produces the symptoms in an alcohol "hang-over."

Molybdenum plays a role as a cofactor in helping break down acetaldehyde to a form that provides the body with energy. Molybdenum plays a large role in the detoxification pathway for acetaldehyde in the human body. There are dozens of known toxins released by yeast in the body. This damages and overworks both the liver and the immune system as the body tries to detoxify these poisons.

In Candida overgrowth, the yeast colonies can dig deep into intestinal walls, damaging the bowel wall in their colonization. The invasive Candida filaments produce disease affecting the entire body in several ways:

Destruction of the intestinal membrane, allowing for:

- Severe leaks of toxins from activity of undesirable microorganisms within the layers of encrusted fecal matter into the bloodstream causing a variety of symptoms and aggravating many pre-existing conditions.
- Absorption of incompletely digested dietary proteins. These are extremely allergenic and may produce a large spectrum of allergic reactions. Food allergies are very common with Candidiasis, as is environmental hypersensitivity (to smoke, auto exhaust, natural gas, perfumes, air pollutants), probably due to Candida filaments infiltrating lung and sinus membranes.
- Migration of Candida itself into the bloodstream. Once in the blood, it has access to all body tissues and may cause various gland or organ dysfunctions, weakening the entire system and further lowering resistance to other diseases.

Candida can also attack the immune system, causing suppressor cell disease, in which the immune system produces antibodies to everything at the slightest provocation, resulting in extreme sensitivities.

Women are more likely to get Candida overgrowth than are men. This is related to the female sex hormone progesterone which is elevated in the last half of the menstrual cycle. Progesterone increases the amount of glycogen (animal starch, easily converted to sugar) in the vaginal tissues which provide an ideal growth medium for Candida. Progesterone levels also elevate during pregnancy. Men are affected less frequently but are by no means invulnerable.

The Relationship Between Candida and Chronic Diseases

Several natural medicine practitioners have long been supporting the notion that intestinal fungi can contribute to chronic diseases.

However, the allopathic medical fraternity has been downplaying the role of intestinal fungi. This is largely since little research has been done; it's difficult to diagnose and it can't be treated properly with pharmaceuticals. New research at Cedars-Sinai Medical Center looked at the connection between fungi and Ulcerative Colitis.

Dr. David M. Underhill and his team at the Inflammatory Bowel and Immunobiology Research Institute have been studying the interaction between Commensal Fungi and the C-Type Lectin Receptor, Dectin-1. In healthy animals Dectin-1 is produced and works as the body's immune response against fungi.

The risk of developing Ulcerative Colitis increases significantly in mice with a defective form of Dectin-1. Dr. Underhill and his team treated these animals with an antifungal drug called Fluconazole and observed that their symptoms moderated.

In humans, a mutated form of Dectin-1 is closely related to Ulcerative Colitis that doesn't respond to medical therapy. When this important receptor isn't working properly, our protection against intestinal fungi is decreased and we are more prone to developing Candidiasis.

It's already known that gut flora in patients with UC differs significantly from healthy individuals. The fungal colonization of the colon may influence the activation of UC, and antifungal treatment causes clinical improvement in most individuals. Patients with Crohn's disease and their healthy relatives are colonized with Candida more commonly than control families.

30 years after, *The Missing Diagnosis* by Orian Truss and, *The Yeast Connection* by William Crook were released, there's growing research in the medical community on the importance of gut flora and intestinal fungi.

Candida has also been correlated with chronic inflammatory diseases such as arthritis and multiple sclerosis. That was the implication of a 2012 study in the prestigious journal *Nature*, conducted by researchers from Charite – Universitatsmedizin, Berlin and the Institute for Research in Biomedicine, Bellinzona, Switzerland.

The study found that cells of Candida seemed to trigger the immune system to produce more inflammation.

The findings are particularly significant because the immune cells being studied play a key role in autoimmune diseases such as multiple sclerosis, rheumatoid arthritis and psoriasis.

"This not only demonstrates that the composition of our microflora has a decisive role in the development of chronic illnesses, but also that the key cells causing illness can develop an anti-inflammatory 'twin'," first author Dr. Christina Zielinski said.

Scientific Research on Candida

The recent research indicates that yeast overgrowth in the intestines does occur and is associated with a variety of symptoms and other health conditions which improve with antifungal treatment. I will quote the scientific references of this research for those that want to look deeper into the topic, at least they will be able to find the research papers.

For example, Candida overgrowth of the GI tract was found in recent studies to:

- Promote the development of food allergies by increasing intestinal permeability and affecting immune function (Gut. 2006 Jul;55(7):954-60; Biosci Microbiota Food Health. 2012;31(4):77-84).
- Aggravate inflammation not only in the gut but in tissues all throughout the body, increasing the risk of allergies and autoimmune diseases. (Med Mycol. 2011 Apr;49(3):237-47; Curr Opin Microbiol. 2011 Aug;14(4):386-91).
- Directly correlate with the amount of inflammation and severity of symptoms in patients with ulcers, Crohn's disease, and ulcerative colitis (J Clin Gastroenterol. 2014 Jul;48(6):513-23; J Physiol Pharmacol. 2009 Mar;60(1):107-18; Curr Opin Microbiol. 2011 Aug;14(4):386-91.
- Increase with the use of antibiotics, especially when there is already inflammation in the intestines (Curr Opin Microbiol. 2011 Aug;14(4):386-91).
- Increase with the use of proton pump inhibitors, otherwise known as anti-acids – drugs that block the production of hydrochloric acid in the stomach (Aliment Pharmacol Ther. 2013 Jun;37(11):1103-11).
- Cause the same symptoms as small intestinal bacterial overgrowth (SIBO) when it occurs in the small intestine (Aliment Pharmacol Ther. 2013 Jun;37(11):1103-11). SIBO symptoms include abdominal pain, chest pain, belching, bloating, fullness, indigestion, nausea, diarrhoea, vomiting, gas, malabsorption, and vitamin deficiencies.
- Promote inflammation in the lungs (Cell Host Microbe. 2014 Jan 15;15(1):95-102).
- Occur more commonly in people with psoriasis and other inflammatory skin disorders (Int J Dermatol. 2014 Dec;53(12):e555-60.).
- Occur more commonly in people with chronic fatigue syndrome (Scan J Gastro. 2007;42(12):1514-1515.).

- Furthermore, people with irritable bowel syndrome (IBS) have more antibodies in their blood to Candida. The severity of IBS symptoms is directly associated with levels of those antibodies (BMC Gastroenterol. 2012; 12: 166).
- People with "medically unexplained symptoms" who also score high on a standardized Candida questionnaire (called the Fungus Related Disease Questionnaire-7) also have higher levels of antibodies against Candida. These people often have a history of frequent or long-term antibiotic use along with symptoms like frequent yeast infections, sugar cravings, and fatigue (J Altern Complement Med. 2007 Dec;13(10):1129-33).
- Higher levels of antibodies against Candida albicans indicates the immune system is hypersensitive to the yeast or may simply reflect greater exposure to it (due to Candida yeast overgrowth) (BMC Gastroenterol. 2012; 12: 166.).

Curing My Own Candida

Before we begin discussing the details of the Candida protocol that I invented some years ago, let me take you on a health odyssey of what motivated me to spend many hundreds of hours investigating Candida and its related problems.

Despite all my knowledge in biology and the workings of the human body, after completing an initial degree in the Biological Sciences in the UK, by the time I had reached the age of 30 my health was a shamble.

I could just about manage to crawl out of bed with excruciating pain in my body and band-type headaches that would last most of the day. I would have a painful breakfast with many digestive issues, drag myself to my office, see patients for a couple of hours then back to bed for 2-3 hours before seeing a few more patients in the afternoon. Painkillers and anti-inflammatories were my main support to get through the day.

At the time, I was working as a Clinical Psychologist and Clinical Sexologist, as apart from the biology degree, I also had qualified in these too. I had not discovered the wonderful world of natural medicine now, but this was all going to change in the next few years.

By evening I was too tired to do anything, and it required a concerted effort just to hold a conversation. I tended to avoid company for this reason and became a recluse – living life close to my devoted family and trying to enjoy the small moments of watching my children develop. I absolutely hated the way I was; by nature, I am a "Type A" personality who loves to be on the go, researching new things. I generally have a very inquisitive mind and like people.

After many months of these persistent symptoms, including chronic headaches that would last for days, accompanied by an unexplainable fatigue, I eventually went to the local G.P. who took some X-rays and found that my frontal sinuses were loaded with fluid – he immediately prescribed antibiotics. Less than two months later I was back there again for more antibiotics as my sinuses were again blocked and causing headaches and pain, not to mention the tiredness, apathy, and on occasions depression. I was quite incapacitated, and this was certainly enough to cause an active person to fall into a depression; otherwise I loved my work. There is nothing more frustrating than waking every morning with band-type headaches that prevented me from concentrating on my work.

The Da Vinci Candida Treatment Protocol

This is a treatment protocol that I developed over many years of study, as well as trial and error with many patients that agreed to experiment – I continue to bow to these patients who helped my learning experience.

I had spent over 11 years trying to treat my systemic Candidiasis which was causing me many health problems and symptoms including chronic fatigue, brain fog, severe digestive disturbances, fibromyalgia, achlorhydria, pancreatic enzyme deficiencies, concentration and mood disturbances.

We have successfully treated over *5,000 patients* with Candida to date at the Da Vinci Center in Larnaca, Cyprus.

Preparing for the Da Vinci Candida Treatment Protocol

<u>Before implementing the Da Vinci Candida Protocol with my patients, I make certain that the rest of the body's physiological systems are as optimized as possible.</u>

I generally check for:

1. Food intolerances – these foods are probably one of the biggest sources of internal inflammation and can be a big burden when eradicating the Candida, so it is important to make certain that the patient avoids these foods. I used VRT Bioresonance testing to test over 100 different foods. We will talk more about the mechanisms of food intolerances a little later.

2. Nutritional deficiencies and heavy metals using a Tissue Hair Mineral Analysis test – this involves taking a small sample of hair and sending it to a laboratory abroad.
3. Using Kinesiology, Autonomic Response Testing, Bioresonance Testing, or any other similar test, the status of the stomach and pancreas – usually you will find many patients will not be secreting enough hydrochloric acid from the stomach and enough pancreatic enzymes from the pancreas.

Here is a table summarizing these preparatory steps:

PREPARATION STEPS BEFORE CANDIDA PROTOCOL

TASK	Supplements needed	Comments
Food Intolerance test		See a Bioresonance practitioner
Hair test for Mineral deficiencies/Heavy metal profile	Supplement what is needed with HMD™ heavy metal detox	Visit: www.worldwideahealthcenter.net
Heavy metal detox	Take HMD™, LAVAGE, CHLORELLA	www.worldwidehealthcenter.net
Constipated?	Take CONSTFORM and OXYGUT, COLFORM	Visit: www.worldwidehealthcenter.net
Digestive issues?	Take DIGESTIZYME & GASTRIC AID	Visit: www.worldwidehealthcenter.net
Bioresonance devices	DEVITA AP, DEVITA RITM, DEINFO USB	Visit: www.deta-elis-uk.com
Begin Candida protocol	CANDA PLUS, HOROPITO, CAPRYLATE, ACIDOPHILUS & BIFIDUS, CANDIDA 30C	Visit: www.worldwidehealthcenter.net

Testing for heavy metals and mineral deficiencies

In clinical work, I have found one test that I use often, and find to be invaluable – is the Hair Tissue Mineral Analysis (HTMA) (131) that we have already mentioned in a previous chapter. This involves taking a small sample of hair by cutting the first inch-and-a-half of growth closest to the scalp at the nape of the neck, or even pubic hair if someone is completely bald. It is then sent to a licensed clinical laboratory where the hair is prepared through a series of chemical and high temperature digestive procedures and is finally analyzed for levels of minerals and toxic metals, using sophisticated measuring devices called spectrometers.

Hair is considered an ideal tissue for sampling and testing[132]. Firstly, it can be cut easily and painlessly and can be sent to the lab without special handling requirements. Secondly, clinical results have shown that a correctly obtained sample can give an indication of mineral status and toxic metal accumulation following long-term or even acute exposure. Hair is used as one of the tissues of choice by the US Environmental Protection Agency in determining toxic metal exposure. Indeed, several studies have concluded that human hair may be a more appropriate tissue than blood or urine for studying a community's exposure to harmful trace elements.

Although our aim is to rid the body of harmful toxic metals, conversely trace minerals are essential in countless metabolic functions in all phases of the life process[133]. For example, zinc is involved in the production, storage, and secretion of insulin and is necessary for growth hormones. Magnesium is required for normal muscular function, especially the heart. A deficiency in magnesium has been associated with an increased incidence of heart attacks; anxiety and nervousness. Potassium is critical for normal nutrient transport into the cell – deficiency can result in muscular weakness, depression and lethargy. Excess sodium is associated with hypertension, but adequate amounts are required for normal health. Even vitamin status can be indirectly assessed from HTMA.

HTMA can detect recent exposure (from the last couple of months) of toxic metals in your blood that ultimately end up in the hair tissues as well. The way I use the test is to take an initial baseline sample to see the levels of minerals and toxic metals that are actively circulating in the blood during the last couple of months – this is basically the time it takes to grow the inch-and-a-half of hair that is taken.

---

131 Bland, J. Hair tissue mineral analysis. an emergent diagnostic technique. Thorsons Publishers, USA, 1983.

132 Watts, DL. Trace Elements and Other Essential Nutrients: Clinical Application of Tissue Mineral Analysis.

133 Wilson, LD. Nutritional Balancing and Hair Mineral Analysis: A Comprehensive Guide. LD Wilson Consultants, Inc., 1993.

I then put my patients on a natural chelator which I researched and invented – it is a natural chelator that has undergone double-blind, placebo-controlled trials with 350 people and is called HMD™. A further HTMA is taken after 2 months to see how many metals have been mobilized from storage sites in the body. Usually we find a percentage increase of metals in the second test.

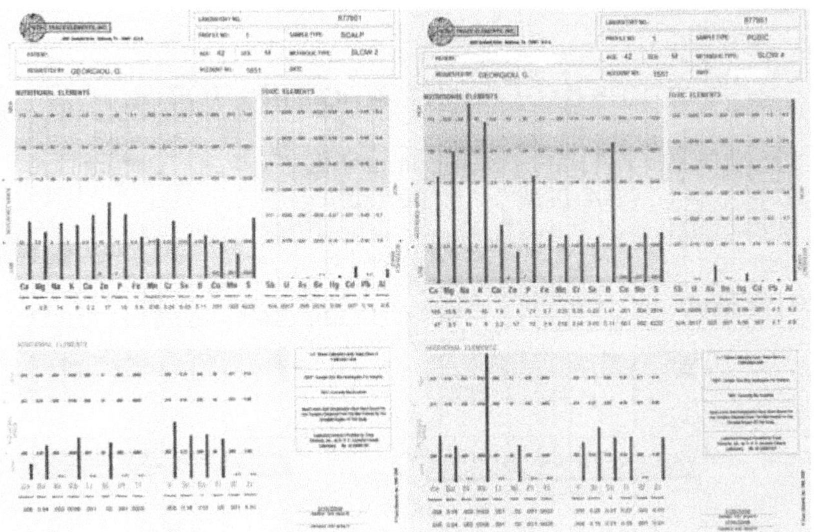

HTMA results two months apart after using HMD™

The two reports above are from the same patient, taken two months apart. On the left is the baseline sample before any natural chelator or minerals were given.

Generally, there is a low level of minerals with a little Cadmium and Aluminium burden. This is what has been circulating in the blood over the last couple of months but is not a reflection of what is stored in the body tissues and organs. On the right are the results of the second hair test, taken two months after the first, while on the HMD™ protocol. Notice that there is a huge increase in the levels of aluminium with some arsenic also appearing – these are the heavy metals that were in the storage organs that were mobilized by the HMD™.

Preparing by Detoxifying

It is very important for the success of the Candida protocol that the internal milieu is balanced and clean. One of the quickest, cheapest and most efficient ways of achieving this is to undergo a 15-day alkaline detox programme using only fresh fruits, vegetables, vegetable juices and soups, steamed vegetables with olive oil and herbs, as well as herbal teas.

Below is a summary table of the steps required to prepare for detoxifying. It is highly recommended that you take the supplements recommended as they are doctor-formulated and have been tried and tested in clinical practice by me personally. These are high quality and pure, but if you can find alternatives then this is fine.

STEPS IN DETOXIFICATION PROTOCOL

TASK	TIME TAKEN	Supplements needed	Comments
Alkaline Detoxification	15 days	HMD MULTIS, KRILL OIL, HEPATO PLUS, VITAMIN C	www.worldwidehealthcenter.net
Parasite detox	15-30 days	PARAFORM PLUS ONE, BLACK WALNUT TINCTURE	www.worldwidehealthcenter.net
Liver/GB cleanse	1 day	MAGNESIUM MALATE, EPSOM SALTS	www.worldwidehealthcenter.net
Heavy Metal Detox	2 months	HMD™, LAVAGE, CHLORELLA	www.detoxmetals.com

There are toxins in the food you eat, the water you drink and the air you breathe. Even your own body produces toxins as a result of its many metabolic processes that keep you alive.

There are several benefits of detoxification:

- The digestive tract is cleansed of accumulated waste and fermenting bacteria.
- Liver, kidney and blood purification can take place, which is not possible during regular eating patterns.

- Mental clarity is enhanced as chemical and food additive overload is reduced.
- Reduced dependency on habit forming substances such as sugar, caffeine, nicotine, alcohol and drugs.
- The stomach size is returned to normal as bad eating habits can be stopped.
- The hormonal system is enhanced which is especially true for growth hormones.
- The immune system is stimulated.

After detoxifying on an alkaline diet for 15 days, patients report higher energy levels, clear and glowing skin, weight loss of several pounds, clear-headedness, reduced cellulite, good body tone and a great feeling of being relaxed.

Before we look at the details, here is a summary table that will help you under the various steps that you need to follow.

Some of these supplements I give to all patients as part of a repair and rejuvenation process; these would include a high-potency multivitamin/mineral formula such as HMD MULTIS, KRILL PLUS, which is a good source of omega 3 fatty acids, but with a lower probability of being high in mercury.

I encounter almost 80% or more of my patient having digestive issues – bloating and distension in the stomach and the intestines - so I will give DIGEST PLUS which are pancreatic enzymes that will help gut digestion, and BETAINE COMPLEX which contains hydrochloric acid for digesting concentrated proteins in the stomach.

For those that are doing the liver and gallbladder cleanse, MAGNESIUM MALATE is important in order to soften the stones before the cleanse as drinking apple juice which contains malic acid is too sweet and will feed the Candida.

TYPICAL DETOXIFICATION & REJUVENTATION SUPPLEMENT SHEET

REMEDY	MORNING	LUNCH	DINNER	COMMENTS
HMD MULTIS Multivitamin/mineral	2	2	0	With food
KRILL OIL Fatty acids – omega 3	1	0	1	With food
DIGESTIZYME Pancreatic enzymes – gut digestion	1	1	1	With main meals only
GASTRIC AID Hydrochloric acid – stomach digestion	1	1	1	With main meals only
HEPATO PLUS Liver detox herbal formula	1	1	1	With food 15 – 30 days only
PARAFORM PLUS ONE Parasite detox herbal formula	1	1	1	Away from food
MAGNESIUM MALATE Softens gallbladder stones	1	1	1	With food, for 15 days only
HMD Heavy metal detox chelator	45 drops	45 drops	45 drops	In a little water or juice
LAVAGE Herbal drainage remedy	25 drops	25 drops	25 drops	Away from food
LUGOL'S IODINE Feeds the thyroid	2 drops	0	2 drops	
WALNUT TINCTURE Parasite detox herbal formula	2 tsp	0	0	
CHLORELLA Clears toxic metals from matrix and gut	2	0	2	With food
Alpha Lipoic acid Water & Fat soluble antioxidant	1	0	1	With food
IF CONSTIPATED:				
CONSFORM Herbal formula for constipation	1	1	1	With food

The Da Vinci Centre Detoxification Diet

These are the foods that are allowed during the detoxification phase, no other family of foods is allowed. You may eat as many of the following foods as you wish, but it is best to eat only when you feel hungry. Wash all fruit and vegetables in a bowl of water with 4-5 tablespoons of grape vinegar added to help wash away any pesticide/ herbicide residues. Rinse afterwards with clean water. Here are the foods that you can eat in plenty:

1. **Salads** – use any type of fresh vegetables you like, in any combination. Use organic vegetables when available and include bean sprouts when in season. Salad dressings should be kept simple - a little virgin olive oil with fresh lemon, or cider vinegar. Add plenty of fresh onion and garlic - these are very detoxifying.
2. **Steamed vegetables** – eat any variety you like, including broccoli, cauliflower, potatoes, beetroot, carrots etc. Steam as opposed to boil, and eat with a little herbal salt, lemon and a little virgin olive oil, with plenty of garlic.
3. **Vegetable soups** - of all kinds, but broccoli, leak and vegetable soups are fine.
4. **Stir-Fried Vegetables** – again, any type of vegetables is fine, cooked in their own juices using a Wok.
5. **Vegetable juices** - drink a minimum of 1-3 per day and try to include one cocktail comprising one-third of a glass of raw green juice (spinach, parsley, cabbage and any other green vegetables), with a small beetroot, topped up with carrot juice. Carrot juice has a strong effect on the digestive system, provides energy, serves as an important source of minerals, promotes normal elimination, has diuretic properties and helps to build healthy tissue, skin and teeth.
6. **Fresh Fruit** - choose the fruit of your choice and eat as much as you like, whenever you like. You could begin the day with 2-3 pieces of fruit, which are gentle on the digestive system. Make a tasty fruit salad. Try to avoid too many juicy fruits as this may overly feed the Candida, and certainly avoid all forms of fruit juices as this will give sugar to the body quickly, again feeding the Candida. Avocados provides a good source of protein. There is tremendous benefit in adding fruit during the detox due to their living enzymes and phytonutrients which are very cleansing to the body. Remember, we are not treating the Candida yet, only helping the body to cleanse and prepare for the 3-month Candida protocol.
7. **Fresh Nuts** – it is generally OK to have some fresh nuts such as almonds and walnuts.

8. **Herbal teas** - any of your choice. Chamomile is a good relaxant; aniseed and mint are good for the digestive system; Kombucha, dandelion tea is excellent for purifying the blood and detoxifying and stimulating liver function; sage tea is a blood cleanser; nettle tea is excellent for driving away excess fluid out of the tissues and is a wonderful cleanser for all the detoxification organs. Drink as many as you like, with a little honey on the tip of a teaspoon if you like.

The purpose of this diet is to detoxify – to remove the toxins from the fat cells and tissues as well as the organs, so that the body can return to its optimum level of functionality.

You will also need to drink at least 8-10 glasses per day of still mineral water to flush out the toxins – this is VERY IMPORTANT, so please take note!

When the 15 days are over, you should carry on eating the above for a couple more days while gently adding a little protein such as fresh steamed or grilled fish, organic chicken, pulses, a soft-boiled organic egg or a little cheese. Go gently on the protein for a couple of days before you begin eating normally again so that you do not overload your digestive system.

Parasites, Heavy Metals and Other Toxins

As part of the detoxification process, the Da Vinci Center also attempts to detoxify heavy metals that can easily be detected using a hair analysis, as already mentioned above.

One of the most researched natural chelators in the world that has undergone double-blind, placebo-controlled trials with 350 people is called HMD™. It has been shown to safely chelate many different types of heavy metals, including uranium, a difficult metal to chelate. It was invented by myself and there are a number of scientific papers written in peer-reviewed journals[134] – Natural Heavy Metal Chelators: Do They Work? and A Natural Heavy Metal Chelator is Born.

Dr. Hulda Clark, Ph.D., N.D., a naturopathic physician, has brought the issue of parasitically-caused diseases and other types of toxicity back into the spotlight in recent years, dealing with this subject at length in her book, *The Cure for all Diseases.* Dr. Hulda describes various methodologies and procedures to cleanse

[134] Georgiou, GJ. Scientific research on natural heavy metal chelators: testing what works. International Journal of Complementary & Alternative Medicine. Volume 11 Issue 5 – 2018.

the body from these nasty creatures. Check out the questionnaire in the Appendix to see whether you are likely to have a parasite load.

The Herbal Parasitic Cleanse

There are some good herbal formulas that are designed to eradicate parasites. One such formula that I use and formulated is called PARAFORM PLUS ONE (one capsule, three times daily, away from food). It contains several powerful anti-parasitic herbs that are suitable for vegetarians, such as:

Magnesium caprylate
Cinnamon powder
Cloves powder
Shiitake mushroom powder
Garlic powder extract (10000mg/g)
Glucomannan (95%)
Pumpkin seed P E 4:1 (40%) (equivalent to 200mg pumpkin seed powder)
Chicory root P.E 4:1 (equivalent to 120mg chicory root powder)
Grapefruit seed P.E 5:1 (equivalent to 100mg grapefruit seed powder)
Cayenne extract 7:1 (equivalent to 100mg cayenne powder)
Fenugreek seed P.E 4:1 (equivalent to 48mg fenugreek seed powder)
Olive leaf extract 15:1, 6% Oleurpein (equivalent to 50mg olive leaf powder)

It is a powerful formula that we have been using with good results in clinical practice, and goes well when combined with **PARAFORM TINCTURE**[135], another powerful anti-parasitic herb – 2 teaspoons in the morning in a little water, away from food.

Bioresonance Devices

As well as using herbal formulas to eradicate parasites, I recently have added other protocols using Bioresonance devices, researched by Russian scientists who developed a powerful, portable, programmable Bioresonance device called the DEVITA AP. This has undergone considerable trials from the Russians who purport its success in eradicating several parasites and microorganisms.

I have been using Bioresonance devices for many years now, but the innovation of the Russian devices is that they are portable, no larger than a mobile phone, and can be programmed to resonate with individual parasites and other microorganisms. There is also the DEVITA RITM that is for upregulating the organ systems.

If we take a crystal wine glass as an example, this has its own resonant frequency, of around 500 Hertz. If we can produce a sound at the same frequency and stand

[135] Available from www.worldwidehealthcenter.net

the glass in front of a speaker, then the glass will absorb this frequency and break. This is the phenomenon of RESONANCE.

In the same way, microbes also have their own resonant frequencies. If we can match these frequencies, the microbes will absorb this energy and burst.

Treatment with the devices is based on the principles of Bioresonance. They are as close as we can get to the Hippocratic Oath that says: *"Do no harm"* when treating people. These gentle devices achieve exactly this – they can heal without being invasive and causing side-effects.

Checkout a presentation at an international conference on YouTube talking about "Alternatives to Antibiotics" https://youtu.be/bYcvs4blUq8

The devices also have the approval of the Ministry of Health of Russia, as well as Israel and Germany where they are presently manufactured with CE approval as wellness devices. These devices also have patents in 73 different countries as well as more than 117 scientific research studies backing it in the last 20 years – see www.deta-elis-uk.com

The Secrets to Success

It is my opinion, if one wants to be successful at eradicating Candida, then you must eradicate the pathogen using natural anti-fungal remedies, while at the same time cleaning up your internal milieu.

One further key to success is the important step of converting the pathogenic, mycelial Candida back to the normal budding yeasts – this is a **crucially important step** often missed by many practitioners of natural medicine. The only remedies that can do this successfully are the Sanum isopathic fungal remedies that have been invented by Professor Enderlein after many years of experimentation using darkfield microscopy.

Many physicians now believe that an interim measure before embarking on any treatment should be a protocol for Candida overgrowth; this possesses such a minor risk and expense that it should be considered in any chronic illness.

One clinical trial a person may try is to avoid certain foods for five days that are known to facilitate the growth of yeast. Such foods include the following:

- **SUGAR and SIMPLE CARBOHYDRATES** such as those found in all sweetened food including honey, molasses, sorghum, maple syrup, sugar, fructose, maltose, dextrose, corn syrup, etc.

- **YEAST PRODUCTS** such as beer, wine, yeast leavened bread, natural B vitamins, brewer's yeast.

- **FERMENTED and MOULDY FOODS** such as mushrooms, cheese, vinegar, mustard, catsup, relish and other condiments made with vinegar.

After avoiding these foods for 5 days, try adding them back into the diet in large quantities. By observing how one feels while off these foods, in comparison to any adverse effects experienced when going back on the foods, one may get a clue as to any possible yeast involvement as a causative factor for any adverse symptoms.

If adverse symptoms are provoked by a return to the yeast enhancing foods, your physician may feel that there is at least a possible reason to suspect Candida overgrowth, which may then warrant more definitive action.

This may not be the best method and personally I do not use it as I will use VRT Bioresonance screening and ART to determine whether there is pathogenic Candidiasis, backed up by the signs and symptoms using Dr. Crook's Candida Questionnaire. However, if you are not a Bioresonance practitioner or use any other form of ANS testing, then this may be a good way to begin.

Detoxification Symptoms – "The Healing Crisis"

When the body detoxifies, it goes through various biochemical and physiological changes (136). Generally, on the first day of fasting, the blood sugar level is likely to drop below 65-70 mg/dl. The liver immediately compensates by converting glycogen to glucose and releasing it into the blood. After a few hours, the basal metabolic rate is likely to fall in order to conserve energy. This means that the heart, pulse and blood pressure will drop. More glycogen may be used from muscles, causing some weakness.

As the body requires more energy, some fat and fatty acids are broken down to release glycerol from the glyceride molecules and are converted to glucose. You may notice the skin becoming quite oily as these fatty acids and glycerol increase in the blood. The skin is one of the largest detoxification organs, so you may get some skin problems such as pimples, acnes or a pussy boil – this is all part of the body trying to cleanse. The complexion may become pallid for a day or two as the wastes accumulate in the blood.

The incomplete oxidation of fats may result in the formation of Ketones, resulting in ketoacidosis. Combined with high levels of urea resulting from protein

---

136 Salloum, TK. Fasting Signs and Symptoms: A Clinical Guide. USA: Buckeye Naturopathic Press, 1992.

metabolism, this state can cause several symptoms which may suppress appetite, as they affect the satiety centre in the hypothalamus. Generally, this takes a few days to happen and you may notice your appetite dwindling. You may get pains in different joints, or organs such as the lungs. There may be a considerable amount of yellow mucus released from the throat and expelled. The sinuses may also begin clearing with more mucus secreted.

Given that the body is releasing these toxins quickly during the first few days of the detoxification process, it should not surprise us to experience some changes in our bodies that may cause certain symptoms. Initially, for the first 2-3 days, these symptoms can be a little unpleasant, SO BE WARNED! A fair number of people will have headaches, nervousness, diarrhea, upset stomach, energy loss, furry tongue, halitosis (bad breath), as well as acne or other skin rashes, a general feeling of malaise, frequent urination due to the toxins irritating the bladder, and some of their existing symptoms may be exacerbated. When the toxic residues enter the blood, they affect mind and body functions.

These may be unpleasant symptoms for the first couple of days, but they are a NORMAL part of the detoxification process, and in natural medicine we call this the HEALING CRISIS or HERXHEIMER REACTION. All these symptoms indicate that the DETOX IS WORKING! This is a temporary and transient crisis, it will pass – so hang on in there and don't worry that there is something wrong with you, apart from the fact that you are loaded with toxins.

There was always something wrong with you, and now you are doing something about it. You are reversing this toxic process that your body has adapted to, but that's not healthy. If you are a coffee drinker, then the symptoms will be more pronounced, as your body will be in a state of withdrawal. Yes, coffee is a drug, and when you come off it you go into withdrawal, meaning that your body will start asking for a dose of what it is addicted to. When it doesn't get it, then it screams for it louder and louder, usually in the form of headaches, migraines, muscle pains, general weakness and lack of concentration.

Enduring a cleansing crisis is the hardest part of the healing process. To stop feeling bad, most people want to eat - but do not eat during a cleansing crisis. The body is overloaded with the work of removing toxins. Digestion makes matters worse. Drinking one or two glasses of sodium bicarbonate (baking soda) – one teaspoon in each glass drunk twice daily - will help to neutralize the ketoacidosis.

Helter-Skelter rides are common. The 'downward slope' is when the body is vigorously cleansing, and the blood gets swamped with toxins causing you to feel down, moody, depressed, achy – like having a bad cold. You feel weak and lethargic. The mind rationalizes: *'I feel horrible: this can't be working.'* You can maintain a normal routine of work on a dip but it requires willpower and determination. It also helps to know that the longer the down period, the greater the fasting high.

Clearing Toxic Metals

Clearing toxic metals, such as mercury that will further aggravate the Candida and cause free radical damage to many organs and tissues, is also a wise step to take.

There are many products on the market that purport to detoxify heavy metals from the body, but none of them are supported by scientific research using correct methodologies.

There is one natural product, however, that has been based on double blind, placebo-controlled research with over 350 people. It has also been used clinically by many practitioners around the world in the last 8 years or so.

This is what I suggest can be used for most cases of heavy metal toxicity. I have called it the HMD ULTIMATE DETOX PROTOCOL and it consists of the following:

- HMD™ – 45 drops x 3 daily for adults[137] – sensitive adults who have chronic diseases or compensated detoxification organs, as well as people with neurological diseases such as multiple sclerosis and the like, as well as autistic people should begin with half this dose or less, and increase by one drop x 3 daily, every day until they reach a comfortable level.

- HMD LAVAGE – this is a herbal formula of wild-crafted and organic herbs such as Silybum marianum (Milk Thistle Seed), Taraxacum officinale (Dandelion Root), Arctium lappa (Burdock Root), Trifolium pratense (Red Clover Tops), Curcuma longa (Turmeric Root), Hydrangea arborescens (Hydrangea Root) and Arctostaphylos uva ursi (Bearberry Leaf). This herbal formula is designed to facilitate detoxification of the liver, kidneys, lymphatics and skin, as well as cleanse the blood and act as a natural anti-inflammatory. Adult dosage: 25 drops x 3 daily for adults, or more as directed by a practitioner.

- NON-TOXIC CHLORELLA – there are many concerns about finding good quality, clean Chlorella that is void of heavy metals and xenobiotics. We have searched and travelled far and wide and found an excellent source that is provided with a Certificate of Analysis with each pot. This chlorella comes from the western coast of Hai-Nan Island, China's southernmost

137 See https://www.detoxmetals.com/hmd-dosage-guidelines/ for full details

island. Hai-Nan Island is a tropical island with an excellent climate and lies on the same latitude as Hawaii. The non-industrialized, pollution-free, tropical island offers favorable growth conditions for chlorella, including intense sunlight, pure water, and clean air. Available in 500mg tabs, adult dosage should be 2 tabs x 3 daily.

Chlorella is required in the gut to take it away toxic metals via the stools. If there is not enough chlorella, the neurotoxins are reabsorbed by the nerve endings in the gut wall and are at risk of being redirected to the spinal cord, and the brain.

Good quality chlorella lines the gut wall and mops up the free toxins found there. High toxicity and increasing symptoms need larger doses. This is very important and differs from the usual advice to reduce supplements if detoxing intensifies symptoms.

- A-LIPOIC ACID – I believe that when metals and other xenobiotics are mobilized in the body, there should be some protection against free radical damage. Lipoic acid is that extraordinary antioxidant which is both water and fat soluble, able to penetrate the brain and other nervous tissues, and is therefore able to protect all parts of the body against free radical damage.

I will often fine-tune this protocol depending on the needs of the patient, but generally this works well for most cases as a basic protocol.

THE DA VINCI CANDIDA PROTOCOL (DCP)

Now that we have completed the preparation by detoxing on many different levels and preparing the internal milieu, we are now ready to begin the Candida protocol in order to eradicate the Candida.

Let's take a conceptual look at the components of the Da Vinci Candida Protocol before we look at the details.

Please note that we are aware that sourcing these products from different companies around the world is difficult and costly on freight charges. Rest assured, however, as you can purchase the complete package online from a one-stop shop at www.worldwidehealthcenter.net.

The Da Vinci Candida Protocol has five basic objectives:

1. Starve the Candida by eliminating the foods that feed it.

2. Kill the Candida using natural anti-Candida products that we will discuss below.

3. Repopulate the bowel flora with a high-potency Acidophilus and Bifidus probiotic that contains 60 billion live bacteria per capsule.

4. Regulate the dysbiosis and convert the pathological, mycelial form of Candida back to the normal form using the SANUM remedies.

5. Restore biochemical balance to the body and strength to the immune system. This will allow the body to regain and maintain control over Candida growth by optimizing the diet. This would involve avoiding food intolerances and following the Metabolic Type Diet by Bill Wolcott. Also, eradicating parasites using herbal formulas that we discussed above as well as chelating heavy metals out of the system.

Here is a summary of the various steps that you need to follow to cure your Candida once and for all. Even though it may be quite detailed, I can guarantee that if you follow it you will succeed, as have more than 5,000 patients that I have treated in the last 15 years or so. The success rate of eliminating the Candida approaches 100%, and by the time you have read all this book you will understand why.

None of these objectives are mutually exclusive, nor can they be addressed in a serial way. They all need to be looked at concomitantly for the treatment protocol to be successful.

Let us now go through the various stages or phases of the Da Vinci Candida Protocol, beginning with a critically important stage – starving the Candida by not feeding it.

First Phase - Starving the Candida

I have found that it is literally impossible to treat Candida if one does not cut out ALL forms of sugar for a period of 3 months. This also includes natural fruit sugars or fructose. The foods that should be strictly AVOIDED for a 3-month period include:

1. **SUGAR** – and all foods that contain sugar. These include white and brown sugar, honey, syrups, liquors, lactose, fructose, all confectionary and sweet cakes, chocolates, ice-creams, home-made sweets and cakes, biscuits, fizzy beverages, all fruit drinks.

2. **YEAST** – all foods that contain yeast including breads, vinegar, ketchups, mayonnaise and pickles.

3. **MUSHROOMS** – all types, including Chinese mushrooms such as Shitake.

4. **REFINED FOODS** – all white flours, white rice, white pasta products, corn flour, custard and white cereal products, unless they are whole-meal or organic.

5. **FERMENTED PRODUCTS** – all alcoholic beverages, vinegar and all vinegar products such as ketchup, mayonnaise and pickles.

STEPS IN CANDIDA PROTOCOL

TASK	TIME TAKEN	Supplements needed	Comments
Starve the Candida	3 calendar months		Need to adhere to this religiously!
Killing the Candida	3 calendar months	CANDA PLUS, HOROPITO, CAPRYLATE, ACIDOPHILUS & BIFIDUS, CANDIDA 30C	www.worldwidehealthcenter.net
Repopulating friendly bacteria in gut	1 day	ACIDOPHILUS & BIFIDUS	www.worldwidehealthcenter.net
Using SANUM remedies to convert pathogenic Candida	2 months	SANUM REMEDIES	www.worldwidehealthcenter.net
Balancing body chemistry		VITAMIN C, BETAINE COMPLEX, DIGEST PLUS	www.worldwidehealthcenter.net

1. **NUTS** – all types of nuts that are cleaned and packaged without their shells – these tend to collect fungal spores and molds from the atmosphere which will antagonize the Candida. Nuts that are fresh with their shells are OK.
2. **FRESH AND DRIED FRUIT** – all fresh fruit should be avoided for the initial **SIX WEEKS ONLY** as again, the fructose they contain will feed the Candida and make it extremely difficult to eliminate.

All other fruit that is not fresh such as cooked, tinned or dried and fruit juices should be avoided for the full 3 months – your health practitioner will advise you when to begin eating fruit again. Obviously, also avoiding fruit juices (vegetable juices are OK).

Second Phase – Killing the Candida

There are several herbal formulas, homeopathics and probiotics that are used in the Da Vinci Candida Protocol. They have been carefully selected after years of experimentation and the fact is they have worked time and time again with hundreds of people. The aim of using these supplements is to kill off the Candida. Here is a table of these supplements in order, taken from one of the handouts that we give our patients, with an explanation on why and how they work later.

Now let us look at the specific remedies in a little more detail to understand why and how they work to eradicate the Candida:

1. CANDA PLUS **(was called KANDIDAPLEX)** - a doctor-formulated compound that contains:

- Calcium undecylenate;
- Pau d'arco (Tabebuia avellanedae) bark extract 100 mg;
- Enlyse™ enzyme blend (cellulase, chitosinase, hemicellulase, protease, serrapeptase, amylase and lipase) 100 mg;
- Berberine (as berberine sulfate) 50 mg;
- Sorbic Acid 25 mg;
- Trans-Resveratrol (from Japanese knotweed (Polygonum cuspidatum) root extract) 10 mg.

Dosage: 2 capsules, 3 x daily

	REMEDY	MORNING	LUNCH	DINNER	COMMENTS
	MAIN PROTOCOL				
R	CANDA PLUS	2	2	2	With meals
R	HOROPITO	1	0	1	With meals
R	ACIDOPHILUS & BIFIDUS	1	1	1	With meals
	CANDIDA 30c	2 pillules	2 pillules	2 pillules	Dissolve in mouth Before meals
	CAPRYLATE	1	1	1	With meals
**	Citricidal drops (Nail Fungus)	1 drop	0	1 drop	Under nails only
*	***Natural Antibiotics***				
	LIQUID SILVER 50	1 tsp	1 tsp	1 tsp	Before food in water
	OLIVE LEAF EXTRACT	1 tab	1 tab	1 tab	With meals
	GRAPEFRUIT SEED EXTRACT	2 tabs	2 tabs	2 tabs	With meals
	VITAMIN C CAPS	1/3tsp - 1/2tsp	1/3tsp - 1/2tsp	1/3tsp - 1/2tsp	Before food in water
	PARAFORM PLUS TWO	1	1	1	With food
	OREGANO OIL	1	1	1	With meals
	TRIFORM	35 drops	35 drops	35 drops	

NOTES:
R = Refrigerate

All the above-named products can be ordered from www.worldwidehealthcenter.net

* The **Natural Antibiotics** are only taken when there is an active infection such as a cold, flu or other infection. Take for 7 days **after** symptom withdrawal to make certain that all the bacteria have cleared from the body.
** Only taken if there is nail fungus

Each individual ingredient in CANDA PLUS has a specific function when it comes to eradicating Candida, as follows:

- Calcium undecylenate; undecanoic acid's ability to alter the composition of fatty acids in the cell membrane leading to an inability to sustain its fungal form.

- Pau D'Arco acts as a powerful antifungal agent. It contains several classes of compounds, lapachol, xyloidone and various napthaquinones. The most important of these is lapachol, which has been shown to inhibit the growth of Candida, similar to Amphotericin B.

- Enlyse™ destroys the BIOFILM of Candida that we previously talked about, which is composed of protein polypeptides, polysaccharide carbohydrates, fibrinogen or fibrin and polynucleotides that contain RNA and DNA material. This structure is bound together with ligands that have stickiness properties.

- Berberine exhibits a broad spectrum of antibiotic activity. Berberine has shown antimicrobial activity against bacteria, protozoa, and fungi and upregulates immunity.

- Sorbic acid inhibits fungi as well as molds often found together in the body.

- Trans-Resveratrol exhibited antifungal activity against Candida. It also inhibited the yeast-to-hyphae morphogenetic transition of C. albicans.

2. HOROPITO (practitioner-strength) – a New Zealand herbal product that contains two powerful anti-fungal agents that have been shown to kill Candida – Pseudowinterata colorata and the synergistic herb Aniseed that boosts effectiveness 6-fold.

Dosage: 1 capsule, twice daily

This natural herb, found mostly in New Zealand, has some amazing properties that have been scientifically researched.

Pseudowintera colorata, or mountain Horopito, is an evergreen shrub or small tree (1–2.5 m) commonly called pepperwood because its leaves have a hot taste.

Used by the indigenous Maori population of New Zealand. Infection due to Candida albicans is documented as once being a major cause of death of Maori babies, due to being fed an "unsatisfactory diet".

3. CAPRYLATE (500 mg) – a derivative of coconut that stops the Candida reproducing as well as killing the Candida. Dosage: 1 capsule, 3 daily

4. CANDIDA 30c - homeopathic – helps to eradicate the Candida but using a different mechanism. Dosage: two pillules or one cap x 3 daily for 2 weeks only. These are stopped just as the Sanum remedies are begun.

Third phase – Repopulating the Friendly Bacteria

This phase runs parallel with phase 2 and uses good quality, human strain probiotics such as the high-potency ACIDOPHILUS and BIFIDUS probiotics by Custom Probiotics, an American company.

The Custom Probiotics formula that we use is a high count, multi strain Acidophilus and Bifidus probiotic dietary supplement containing 60 billion cfu's per capsule at the time of expiration; resistant to stomach acids, with a slow die-off with temperature.

The Ingredients include 5 different strains of probiotics such as L. Acidophilus, L. Rhamnosus, L. Plantarum, B. Lactis, and B. Bifidum.

There is considerable scientific evidence for activity of probiotics against a wide range of intestinal pathogens, including Candida species. Despite this, the mechanisms of effect have been poorly defined. However, it can be speculated that one or more of the following possible effects are in operation:

- competition for nutrients
- secretion of antimicrobial substances (e.g. bacteriocins, peroxides)
- reduction of gut pH
- blocking of adhesion sites (Kennedy et al, 1985)
- repression of virulence
- blocking of toxin receptor sites
- immune stimulation (local and systemic)
- suppression of toxin production

To these supplements, we add a good-quality multivitamin such as HMD MULTIS to provide all the vitamins and minerals that the immune system requires for optimal functioning. Also, taking KRILL PLUS is helpful as this acts as a natural anti-inflammatory.

Phase 4 – Using SANUM Isopathic Remedies to Normalize Pathogenic Candida

All the above must be taken for the full 90 days of the protocol, with the exception of the Candida 30c. After two weeks of the anti-Candida diet, certain specialized isopathic remedies are introduced, known as SANUM remedies from Germany, after the work of the famous Prof. Enderlein.

SANUM therapy is widely recognized to positively influence the regulatory processes, the internal milieu, immune response capacity and the symbiotic bacterial ecology within the body.

Each of these isopathic remedies are only taken a couple of times per week, except for the Albicansan remedy that is taken day by day. The reason that we have spaced them out in the table below is that they tend to clash and antagonize each other and cannot all be taken at the same time. So, if you follow the sequence in the table below, beginning from the specific day that you begin taking them, whether this is Monday, or Tuesday or Wednesday and so forth:

	Mon am	Mon pm	Tues am	Tues pm	Wed am	Wed pm	Thur am	Thur pm	Fri am	Fri pm	Sat am	Sat pm	Sund am	Sund pm
Albicansan Capsules or/& Suppositories		■		⊘		■		⊘		■		⊘		■
Mucokehl Tablets	■							■						
Pefrakehl Capsules				■					■					
Nigersan Tablets					■							■		
Fortakehl Tablets							■						■	
Notakehl Tablets			■								■			

Specifically, each of the 6 remedies is taken as follows:

- ✓ Albicansan ® (Candida albicans) – caps 4X - **1 cap every second day**.
- ✓ Fortakehl ® (Penicillium roquefortii) – tabs 4X - **1 tab twice weekly**.
- ✓ Mucokehl ® (Mucor racemosus) – tabs 5X - **1 tab twice weekly.**
- ✓ Nigersan ® (Aspergillus niger) – tabs 5X - **1 tab twice weekly.**
- ✓ Notakehl ® (Penicillium chrysogenum) – tabs 5X - **1 tab twice weekly.**
- ✓ Pefrakehl ® (Candida parapsilosis) – Caps 4X - **1 cap twice weekly.**

If there is vaginal discharge, or anal Candida, then vaginal or anal pessaries of Albicansan D3 must also be used to eliminate this topical infection. These can be used every second day last thing at night, after sex and are shown on the table above with the symbol ⦸.

The SANUM remedies are continued for 10 weeks until the end of the Candida protocol.

These remedies are taken BEFORE or AWAY from food. Therefore it is best to store them in the bedroom, away from electrical equipment, and take them as soon as you wake in the morning and last thing at night.

There are both capsules and tablets. The capsules you need to open and pour the powder that they contain under the tongue and allow it to absorb for a few minutes. The tablets dissolve under the tongue for a few minutes. No water needs to be drunk, as they will absorb directly into the blood stream from the blood vessels under the tongue.

1. **ALBICANSAN** – There are capsules as well as suppositories of this remedy. Women can use the suppositories in case of vaginal Candidiasis which is usually very common. European health practitioners report that this remedy may be useful as supportive therapy in.:

   ✓ intestinal overgrowth of Candida
   ✓ mycosis
   ✓ resistant skin infections of mouth
   ✓ stomatitis
   ✓ gingivitis
   ✓ urogenital mycosis
   ✓ vaginitis
   ✓ urethritis with subsequent adnexitis
   ✓ cholecystitis
   ✓ colitis of fungal origin
   ✓ allergies

2. **FORTAKEHL** - European practitioners report that Fortakehl promotes normal bowel flora in the gastro-intestinal tract (especially after antibiotic therapy) which could be helpful for such conditions as gastritis, enteritis, colitis, gall bladder problems, pancreatitis, diarrhea, constipation, ulcers, yeast infections of the intestines, the vagina, and the skin.

3. **MUCOKEHL** - European health practitioners report that this remedy is useful as supportive therapy in chronic and acute disturbances of circulatory system, such as:

- ✓ thrombosis
- ✓ embolism
- ✓ angina pectoris
- ✓ post infarct
- ✓ varicosities
- ✓ hemorrhoids
- ✓ diabetic gangrene and neuropathy
- ✓ constipation.

4. **NIGERSAN** - European health practitioners report that this remedy is useful in disorders that have to do with disturbed calcium metabolism which could involve bone and tooth rehabilitation. European reports further indicate that Nigersan, also known as Pleo™ Nig, has been successfully used for urogenital tract problems in men and women such as prostate, ovaries, kidney and bladder complaints. It appears to be helpful for enhancing lymph circulation which in turn leads to increased detoxification, especially after illness.

5. **NOTAKEHL** - European practitioners report that Notakehl, otherwise known as Pleo™ Not, is very useful to enhance the immune system, and as a supportive therapy for infections of bacterial origin and inflammations such staph, strep, acne, ear infections, tonsil infections, sore throat, neuritis, neuralgia, urinary tract infections, prostate irritation, respiratory infections and neuropathy.

6. **PEFRAKEHL** - European health practitioners report that Pefrakehl, otherwise known as Pleo™ Pef, may be useful as a supportive therapy in relieving the symptoms of intestinal overgrowth of Candida, yeast infections, mycosis, fungal, bacterial and viral infections of the mouth and the teeth, ear infections, gingivitis, urogenital yeast infections, vaginal yeast infections, anal inflammations and irritations.

N.B. Please note that if you are allergic to PENICILLIN, you should NOT take the NOTAKEHL (Penicillium chrysogenum) and FORTAKEHL (Penicillium roquefortii) as these are likely to cause unpleasant symptoms such as lethargy, fatigue, brain fog, muscle pains and a general feeling of unwellness. The treatment will still work without these two SANUM remedies.

Phase 5 - Balancing Body Chemistry

It is a commonly recognized and accepted fact that immune system efficiency is highly dependent on the proper biochemical balance in the body. This of course, is dependent on proper and adequate nutrition to supply the body with all the required biochemical constituents (vitamins, minerals, enzymes, intrinsic factors, etc.).

Different people require different amounts of nutrients for optimum health. The criteria for the determination of these differing nutritional requirements lies within the definition of one's metabolic type, i.e. the genetically determined metabolic and nutritional parameters that define each person's individuality on every level.

It is precisely because different people have different metabolic types, and therefore different needs for nutrition, that the allopathic, symptom-treatment approach in nutrition is baseless and so often ineffective. This further explains why what (nutritionally) helps make one person better, may have little or no effect on another, or even make a third person worse.

I have not tried to modify this protocol as I have found it to be so successful in the treatment of over 5,000 patients to date, that I dare not juggle with it in case it loses its effectiveness. I'm sure that it can be improved upon and would welcome comments from other practitioners working with Candida. It is only through sharing that we will grow and become better practitioners.[138, 139]

Package of all supplements required for the Da Vinci Candida Protocol

If you purchase the DA VINCI CANDIDA PROTOCOL – COMPLETE PACKAGE of supplements from www.worldwidehealthcenter.net you will receive the following products to last you throughout the complete treatment over 3 months:

- 6 containers of CANDA PLUS
- 3 containers of HOROPITO
- 6 containers of CAPRYLATE
- 3 containers of ACIDOPHILUS AND BIFIDUS
- 1 bottle of CANDIDA 30 C
- SANUM REMEDIES – complete set for 3 months (7 packs in total) containing Nigersan D5, Pefrekehl D4, 2 x Albicansan D4, Fortakehl D5, Notakehl D5, Mucokehl D5 – Albicansan suppositories can be ordered extra for women with vaginal discharge.

You may also email admin@worldwidehealthcenter.net

---

[138] Georgiou, G.J. Scourge of the 21st Century: Systemic Candidiasis – Part 1 & 2. British Naturopathic Journal, Vol. 25, No. 1, 2008.

[139] Georgiou, G.J. Systemic Candidiasis: Scurge of the 21st Century. Semmelweis- Institut GmbH, 27318 Hoya (Weser), Germany, 2015.

Reintroducing Fruit

Fruit can be re-introduced back into the diet **FOUR WEEKS** after you begin taking the SANUM remedies, or 6 weeks after beginning the Candida protocol.

Stay with two SOLID portions of fruit daily for the remainder of the protocol. One medium apple would be considered as one portion, or ½ teacup of berries would be one portion, or 2 small plums would be one portion.

All JUICY fruits such as watermelon, grapes, oranges, grapefruit, tangerines, mangos, pineapple and sweet figs should be avoided throughout the 3 months of the treatment as they give their sugars to the blood too quickly. Stick with apples, pears, plums, ½ cup of berries, kiwi, and paw-paw. Have these in between meals as snacks, one mid-morning and one mid-afternoon.

Herxheimer Reactions

Depending on the severity of Candida overgrowth and the amount of the agents taken, the Candida can be killed off in vast numbers in a very short period. As the fungi are killed, they release substances that are toxic to the body called mycotoxins. If the elimination organs such as the kidneys, liver, lymphatics, gut and skin cannot clear these mycotoxins quickly and they accumulate in the tissues, then a temporary toxic or allergic-type reaction can occur. The technical name for this experience is a 'Herxheimer reaction'; it is more commonly referred to as "die off."

Usually die-off lasts about 12 – 24 hours, though on rare occasions it can last several days. It can usually be controlled by reducing the dosage of the remedies used to kill the Candida, as well as taking drainage herbs and homeopathics that your practitioner will advise you of.

Signs of Herxheimer reaction can be many and varied but generally involve such discomfort as aching, bloating, dizziness, nausea, and an overall "goopy sick" feeling, or a worsening of original symptoms. Fortunately, die off is generally short in duration, and although uncomfortable, is at least a confirmation of the presence of Candida and that something "good" is happening.

Exercise as well as ensuring proper, daily bowel evacuation has been reported as being helpful in countering the adversities of die off. Maintaining a high daily intake of pure water is also important to keep the channels of elimination open. Sometimes taking a teaspoon of baking soda (sodium bicarbonate) in a glass of water can help to quickly neutralize acidic reactions in the body that lead to inflammation and pain.

It may be possible to slow down these symptoms, many of which are caused by acetaldehyde, one of the main toxins produced by yeast. Taking Molybdenum – 10 drops x 2 times daily in water, away from food - can break down this toxin into something far less harmless. It may be worth considering adding these to the Candida protocol if Herxheimer reactions are bad.

The Blocking Factors of Recovery – Reasons for Failing

Many times, people who have Candidiasis don't follow the Candida protocol precisely, consistently, and for a long enough period. Often when people feel better while they are on the Candida diet, they tend to go off it too quickly.

When people have Candida or CRC, they usually have weakened immune systems. When the immune system is suppressed, it is prone to more infections and disease, making it impossible for a person to fully recover. Therefore, it is important to help boost the immune system by using a variety of supplements. One of the most powerful ones that is so simple to take is VITAMIN C. Taking a couple of grams, twice per day really helps to keep the immune system working well.

Some of the factors responsible for failure to achieve a total cure could be:

1. Lack of hydrochloric acid (HCL) in stomach

Hydrochloric acid is produced in the stomach to aid in activating digestion of foods and protection of the intestinal flora, but mostly to help digest proteins and help absorb nutrients such as vitamin B12, calcium, iron and intrinsic factor.

One of the most common causes of HCL imbalances is past antibiotic use. Antibiotics destroy the beneficial bacteria that synthesize B vitamins necessary for HCL production in the stomach. Proper HCL levels in the stomach kill off many pathogens that otherwise would enter the intestinal tract and potentially create problems.

HCL's important functions include:

- ✓ Breaking down proteins into essential amino acids and nutrients
- ❖ Stimulating your pancreas and small intestines to produce the digestive enzymes and bile necessary to further breakdown the carbohydrates, proteins and fats
- ❖ Preventing disease by killing pathogenic bacteria and yeast normally present in foods
- ❖ Low stomach acid leads to a cascade of digestive problems such as bloating, gas and constipation.

- Low gastric acid causes a variety of intestinal problems such as bloating, flatulence and indigestion. So, if the patient suffers from hypochlorhydria or low production of hydrochloric acid from the stomach, then add BETAINE COMPLEX.

It is only those very rare cases where we have a case of antifungal-resistant Candida that is a problem. This usually happens when the patient has been treated time and time again with medicinal anti-fungals and the Candida have now become a 'super Candida'. This again can be eliminated using this protocol, but the time required will be stretched to 4-5 months.

I have never had an antifungal-resistant case that was not cured in a maximum of 5 months, but as I said earlier, these are very rare occurrences and personally I have not seen more than a handful of cases in my career.

Natural Antibiotics During the Candida Protocol

It is critical that anyone on the 3-month Candida protocol stock-up on NATURAL ANTIMICROBIAL PACK that they might require if they come down with a cold, flu, sore throat or any kind of infection while they are still on the Candida protocol.

These natural antibiotics have been tried and tested for many years and seem to work fine with most infections. However, it is very important to take these immediately when the first symptoms appear. If you leave the infection for a couple of days, the microbes will spread quickly, and it will be more difficult to shift it with the natural antibiotics.

Therefore it is critical to have these natural antibiotics in your medical dispensary BEFORE beginning the Candida protocol. They have an expiry date of between two and five years, so you will no doubt use them during this time.

The dosages mentioned below are for adults. For maximum effectiveness it is good to use at least four of the natural antibiotics mentioned below, all in combination together.

These natural antibiotics and herbal supplements include the following that have been used successfully in clinical practice, and in fact have been used by all my family for over 30 years, given that none of my 4 children have ever taken antibiotics in their lives!

1. GRAPEFRUIT SEED EXTRACT **(Citricidal™)**: Is a very effective anti-fungal, available in tablet form as well as liquid form which can be placed under nails with fungus. Take 2 tablets 3 times daily. For nails, one drop under each nail morning and evening.

2. OREGANO OIL: If one is citrus intolerant, then you can use Oregano oil gel capsules instead – 1 gel capsule 3 times daily.

3. NANO SILVER LIQUID 50 ppm (colloidal silver) – You can take 1-3 teaspoons, 3 times daily.

4. VITAMIN C – Take either 2 caps (1000 mg each) 3 times daily, or ½ teaspoon 3 times daily of the calcium ascorbate powder form.

5. PARAFORM PLUS TWO – this contains a broad spectrum of active herbals, probiotics and other natural cleansing and protective agents, which have anti-bacterial, anti-fungal, anti-microbial and anti-inflammatory actions. Take one cap x 3 times daily.

There is no reason why ALL these should not be combined, but at least 4 of the 5 should be combined for maximum effectiveness. Please do not underestimate the importance and value of stocking up on these natural antimicrobials.

We have prepared a NATURAL ANTIMICROBIAL PACK in our one-stop shop for your convenience (www.worldwidehealthcenter.net).

On a few occasions I have seen patients that I was treating for Candida not stocking these natural antibiotics and they came down with a nasty bug that went deep into the lungs within days. By the time they could obtain all these remedies, their symptoms had reached a level where they had to see a medical practitioner, who rightly so, prescribed antibiotic drugs.

It is touch and go whether the Candida protocol will succeed or not when taking antibiotic drugs. The problem is that the antibiotics will inevitably kill off the good bacteria in the gut as well as the bad, and if this creates a severe enough dysbiosis, then the pathogenic, hyphal forms of Candida will begin to proliferate again.

This is very sad when you have to announce to the patient that they have to extend their Candida protocol for another month or longer – very frustrating!

My Own Case Studies from Patients Cured

There is still a lot of controversy around the topic of Candida, and I am the first to agree that we do not have all the answers. One thing that I have witnessed in clinical practice, however, is the astounding recovery that many of these so-called Candidiasis patients make when placed on the Da Vinci Candida Protocol (DCP).

Personally, I have seen many different skin problems clear when the systemic Candidiasis is treated including psoriasis, as well as chronic sinusitis, joint pains, cheloids or scar formations, splitting skin on hands, chronic coughs and sore throats of many years standing, chronic thrush and vaginal discharge, headaches and migraines, chronic fatigue or myalgic encephalomyelitis (ME) and many other rather atypical symptoms that were labeled as "Idiopathic" which basically means "unknown etiology." Here are a few case histories for your interest:

Case 1

This is a case of a woman who went in for a D&C scrape of the uterus and the gynecologist ruptured the uterus and she required emergency surgery due to heavy internal hemorrhage. She received several IV antibiotics and a couple of months after being discharged she suffered from splitting hands along with chronic thrush, fatigue and other skin rashes of unknown origin. She made a dramatic improvement in all these symptoms after completing the Da Vinci Candida Protocol.

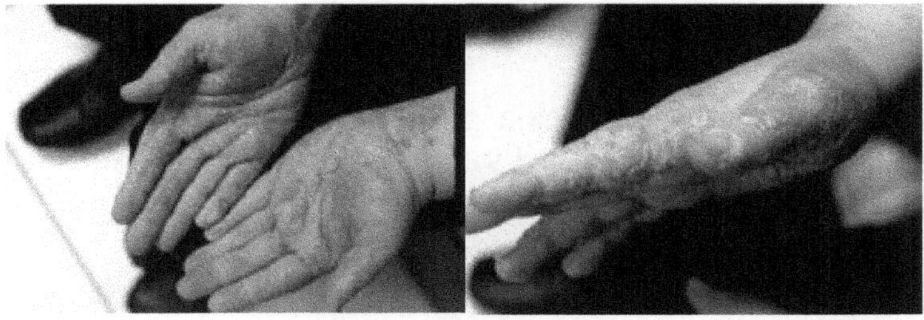

Case 1: Bad case of splitting hands after IV antibiotics

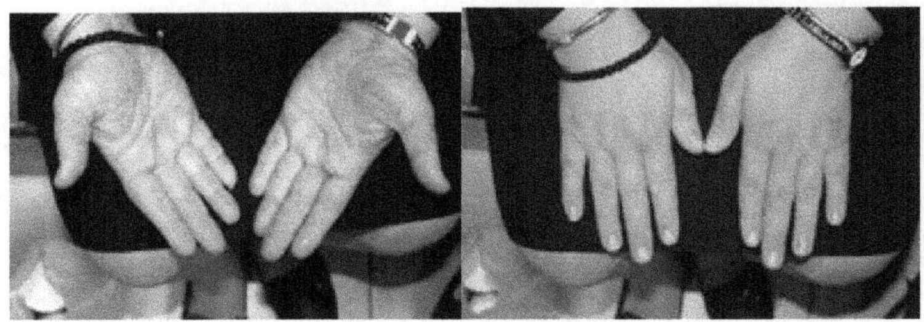

Case 1: Two-months into the Da Vinci Candida Treatment

Case 2

This is a lady that had suffered from chronic psoriasis for over 20 years. This had spread to most of her torso as well as limbs. One of the underlying problems of the skin problem was systemic Candidiasis which cleared after three months of the Da Vinci Candida Protocol.

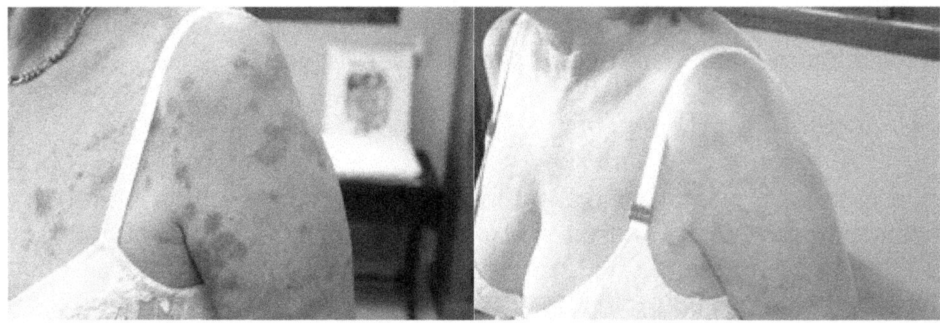

Case 2: Chronic psoriasis (left) and 3-months after completion of Da Vinci Candida Treatment

Case 3

A complex case of an idiopathic skin problem of 20 years' duration. Using the Candida Treatment Protocol resulted in over 75% improvement, but there was a bacterial element that needed further treatment to eliminate it.

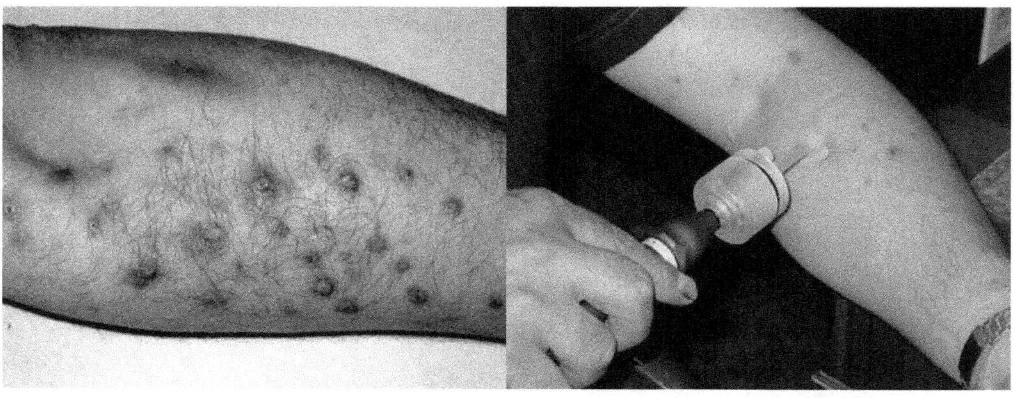

Case 3: Idiopathic skin problems of 20-years duration (left) and after treatment (right)

Case 4

A young adult who had contracted herpes and Steven-Johnson Syndrome during blood infusions – when presented for treatment he was in excruciating pain, had lost 8 kg and was tube feeding. Treatment using the Candida Treatment Protocol eliminated this difficult problem.

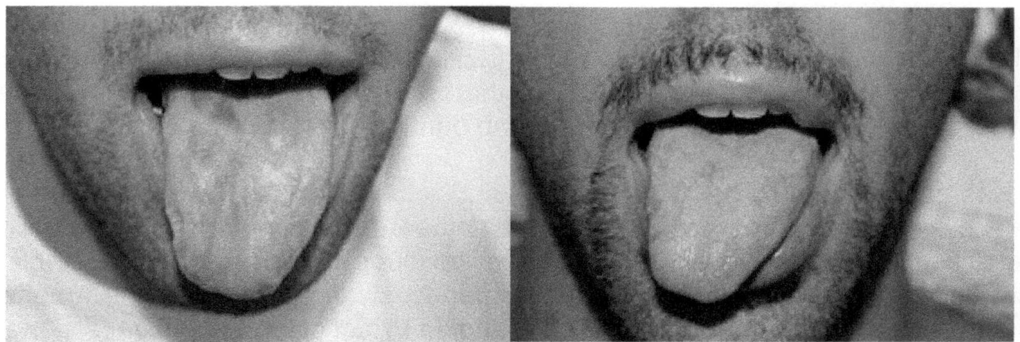

Case 4: Complex case with underlying Candida (left) and one month into treatment (right)

Other Clinical Cases

Here are a few more cases that I have seen in clinical practice – each has different symptoms, yet one of the major underlying factors was Systemic Candidiasis.

Case No. 1: Mrs. A, Age 44

Mrs. A's presenting symptoms were somewhat unusual in that she continually complained that she frequently had the sense of a strong fishy odor in her nostrils over the last 7 years.

She remembers that this began when she had cleaned mold in her house with chlorine – the mold had appeared after a flood.

She also suffered from many allergies which included allergy to flowers, bananas and melon.

Her main symptoms apart from the annoying fishy odor was, constant intermittent coughing as well as a heavy pressure-type sensation in the chest and lungs. She had clear signs of nail fungus as well as frequent vaginal discharge.

She had consulted several medical doctors and dermatologists, but with no success. The dermatologist gave her antifungal cream for the nails. The condition remained as before.

She underwent Bioresonance diagnosis using the VEGA system and was found to have a number of food intolerances too such as: wheat, lactose and milk products, bananas, caffeine, sugar, chicken, pork, nightshade family of vegetables (potatoes, tomatoes, peppers, and aubergines), olive oil and olives.

The VEGA test also showed that she was resonating with pathological, mycelial forms of Candida albicans, indicating that she was suffering from systemic Candidiasis – mixed molds were also found during this testing protocol.

It was decided to help her body to detox and return to an alkaline pH, as well as help eliminate inflammatory chemicals and other toxins. She followed an alkaline detoxification diet for 2 weeks based on alkaline foods such as fruit and vegetables. Her energy levels after the detox had tremendously increased and she reported clarity of mind. She began the Da Vinci Candida Protocol for 3 months – see main text for details.

The smell of fish had decreased by 30% in intensity and the frequency to cough had also decreased by 40% within the first 3 weeks of the protocol treatment. After two months of treatment, the cough had improved 60%.

Previously she would cough for one hour, now she coughs less than one minute. The smell of fish has improved by 70%.

After the completion of the Candida protocol (3 months), the Candida finally disappeared, and the cough had improved by 100%. This was the first time that the cough had improved in the past 7 years. The smell of fish had also vanished as well as the nail fungus on her toes – this was also helped by adding grapefruit seed extract liquid – one drop per nail morning and evening. She was a very happy woman!

Case No. 2: Mr. M, Age 45

Mr. M presented with a chronic cough that he had for the past 7-8 years, accompanied by whitish phlegm. He was diagnosed with H. Pylori for which the medical doctor prescribed antibiotics which were taken on and off for a period of 2 years. The coughing however persisted even though he had consulted many doctors, including ENT (otolaryngologists) and pneumologists with no results.

Before coughing began, he lived in a moldy apartment.

He underwent VEGA food intolerance testing that showed intolerance to several foods such as: wheat, soya, lactose and milk products, beans, caffeine, almonds and walnuts, pork, citrus (lemon, grapefruit, and oranges), olive oil and olives. He is a vegetarian but includes lactose and fish in his diet.

The VEGA testing also showed that he was suffering from systemic Candida albicans. He followed an alkaline detoxification diet for 15 days based on fruit and vegetables. During the detox the cough had decreased by 50% in frequency and 70% decrease in intensity. The white phlegm had stopped completely.

Immediately after the detox he began the Da Vinci Candida protocol for 3 months. During the Candida protocol his energy levels had massively increased, and he had incredible clarity of mind.

After the Candida treatment, his cough had completely vanished, and the phlegm decreased to minimum.

Case No. 3: Mrs. S, Age 49

Mrs. S complained that she had bronchial asthma and suffered from allergies. Medical doctors gave her cortisone sprays. She also suffered from obesity (147 kg) and whenever she tried to diet, she suffered from hypoglycemia.

Other health issues included atrial fibrillation (cardiac arrhythmia) and GERD-gastroesophageal reflux disease. She was taking Warfarin, an anticoagulant, to prevent blood clots from forming. She was also taking medication to control her arrhythmia.

She had also removed her thyroid nodules and was taking thyroxine daily.
It was recommended that she begin with a compromised alkaline detoxification diet lasting 1 month. This means that the body will be detoxing slower than the 15-day alkaline detox diet by leaving in protein foods the first two weeks. This procedure is recommended when there are chronic degenerative diseases, in order to prevent any possible adverse reactions caused by the elimination of inflammatory chemicals.

So, the first week of detox she could eat fish and pulses along with fruit and vegetables. The second week the fish was eliminated and only the pulses remained along with the fruit and vegetables. During the final two weeks, she only ate fruit and vegetables.

During the detox her stomach digestion improved, and she was feeling much better; edema had also disappeared after some heavy urination initially, and she had lost noticeable inches around her waist – to her delight as weight loss had been blocked for a long time.

During Bioresonance testing it was shown that she was intolerant to several foods such as: wheat, lactose and milk products, citrus (oranges, lemons, grapefruits), caffeine, sugar, hazelnut, walnuts, almonds, pork, chicken, and nightshade family of vegetables (potatoes, tomatoes, aubergines, peppers).

In addition, the Vega Bio-dermal testing also showed that she was suffering from systemic Candidiasis. She therefore began the Da Vinci Candida protocol for 3 months. During the Candida protocol, she had lost a total of 12 kg, her asthmatic symptoms had gone completely, and she could now climb steps without wheezing and panting, being much quicker on her feet. As an added gift, her chronic sinusitis had also completely cleared.

APPENDIX

If you would like to know if your health problems are yeast-related, take this comprehensive test. Questions in Section A focus on your medical history-factors that promote the growth of Candida and that are frequently found people with yeast-related health problems. In Section B, you will find a list of 23 symptoms that are often present in patients with yeast-related health problems. Section C consists of 33 other symptoms that are sometimes seen in people with yeast-related problems – yet they may also be found in people with other disorders.

Fill out and score the questionnaire should help you, and your physician, evaluate the possible role that candida plays in your health problems.

SECTION A: HISTORY

- Have you ever taken tetracycline, or other antibiotics, for acne for one month or longer? (points 35)
- Have you, at any time in your life, taken broad-spectrum antibiotics or other antibacterial medication for respiratory, urinary or other infections for two months or longer, or in shorter courses four or more times in a one-year period? (Points 35).
- Have you taken a broad-spectrum antibiotic drug even in a single dose? (points 6)
- Have you at any time in your life been bothered by persistent prostatitis, vaginitis or other problems affecting your reproductive organs? (points 25)
- Are you bothered by memory or concentration problems do you sometimes feel spaced out? (points 20)
- Do you feel "sick all over", yet despite visits to many different physicians the cause has not been found? (points 20)
- Have you been pregnant two or more times? (points 5)
- One time? (points 3)
- Have you taken birth control pills for more than two years? (points 15)
- For six months to two years? (points 8)
- Have you taken steroids orally, by injection or inhalation for more than two weeks? (points 15)
- For two weeks or less? (points 6)
- Does exposure to perfume, insecticides, fabric shop odours and other chemicals provoke symptoms? Moderate to severe (points 20) Mild (points 5)
- Does tobacco smoke really bother you? (points 10)
- Are your symptoms worse on damp, muggy days or in mouldy places? (points 20)
- Have you had athlete's foot, ring worm, jock itch or other chronic fun-gal infections of the skin or nails? Severe or persistent (points 20) Mild to moderate (points 10)
- Do you crave sugar? (points 10)

Total Score, Section A _______________

SECTION B: MAJOR SYMPTOMS

For each of your symptoms, enter the appropriate figure in the pint score column.

1. If a symptom is occasional or mild **3 points**
2. If a symptom is frequent and/ or moderately severe **6 points**
3. If a symptom is severe and/ or disabling **9 points**

Add total score and record it at the end of this section.

- Fatigue or lethargy ________
- Feeling of being "drained" ________
- Depression or manic depression ________
- Numbness, burning or tingling ________
- Headache ________
- Muscle aches ________
- Muscle weakness or paralysis ________
- Paint and/ or swelling in joints ________
- Abdominal pain ________
- Constipation and/ or diarrhoea ________
- Bloating, belching or intestinal gas ________
- Troublesome vaginal burning, itching or discharge ________
- Prostatitis ________
- Impotence ________
- Loss of sexual desire or feeling ________
- Endometriosis or infertility ________
- Cramps and/ or other menstrual irregularities ________
- Premenstrual tension ________
- Attacks of anxiety or crying ________
- Cold hands or feet, low bode temperature ________
- Hypothyroidism ________
- Shaking or irritable when hungry ________
- Cystitis or interstitial cystitis ________

TOTAL SCORE, SECTION B ________

SECTION C: OTHER SYMPTOMS

For each of your symptoms, enter the appropriate figure in the point score column.

1. If a symptom is occasional or mild **3 points**
2. If a symptom is frequent and/ or moderately severe **6 points**
3. If a symptom is severe and/ or disabling **9 points**

Add total score and record it at the end of his section.

- Drowsiness, including inappropriate drowsiness ________
- Irritability ________
- In coordination ________
- Frequent mood swings ________
- Insomnia ________
- Dizziness/ loss of balance ________
- Pressure above ears, tenderness of cheekbones or forehead ________
- Tendency to bruise easily ________
- Eczema, itching eyes ________
- Psoriasis ________
- Chronic hives (urticaria) ________
- Indigestion or heartburn ________
- Sensitivity to milk, wheat, corn or other common foods ________
- Mucus in stools ________
- Rectal itching ________
- Dry mouth or throat ________
- Mouth rashes, including "white" tongue ________
- Bad breath ________
- Foot, hair or body odour not relieved by washing ________
- Nasal congestion or postnasal drip ________
- Nasal itching ________
- Sore throat ________
- Laryngitis, loss of voice ________
- Cough or recurrent bronchitis ________
- Pain or tightness in chest ________
- Wheezing or shortness of breath ________
- Urinary frequency or urgency ________
- Burning on urination ________
- Spots in front of eyes or erratic vision ________
- Burning or tearing eyes ________
- Recurrent infections or fluid in ears ________
- Ear pain or deafness ________

TOTAL SCORE, SECTION C ________

GRAND TOTAL (SECTION A, B AND C) ________

The **Grand Total Score** will help you and your physician decide if your health problems are yeast-connected. Scores in women will run higher, as seven items in the questionnaire apply to women, while only two apply exclusively to men.

- Yeast –connected health problems are almost certainly present in women with scores of **more than 180,** and in men with of **more than 140.**
- Yeast-connected health problems are probably present in women with scores of **more than 120,** and in men with scores **more than 90.**
- Yeast-connected health problems are possibly present in women with scores of **more than 60,** and in me of **more than 40.**
- With scores of less than 60 in women and 40 in men, yeasts are less apt to be the cause of health problems.

Score of **60-99** yeast a possible cause of health problems
Score of **100-139** yeast a probable cause of health problems.
Score of **140 or more** yeast **almost certainly** a cause of health problems.

PARASITE QUESTIONNAIRE

These are many causes for each symptom listed below. Assign points to each symptom and see if a pattern develops.

A= Symptom never occur

B= Symptom occurs occasionally

C= Symptom occurs frequently

D= Symptom occurs regularly

10-14 points = maybe parasite infestation
15- 20 points = suspect parasites
22-25 points = likely- (Further testing helpful)
25 or more = parasites involvement high likely

Questions		A	B	C	D
	Restless sleep	0	1	2	3
	Skin problems, rashes, itches	0	1	2	3
	Increased appetite, hungry after meals	0	1	2	3
	Frequent diarrhea, loose stools	0	1	2	3
	Grinding of teeth when asleep	0	1	2	3
	Variable, changeable consistency of stools	0	1	2	3
	Picking of nose, boring nose with finger	0	1	2	3
	Abdominal pains	0	1	2	3
	Vertical wrinkles around mouth	0	1	2	3
	Rectal, anal itching	0	1	2	3
	Parallel lines (tracks) in soles of feet	0	1	2	3
	Intestinal cramps, burning	0	1	2	3
	Irritability (no apparent reason)	0	1	2	3
	Feeling bloated, gaseous	0	1	2	3
	Diarrhea alternating with constipation	0	1	2	3
	Bowel urgency, occasional accidents	0	1	2	3
	Hyperactive tendency (nervous)	0	1	2	3
	Dark circles under eyes	0	1	2	3
	Need for extra sleep, waking unrefreshed	0	1	2	3
	Allergies, food sensitivities	0	1	2	3

	Fevers of unknown origin	0	1	2	3
	Night sweats (not menopausal)	0	1	2	3
	Kissing pets, allowing them to lick your face	0	1	2	3
	Anaemia	0	1	2	3
	Frequent colds, flu, sore throats	0	1	2	3
	Going barefoot in parks, public streets	0	1	2	3
	Travelling in 3rd countries	0	1	2	3
	Eating lightly cooked pork products	0	1	2	3
	Eating sushi, sashimi	0	1	2	3
	Sleeping with pets on bed	0	1	2	3
	Bed wetting	0	1	2	3
	Men: sexual dysfunction	0	1	2	3
	Forgetfulness	0	1	2	3
	Slow reflexes	0	1	2	3
	Loss of appetite	0	1	2	3
	Yellowish face	0	1	2	3
	Heart beat rapid	0	1	2	3
	Heart pain	0	1	2	3
	Pain in the umbilicus	0	1	2	3
	Blurry, unclear face	0	1	2	3
	Pain: back, thighs, shoulders	0	1	2	3
	Lethargy, apathy	0	1	2	3
	Numbness, tingling in hands, feet	0	1	2	3
	Burning pains in the stomach, intestines	0	1	2	3
	Menstrual problems	0	1	2	3
	Dry lips during day, damp at night	0	1	2	3
	Drooling while asleep	0	1	2	3
	Occult blood in stool (shown from lab tests)	0	1	2	3

	History of giardia, pin worms, other worms	0	1	2	3
	Swimming in creeks, rivers, lakes	0	1	2	3

Total score ___________

REFERENCES

Al-Doory Y. 1969. The mycology of the freeliving baboon (Papio sp.). Mycopathologia et Mycologia Applicata 38: 7–15.

Anderson KE, Kappas A. Dietary regulation of cytochrome P-450. Annu Rev Nutr. 11:141-167, 1991.

Ballie-Hamilton, P. The Detox diet. UK: Penguin, 2002.

Banerjee, M., D.S. Thompson, A. Lazzell, P.L. Carlisle, C. Pierce, C. Monteagudo, J.L. Lopez-Ribot, and D. Kadosh. 2008. UME6, a novel filament-specific regulator of Candida albicans hyphal extension and virulence. Mol. Biol. Cell 19, 1354-1365.

Barclay GR, McKenzie H, Pennington J, Parratt D, Pennington CR. The effect of dietary yeast on the activity of stable chronic Crohn's disease. Scand J Gastroenterol 1992; 27 :196–200.

Bartlett JG, Gilbert DN, Spellberg B. Seven ways to preserve the miracle of antibiotics. Clin Infect Dis. 2013;56(10):1445–1450.

Bartlett JG, Gilbert DN, Spellberg B. Seven ways to preserve the miracle of antibiotics. Clin Infect Dis. 2013;56(10):1445–1450.

Bastidas RJ, Heitman J: Trimorphic stepping stones pave the way to fungal virulence. PNAS 2009; 106: 351–2.

Bastidas RJ, Heitman J: Trimorphic stepping stones pave the way to fungal virulence. PNAS 2009; 106: 351–2.

Berman J: Morphogenesis and cell cycle progression in Candida albicans. Curr Opin Microbiol 2006; 9: 595–601.

Bernhardt H, Knoke M. Mycological aspects of gastrointestinal microflora. Scand J Gastroenterol 1997; 32(suppl 222) :102–106.

Bland JS, Bralley JA. Nutritoinal upregulation of hepatic detoxification enzymes. J Appl Nutr. 44(3&4):2-15, 1992.

Blankenship, J.R. and A.P. Mitchell. 2006. How to build a biofilm: a fungal perspective. Curr. Opin. Microbiol. 9, 588-594.

Brandtzaeg P. The mucosal B cell and its functions. In: Brostoff J, Challacombe S (eds): Food Allergy and Intolerance. London: Saunders; 2002:127-171.

Budtz- Jorgensen, E. Cellular immunity in acquired Candidiasis of the palate. Scand. J. Dent. Res. 81, 372, 1973

Cabot, S. Juice Fasting Detoxification. USA: The Sprout House, 1992.
Calderone RA, Fonzi WA: Virulence factors of Candida albicans. Trends Microbiol 2001; 9: 327–35.

Calderone, R.A., and R.L. Cihlar (e.d.). Fungal pathogenesis: principles and clinical applications. Marcel Dekker, Inc., New York, N.Y, 2002

Carlisle PL, Banerjee M, Lazzell A, Monteagudo C, Lopez-Ribot JL, Kadosh D: Expression levels of a filament-specific transcriptional regulator are sufficient to determine Candida albicans morphology and virulence. PNAS 2009; 106: 599–604.

Carlisle, P.L., M. Banerjee, A. Lazzell, C. Monteagudo, J.L. LopezRibot, and D. Kadosh. 2009. Expression levels of a filament-specific transcriptional regulator are sufficient to determine Candida albicans morphology and virulence. Proc. Natl. Acad. Sci. USA 106, 599-604.

Centers for Disease Control and Prevention, Office of Infectious Disease Antibiotic resistance threats in the United States, 2013. Apr, 2013. Available at: http://www.cdc.gov/drugresistance/threat-report-2013. Accessed January 28, 2015.

Crampin, H., K. Finley, M. Gerami-Nejad, H. Court, C. Gale, J. Berman, and P.E. Sudbery. 2005. Candida albicans hyphae have a Spitzenkorper that is distinct from the polarisome found in yeast and pseudohyphae. J. Cell. Sci. 118, 2935-2947.

Crandall M. The pathogenetic significance of Intestinal Candida Colonization, 2004

Crook WG: The yeast connection, A medical Breakthrough 2nd Addition Professional Books, Jackson, TN, 1984

Crook WG: The Yeast Connection, A Medical Breakthrough 2nd Addition Professional Books, Jackson, TN, 1984.

Crook, WG. The Yeast Connection and the Woman. Professional Books, Jackson TN 1987.

Dalkilic E, Aksebzeci T, Kocatürk I, Aydin N, Koculu B: The investigation of pathogenity and virulence of Candida. In: Tümbay E, Seeliger HPR, Ang Ö (eds.): Candida and Candidamycosis. New York: Plenum Press 1991; 50: 167–74

Davies MH, Gough A, Sorhi RS, Hassel A, Warning R, Emery P. Sulphoxidation and sulphation capacity in patients with primary biliary cirrhosis. J Hepatol. 22(5):551-560, May 1995.

Enderlein, G. (1925). Bakterien-Cyclogenie, Verlag de Gruyter & Co, Berlin.

Fitzsimmons N, Berry DR. Inhibition of Candida albicans by Lactobacillus acidophilus: evidence for the involvement of a peroxidase system. Microbios 1994; 80 :125–133.

Gail Burton. Candida - The Silent Epidemic, Candida Causative factors, 4-9, 2003

Georgiou, G.J. (2005) Explore! Volume 14, No. 6.

Georgiou, G.J. (2008) British Naturopathic Journal, Vol. 25., No. 1 & 2.

Grant DM. Detoxification pathways of the liver. J Inher Metab Dis. 14;421-430, 1991.

Grubb SEW, Murdoch C, Sudbery PE, Saville SP, Lopez-Ribot JL, Thornhill MH: Candida albicans-endothelial cell interactions: a key step in the pathogenesis of systemic candidiasis. Infect Immun 2008; 76: 4370–7.

Hesseltine HC, Campbell LK. 1938. Diabetic or mycotic vulvovaginitis. American Journal of Obstetrics and Gynecology 35:
272–283.

Hornby, J.M., E.C. Jensen, A.D. Lisec, J.J. Tasto, B. Jahnke, R. Shoemaker, P. Dussault, and K.W. Nickerson. 2001. Quorum sensing in the dimorphic fungus Candida albicans is mediated by farnesol. Appl. Environ. Microbiol. 67, 2982-2992

Hube B: From commensal to pathogen: stage- and tissue-specific gene expression of Candida albicans. Curr Opin Microbiol 2004; 7: 336–41.

Hulda Regehr Clark, Ph.D., N.D., The Cure for all Diseases 1995
Hussein, H.S., and J.M. Brasel. Toxicity, metabolism, and impact of mycotoxins on humans and animals. Toxicology 167, 2001

Iwata, K.; Yamamoto, Y "Glycoprotein Toxins Produced by Candida albicans." Proceedings of the Fourth International Conference on the Mycoses, PAHO Scientific Publication #356, June 1977.

John Parks Trowbridge, M.D., and Morton Walker, D.P.M., The yeast syndrome- Antibiotics Encourage Yeast Overgrowth, 45-46, 1986

Kanda N, Tani K, Enomoto U, Nakai K & Watanabe S. The skin fungus-induced Th1- and Th2-related cytokine, chemokine and prostaglandin E 2 production in peripheral blood mononuclear cells from patients with atopic dermatitis and psoriasis vulgaris. Clinical & Experimental Allergy; 32(8):1243-50.

Kennedy MJ, Volz PA. Ecology of Candida albicans gut colonisation: inhibition of Candida adhesion, colonisation and dissemination from the gastrointestnal tracy by bacterial antagonism. Infect Immun 1985; 49: 654–63.

Koivikko A, et al. Allergenic cross-reactivity of yeasts. Allergy 1988; 43:192-200.

Kubo I, Fujita K, Lee SH, Ha TJ. Antibacterial activity of polygodial. Phytother Res. 2005 Dec;19(12):1013-7.

Kumamoto CA, Vinces MD: Alternative Candida albicans lifestyles: growth on surfaces. Annu Rev Microbiol 2005; 59: 113–33.
Douglas LJ: Candida biofilms and their role in infection. Trends Microbiol 2003; 11: 30–6.

Kumamoto CA, Vinces MD: Alternative Candida albicans lifestyles: growth on surfaces. Annu Rev Microbiol 2005; 59: 113–33.

Lee SH, Lee JR, Lunde CS, Kubo I. In vitro antifungal susceptibilities of Candida albicans and other fungal pathogens to polygodial, a sesquiterpene dialdehyde. Planta Med. 1999 Apr;65(3):204-8.

Leon Chaitow N.D, D.O, Candida Albicans- Could yeast be your problem? How Candida gets out of hand. Chapter 3- Immune System Deficiency, 24-26, 1991

Lushniak BD. Antibiotic resistance: a public health crisis. Public Health Rep. 2014;129(4):314–316.

Luyt CE, Brechot N, Trouillet JL, Chastre J. Antibiotic stewardship in the intensive care unit. Crit Care. 2014;18(5):480.

Magee PT, Chibana H: The genomes of Candida albicans and other Candida species. In: Calderone RA (ed.): Candida and candi - diasis. Washington: ASM Press 2002; 293–304

Michael T. Murray, N.D., Chronic Candidiasis, Dietary factors, sugar and the yeast syndrome: 43,44, 1997

Morita E, Hide M, Yoneya Y, Kannbe M, Tanaka A, Yamamoto S: An assessment of the role of Candida albicans antigen in atopic dermatitis. J Dermatol 1999; 26: 282–7. 20. Pappas PG, Rex JH, Sobel JD, et al.: Guidelines for treatment of Candidiasis. CID 2004; 38: 161–89. 21.

Morschhäuser J, Köhler G, Ziebuhr W, Blum-Oehler G, Dobrindt U, Hacker J: Evolution of microbial pathogens. Phil Trans R Soc Lond 2000; 355: 695–704.

Netea MG, Brown GD, Kullberg BJ, Gow NAR: An integrated model of the recognition of Candida albicans by the innate immune system. Nat Rev Immunol 2008; 6: 67–78.

Nieuwenhuizen WF, Pieters RH, Knippels LM, Jansen MC, Koppelman GJ. Is Candida albicans a trigger for the onset of coeliac disease? Lancet 2003; 361 :2152–2154.

Nobile, C.J. and A.P. Mitchell. 2006. Genetics and genomics of Candida albicans biofilm formation. Cell. Microbiol. 8, 1382-1391

Noverr MC, Falkowski NR, McDonald RA, McKenzie AN, Huffnagle GB: Development of allergic airway disease in mice following antibiotic therapy and fungal microbiota increase: role of host genetics, antigen, and interleukin-13. Infect Immun 2005; 73: 30–8.

Noverr MC, Phare SM, Toews GB, Coffey MJ, Huffnagle GB: Path - ogenic yeasts Cryptococcus neoformans and Candida albicans produce immunomodulatory prostaglandins. Infect Immun 2001; 69: 2957–63.

Noverr MC, Noggle RM, Toews GB, Huffnagle GB: Role of antibiotics and fungal microbiota in driving pulmonary allergic responses. Infect Immun 2004; 72: 4996–5003.

Odds FC. 1988. Candida and Candidosis, 2nd edn. Bailli`ere Tindall: London.

Piddock LJ. The crisis of no new antibiotics—what is the way forward? Lancet Infect Dis. 2012;12(3):249–253.

Piispanen AE, Hogan DA: PEPped up: induction of Candida albicans virulence by bacterial cell wall fragments. Cell Host Microbe 2008; 4: 1–2

Polakova S, Blume C, Zarate JA, Mentel M, Jorck-Ramberg D, Stenderup J, et al.: Formation of new chromosomes as a virulence mechanism in yeast Candida glabrata. PNAS 2009; 106: 2688–93

Poulain D, Hopwood V, Vernes A. Antigenic variability of candida albicans. CRC Crit Rev Microbiol 1985; 12:223-70.

Raska M, Belakova J, Krupka M, Weigl E: Candidiasis – Do we need to fight or to tolerate the Candida fungus? Folia Microbiol 2007; 52: 297–312.

Reinel D, Plettenberg A, Seebacher C, et al.: Orale Candidose. Leitlinie der Deutschen Dermatologischen Gesellschaft und der Deutschsprachigen Mykologischen Gesellschaft. JDDG 2008; 7: 593–7.

Reinholdt J, Krogh P, Holmstrup P. Degradation of IgA1, IgA2, and S-IgA by candida and torulopsis species. Acta Path Microbiol Immunol Scand, Sect C 1987; 95:65-74.

Romani L, Bistoni F, Puccetti P. Initiation of T-helper cell immunity to Candida albicans by IL-12: the role of neutrophils. Chem Immunol. 1997; 68:110-35.

Romani L, Bistoni F, Puccetti P: Adaptation of Candida albicans to the host environment: the role of morphogenesis in virulence and survival in mammalian hosts. Curr Opin

Microbiol 2003; 6: 338–43.

Salloum, TK. Fasting Signs and Symptoms: A Clinical Guide. USA: Buckeye Naturopathic Press, 1992.

Scrivner, J. Detox Yourself. UK: Judy Piatkus (Publishers) Ltd., 1998.

Seelig MS. Mechanisms by which antibiotics increase the incidence and severity of candidiasis and alter the immunological defences. Bacteriol Rev 1 1966; 30 :4442–4459.

Shah DT, Jackman S, Engle J, Larsen B. Effect of gliotoxin on human polymorphonuclear neutrophils. Inf Dis Obster Gynecol 1998; 6 :168–175.

Shen J, Cowen LE, Griffin AM, Chan L, Kohler JR: The Candida albicans pescadillo homolog is required for normal hypha-to-yeast morphogenesis and yeast proliferation. PNAS 2008; 105: 20918–23.

Soll DR: Phenotypic switching. In: Calderone RA (ed.): Candida and Candidiasis. Washington: ASM Press 2002; 123–42.

Sudbery, P.E., N.A.R. Gow, and J. Berman. 2004. The distinct morphogenic states of Candida albicans. Trends Microbiol. 12, 317- 324

The Chronic Candidiasis Syndrome: Intestinal Candida and its relation to chronic illness OAM 1996-1997, 16. Gutierrez, J.; Maroto, C. et al: Circulating Candida antigens and antibodies: useful markers of candidemia. Journal of Clinical Microbiology. 31(9):25502, 1993.

Thewes S, Kretschmar M, Park H, Schaller M, Filler SG, Hube B: In vivo and ex vivo comparative transcriptional profiling of invasive and noninvasive Candida albicans isolates identifies genes associated with tissue invasion. Mol Microbiol 2007; 63: 1606–28.

Trowbridge JP and Walker M The Yeast Syndrome Bantam Books, New York, New York 1986.

Trowbridge JP and Walker M. The yeast Syndrome Bantam Books, New York, N.Y, 1986
Truss C: The Missing Diagnosis Birmingham Alabama (The author) 1983.

Truss C: The missing Diagnosis Birmingham Alabama (The Author), 1983

Truss, CO. Metabolic abnormalities in patients with chronic Candidiasis - the acetaldehyde hypothesis, Journal of Orthomolecular Medicine, 13:63- 93, 1984

Viswanathan VK. Off-label abuse of antibiotics by bacteria. Gut Microbes. 2014;5(1):3–4.

Vojdani A, Rahimian P, Kalhor H and Mordechai E. Immunological cross reactivity between candida albicans and human tissue. J Clin Lab Immunol 1996; 48:1-15.

Wade, C. Inner Cleansing: How to Free Yourself from the Joint-Muscle-Artery-Circulation Sludge. New York: Parker Publishing Co., 1992.

Walsh, TJ.; Lee, JW.; et al: "Serum Darabinitol measured by automated quantitative enzymatic assay for detection and therapeutic monitoring of experimental disseminated candidiasis: correlation with tissue concentrations of Candida albicans." Journal of Medical & Veterinary Mycology. 32(3):20515, 1994.

Weig M, Werner E, Frosh M, Kasper H. Limited effect of refined carbohydrate dietary supplementation on colonization of the gastrointestinal tract of healthy subjects by Candida albicans. Am J Clin Nutr 1999; 69 :1170–1173.

William G. Crook, M.D., Chronic Fatigue Syndrome and the yeast connection, Probiotics: 260,261, 1992

William G. Crook, M.D., The yeast connection - Candida questionnaire and score sheet - Diagnosis of a yeast-Related disorder, 29-33, Food allergies: 122, 1986

Xu XL, Lee RTH, Fang HM, Wang YM, Li R, Zou H, et al.: Bacterial pepti doglycan triggers Candida albicans hyphal growth by directly activating the adenylyl cyclase cyr1p. Cell Host Microbe 2008; 4: 28–39

VIDEOS

If you wish to watch some webinars and videos that I have done on the subject of Candida and others, here they are (if you cannot see the link, just search on YouTube for "Dr. Georgiou and Candida":

Candida Videos:

https://www.youtube.com/watch?v=nOYIFKrGbrM&t=620s

https://www.youtube.com/watch?v=VQnE8VQXEpc

Heavy Metals Video:

https://www.youtube.com/watch?v=lZNFPWPWNnc&index=7&list=PLXDVp62iaBwzezTyezZ4M8ZFhL5szJ-hR

In the next chapter we will examine how we can use energetic medicine and bioresonance to cure different diseases in general.

Chapter 7

Curing with Energetic Medicine and Bioresonance

Everything is vibration

The human body is a symphony of sounds. Every chakra, organ, bone, tissue and cell has its own resonant frequency; its own sound. Together, they create a unified or composite frequency with its own sound, like the instruments of an orchestra coming together. Ideally, the individual sounds and frequencies comprise a harmonious whole. That is, when the body is functioning as it should. However, when an organ is out of time or out of tune with the rest, then the entire body is affected. This disharmony leads to states of disease and disintegration.

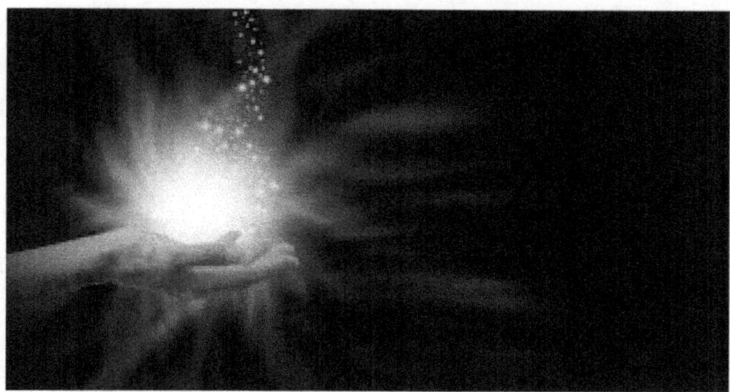

Every living and none living thing has its own resonant frequency – everything is vibration. Every organ of the body has its own individual resonant frequency, much like the note of a tuning fork. All bacteria, viruses, parasites and fungi also have their own frequencies.

It's interesting that the latest quantum physics theory, born only a decade or so ago, arrives at a similar conclusion. It's called String Theory and it basically suggests that the physical universe is built out of sound vibrations, kind of as if everything is the result of some huge cosmic guitar being played somewhere. It's a mind-blowing concept that is held by some of the sharpest minds in the physics community, including Steven Hawking.

Everything in the world is made up of energy. We are all constantly vibrating masses of microscopic particles that are always in motion. Every object, person and organ have a healthy vibration rate called resonance. If that vibration is out of resonance, disease results.
Every organ, every bone, every tissue, every system, all are in a state of vibration. Now, when we are in a state of health, the body puts out an overall harmonic of health. However, when a frequency that is counter to our health sets itself up in some portion of the body, it creates a disharmony that we call *dis-ease.*

When an organ such as the liver gets sick, the frequency usually drops. The lungs resonate at a frequency of 72 cycles per second, also known as Hertz. If the lungs develop an infection, then the frequency will change, usually dropping a few Hertz.

At the University of California, Los Angeles, nanotechnologist Jim Gimzewski is pioneering a new science he calls sonocytology - the study of cell sounds. His first experiments began with yeast cells, using a nanotechnology tool called an atomic force microscope to detect sound-generating vibrations and then using a computer to enhance the volume. The yeast cells were heard to produce harmonics of around 1,000 Hz.

In musical terms, they were "singing" in the range of C-sharp to D above middle C. Killing the yeast cells with alcohol made the pitch rise dramatically, as if the cells were screaming. Cellular harmonics were also affected by temperature, speeding them up or slowing them down. Genetic mutations were found to make a slightly different sound than normal cells. Dead cells emitted a low rumbling like radio static.

Distinguishing between the sound signatures of healthy and diseased cells may be a part of the medicine of the future.

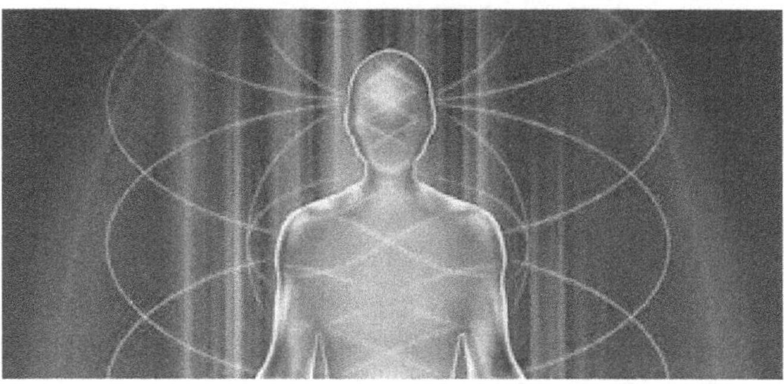

Healing Frequencies

The healing nature of the frequency spectrum lies in the ability of a living organism to absorb a very precise range of frequencies that can physically create a healing effect on certain organs and organic systems.

In many cases the healing effect of frequencies is achieved by the ability of the frequency to create a very accurate effect on specific bacteria and viruses by sending highly matched Healing Frequencies capable of neutralizing their chemical structure.

"Put a cat and a bunch of broken bones in the same room" some veterinary schools joke, *"and the bones will heal."* Only two years ago, scientists discovered that vibrations between 20-140 Hz are anabolic for bone growth and will also help to heal fractures, mend torn muscles and ligaments, reduce swelling, and relieve pain. Fauna have found that a cat's purr not only matches this vibration, but its dominant frequencies are 25 and 50 Hz - the optimum frequencies for bone growth and fracture healing. All cats, including larger ones such as pumas, ocelots and lions, have further sets of strong harmonics at the exact Hertz that generate muscle strength, increase joint mobility and provide therapeutic pain relief.

Richard Gerber, M.D. states in his book, *Vibrational Medicine:*

> *"When viral and chemical environmental stressors are introduced into the human biological system, the place where they will cause the most damage will be partially determined by the weakest link in the physiologic/subtle energy chain.*
>
> *From an energetic standpoint, the human body, when weakened or shifted from equilibrium, oscillates at a different and less harmonious frequency than when healthy. This abnormal frequency reflects a general state of cellular energetic imbalance within the physical body.*
>
> *When a weakened individual is unable to shift their energetic mode to the needed frequency a certain amount of subtle energetic help may be needed. When supplied with a dose of the needed energetic frequency, it allows the cellular bioenergetic systems to resonate in the proper vibrational mode, thereby throwing off the toxicities of the illness."*

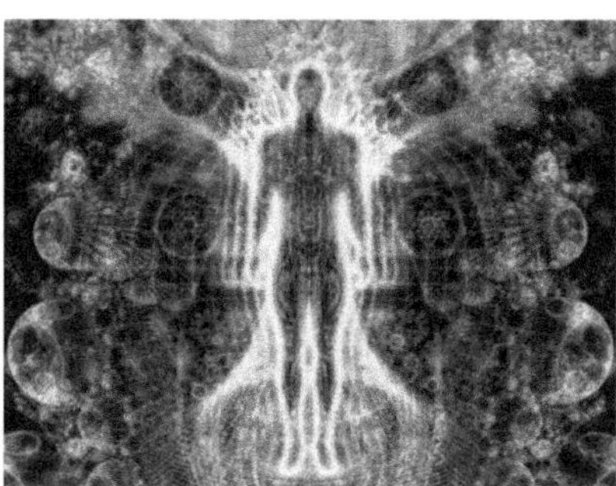

Bioresonance

Each body has its own unique frequency. When the interaction of these frequencies is balanced, you feel peaceful and at perfect harmony with yourself as well as towards other people. When they are off balance, it can have significant negative effects.

An unbalanced body is unable to fulfil its energy contribution to the system. This can have negative psychological and physical consequences on an individual. Anger, depression, constipation, lack of concentration, and sexual dysfunctions are just a few examples of symptoms due to unbalanced internal frequencies.

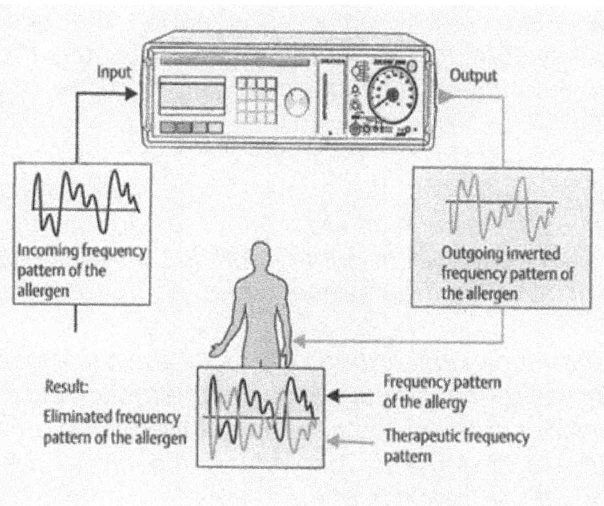

If we can produce the same frequency as a healthy lung using a frequency generator, then we can help the lung to recuperate its normal functioning. The body heals and rebalances itself when it is connected to healthy frequencies. This is the principle of BIORESONANCE.

If we take a crystal wine glass as another example, this also has its own resonant frequency of around 500 Hertz. If we can produce a sound at the same frequency and stand the glass in front of a speaker, then the glass will absorb this frequency and break. This is the phenomenon of RESONANCE.

In the same way, microbes also have their own resonant frequencies – if we can match these frequencies then the microbes will absorb this energy and burst.

There have been many researchers that have worked on energy medicine and Bioresonance this century, such as Dr. Rife, Dr. Voll, Dr. Schimmel, Dr. Morell and others. In addition, unknown to the West, the Russians have worked in the background and made ground-breaking discoveries in this field.

The Russians conducted extensive studies on over 25,000 people. They established an accurate system of analysing and reinforcing energetic health of the organs and their connection to specific areas on the skin (dermal-visceral zones). The Russian space program uses this technology because it enables convenient and non-invasive monitoring and enhancing of the health of their cosmonauts.

Over the last 17 years, Russian scientists, spearheaded by Dr. Konoblov, a medical doctor and Ph.D. physicist, have developed small, portable devices that are innovative and cutting-edge, at only a fraction of the cost of previous generation machines.

These devices produce weak electromagnetic fields at varying frequencies that can penetrate the body's cells and bring them back to optimal balance and health.

Deta Elis Bioresonance Devices

The Russian company initially called DETA ELIS and now DEHOLDINGS, has developed a number of therapeutic devices. One of these is called the DEVITA AP (Fig. 1) and is designed to resonate with different microorganisms to destroy them. It is no bigger than a mobile phone and can comfortably be carried in one's pocket or placed under the pillow and ran at night while sleeping.

The other device (Fig 1) is called the DEVITA RITM and is designed to resonate at the same frequencies as normal organ systems, hence helping to upregulate these organs, bringing them back to normal functioning.

Both these devices can be programmed using the DEINFO USB (Fig 1) which contains more than 3,000 programmes for eradicating many microorganisms including parasites, protozoa, bacteria, fungi and viruses, as well as many other programmes for all the organ systems of the body.

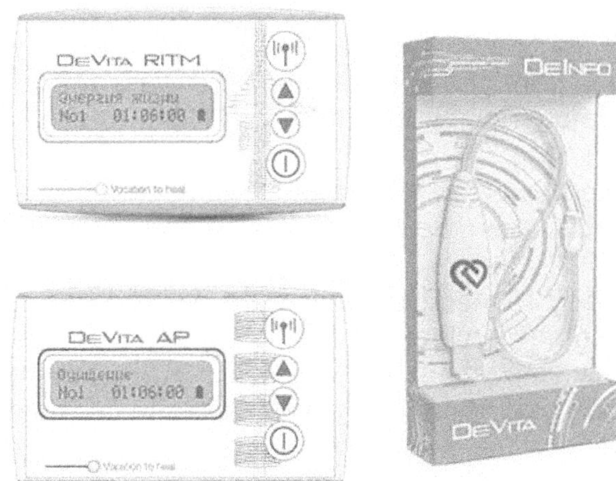

Fig 1. The DEVITA AP and RITM portable Bioresonance devices
www.deta-elis-uk.com

The Hippocratic Oath states, "*Do no harm*" when treating people. These gentle devices achieve exactly this – they can heal without being invasive and causing side-effects. The devices can be used with children and pets and can therefore act as your "family doctor".

The devices have undergone clinical trials with many thousands of patients suffering many different health problems, as well as being certified by the Ministry of Health of the Russian Republic. These devices have also been patented in 73 different countries and have won many certificates and awards.

They are presently manufactured in Germany and have a CE as an electromagnetic wellness device.

MINI Bioresonance Device

Recently, the DETA ELIS company discovered a new device for conducting bioresonance therapy in the comfort of your own home. No need to visit practitioner's offices and pay for every treatment – this is the MINI Bioresonance device or MINI BRT.

The NEW Devita BRT device is easy to use and is designed for a wide range of users. It is basically a hand-held, portable bioresonance therapy (BRT) device that is very user friendly. It contains two brass
hand electrodes and two brass foot electrodes.

The patient's body signals are conducted from the right hand into the input of the device using a hand electrode. In the Devita BRT device, the disharmonious frequencies are filtered out and inverted. These inverted therapeutic oscillations are now given back to the patient via the left hand using another electrode.

These returning oscillations help to balance the patient electromagnetically and are again fed into the Devita BRT device for further analysis. The process is repeated constantly in fractions of a second. The pathological signals in the body are consequently reduced and finally extinguished, and the physiological endogenous regulatory forces can regulate the biological process unhindered.

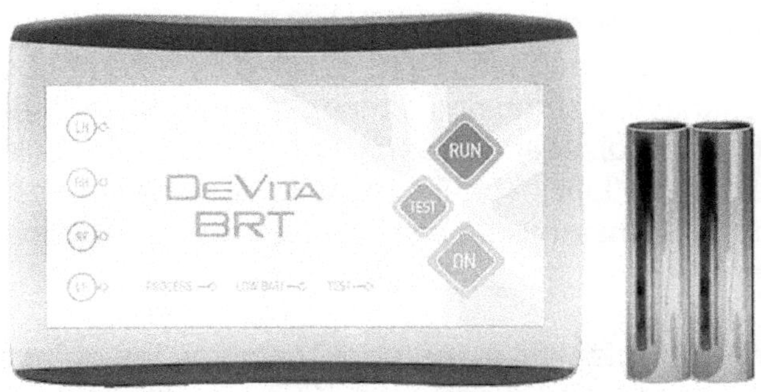

I strongly believe that bioenergetic and informational medicine is going to be the medicine of the future. These discoveries on energetics are now gradually percolating into the consciousness of medical practitioners. Researchers, healthcare professionals and the public are realizing that these energetic healing modalities are here to stay.

In clinical practice, I have used various energetic diagnostic and healing modalities that have completely cured difficult chronic diseases, where more orthodox approaches could not help. Other users of the Deta Elis devices are getting good results in different diseases, so this is encouraging.

Having said this, however, these devices are not a cure-all for all diseases – nothing is! We can use and respect the technology knowing that it will do us no harm with the potential to heal on levels that other remedies and drugs cannot.

A Little History

In 1923, George's Lakhovsky[140], a Russian engineer working in France, built a simple apparatus capable of registering microvoltage measurements from human

[140] Lakhovsky, G. The Waves Which Cure (Gauthier-Villars and Co), 1929.

cells, plants and microbes. In his studies of normal and diseased cells, Lakhosvky found that there were marked differences in their oscillation patterns.

Each group of cells emitted frequencies specific to its organ or tissue of origin. Cancerous cells emitted a different, abnormal pattern. Lakhovsky also discovered that harmful factors such as faulty nutrition, environmental pollutants such as toxic chemicals or heavy metals, bacteria or viruses weaken and distort cellular electro-magnetic fields prior to the onset of illness and death.

A little later, Professor Harold Saxton Burr[141], of Yale Medical School, carried out his own investigation of human-energy related phenomenon. His systematic measurements of the electromagnetic fields emitted by different bodily tissues and organs confirmed Lakhovsky's findings concerning the difference in the electrical emissions of healthy and diseased organs and tissues. He called these the 'L-fields' with 'L' representing "Life." Thanks to the controlling L-fields, new molecules and cells in the body are constantly being rebuilt, arranging themselves in the same pattern as the old ones.

With the advancement of scientific research technology, the number of discoveries regarding the human energy field grew. In 1967, the magnetic field around the human heart was observed and recorded using a sophisticated Superconducting Quantum Interference Device (SQUID) at the Massachusetts Institute of Technology in Cambridge, Massachusetts by Zimmermann and his colleagues.[142,143]

Professor Tiller[144] believes that the magnetic elements in living cells are repositories for voluminous amounts of information, the pathological content of which contributes to the development and sustainment of chronic diseases. All of the major assaults that the body is not able to overcome (toxins, infectious agents and physical or emotional traumas) become imprinted onto these cellular recordings in a CD-like fashion and then continuously feed back into the body's chemistry, negatively altering it.

German physicist Professor Herbert Frohlick[145] of the University of Liverpool, a world-renowned authority on human energy research, summarized his fifty years of research in the field by concluding that every structure in the body, including the

---

[141] Burr, H.S. Bluprint for Immortality, Neville Spearman Publishers, 1972.

[142] Zimmermann, J.E. Josephson effect devices and low frequency filed sensing. *Cryogenics* 12:19-31, 1972.

[143] Zimmermann, J.E., Thiene P, Harding J T. Design and operation of stable rf-biased superconducting point-contact quantum devices, and a note on the properties of perfectly clean metal contacts. *Journal of Applied Physics*. 41:1572-1580, 1970.

[144] Tiller, W. Energy Fields and the Human Body. Frontiers of Consciousness, edited by J. White. New York, Avon Books, 1974.

[145] Hyland, GJ and Rowlands, P (ed). *Herbert Frohlich FRS: A Physicist Ahead of his Time.* (2nd edition), UK: University of Liverpool, 2008.

entire chemistry of the body down to the chromosomes, is energy-operated and driven by electromagnetic fields that are created by flows of charged ions. He received the Max Planck Medal, the highest award for physics in Germany.

How does the body work energetically?

When students of medicine and biology study the cell, the diagrams that they study are very simplistic in the sense that they only look at the structural components; the different organelles contained inside the cell and their function. However, to be able to understand the energetic systems of the body, we need to understand the basic anatomy of the body's Living Matrix.

It is the living matrix or extracellular matrix (ECM) that communicates with each cell of the body forming a complex web of interconnectedness. Figure 2 is a summary of these interconnections – notice how the tissues surrounding the digestive tract, nerves, bones, blood vessels, muscles and underlying the skin contain a sparse but active number of generative cells that form and continuously modify the extracellular matrix and play an important role in injury repair and defense against disease.

These cells are part of a structural, energetic and informational continuum. This fibre system is now recognized by many scientists as an important communication system that affects all metabolic systems as well. It is part of a semiconducting, oscillatory continuum that allows all parts of the biological organism to communicate with each other. One research scientist, Adey, in 1993 referred to this as *"whispering between cells."*[146]

---

[146] Adey, WR. Whispering between cells: electromagnetic fields and regulatory mechanisms in tissue. *Frontier Perspectives*. 3:21-25, 1993.

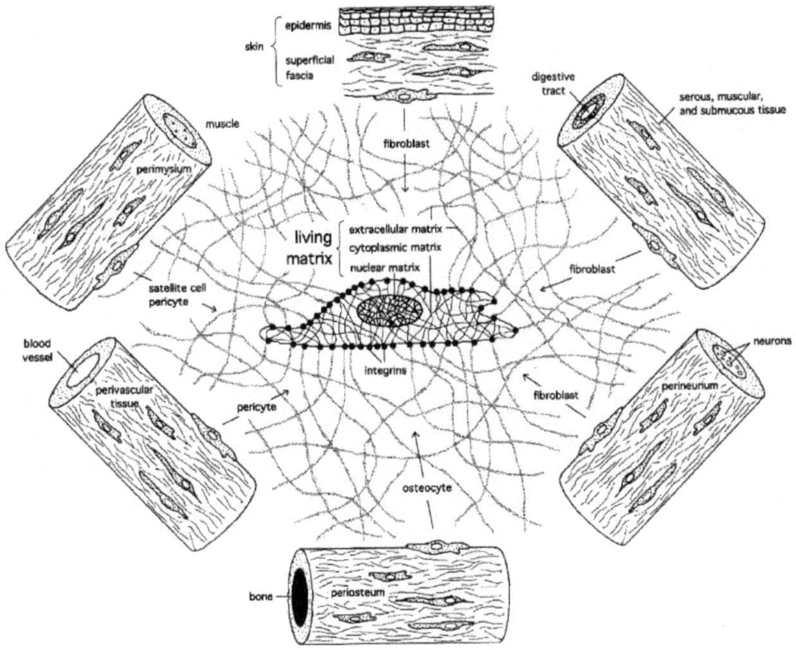

Fig. 2 The Living Matrix

In trying to understand the energy dynamics of the living matrix, the field of physics plays an important role. In the structure of the living matrix there is a degree of coherent crystallinity – this is like an ordered crystal matrix that is very important to the structure-energy-communication model of living tissue.

Interestingly, many of the key molecules that make up the living matrix such as collagen, elastin, keratin, DNA, actin and myosin are all helical, much like a helical spring. If we can understand how the helical spring can convert energy from one form to another, then we will better understand how the living matrix can respond to different energies.

This system is comprised of two main structures: the visible and invisible connective tissue that extends from the molecular level of our body throughout our energy field and the element of water.

It was back in 1941 that Albert Szent-Györgyi,[147] who had received the Nobel Prize in 1937 for the synthesis of Vitamin C, gave the Korányi Memorial Lecture in Budapest, Hungary. He said:

[147] Szent-Györgyi, A. The Study of Energy Levels in Biochemistry) *Nature* 148:157-159, 1941.

"If a great number of atoms are arranged with regularity in close proximity, as for instance, in a crystal lattice, the electrons cease to belong to one or two atoms only and belong to the whole system...A great number of molecules may join to form energy continua, along which energy, excited electrons may travel a certain distance."

What this means is that free electrons can move around the body quickly and transfer energy and information wherever they wish. This is clarified further by Dr. Donald Coffey and an eminent group at Johns Hopkins School of Medicine.[148] They were studying the nuclear matrix and its interconnections with both DNA and with molecules that extend across the nuclear envelope and connect to the cytoskeleton.[149]

In 1991, the same group produced an inspiring report on the way signals propagate through this matrix, which they termed a tissue tensegrity matrix system.[150] The tensegrity aspect had evolved from the work of Buckminster, Fuller and others.[151] Tensegrity is defined as a continuous tensional network (called tendons) supported by a discontinuous set of compressive elements (called struts).
The 1991 report by Pienta and Coffey gave precise language and experimental validation to the transfer of energy and information through the living matrix:

"Cells and intracellular elements are capable of vibrating in a dynamic manner with complex harmonics, the frequency of which can now be measured and analysed in a quantitative manner...a tissue-tensegrity matrix system...is poised to couple the biological oscillations of the cell from the peripheral membrane to the DNA."

The helical molecules in living systems are piezoelectric semiconductors which have the ability of emitting and absorbing and converting light energy into vibrations that can travel through the living matrix. Due to the transverse Hall effect, these helical molecules can also respond to magnetic and biomagnetic fields.

---

148 Presented by James L. Oschman, Ph.D.in a lecture entitled "The development of the living matrix concept and its significance for health and healing in a speech commemorating the London premier of The Living Matrix: a new film on the science of healing and the Science of Healing Conference at Kings College, London on March 13, 2009.
149 Berezney, R., Coffey, D.S. Isolation and characterization of a framework structure from rat liver nuclei. *Journal of Cell Biology* 73:616-637, 1977.
150 Pienta K.J., Coffey D.S. Cellular harmonic information transfer through a tissue tensegrity-matrix system. *Medical Hypotheses* 34:88-95, 1991.
151 Tensegrity is a naturally occurring construct first recognized and developed by sculptor Ken Snelson and visionary R. Buckminster Fuller. For a detailed discussion, go to Dr. Stephen M. Levin's web site, http://www.biotensegrity.com

Whenever a therapist applies any type of stimulus to the living matrix, whether it is by touch on the skin, inserting an acupuncture needle, using a pulsing electromagnetic field such as the PAPIMI that we will discuss below, the vibratory energy from these stimuli will be converted by the helical molecules of the living matrix into signals that will travel throughout the living matrix.

Informational Medicine

There are also many phenomena in healing that are not governed by quantity, space and time. These phenomenon and related treatment modalities are outside modern-day medicine since they are not covered and explained by modern-day physics. These can be placed into the category of 'Informational Medicine' and would include homeopathy, psychology, emotional freedom technique, distant healing, prayer healing, radionics, Hellinger Family Constellations and more. Of these, homeopathy was the first systemically developed form of informational medicine in recent history.

Informational medicine consists of words, signs, symbols, rituals and pictures – the use of information in all its forms. Even though this has not been recognized formally by modern medicine, it no doubt exists and is a powerful healing modality that goes beyond the placebo effect.

There are many informational modalities that are often misunderstood as being energetic. Since these modalities do not use substance or energy to diagnose or heal, there is no way that atomic physicists using quantum mechanics can measure the energy, as it does not exist as an energy system but an information system.

Alongside the levels of matter and energy, information forms a third level of existence that is guided by its own laws which differ in many aspects from those of matter and energy. They can, however, co-exist. Matter and energy can be transformed into each other, as can information be transformed into energy or vice versa. Information can also be *transported* via energy.

However, a new aspect that is unknown in modern physics, maybe except for Global Scaling[152], is that information can be transmitted *without* energy. This is possible because pure information is not ruled by time and space. It may be difficult to conceive, but our world is holographic in its structure, which means that every

[152] The Theory of Global Scaling assumes that matter resonates harmonically at its lowest level of energy. This lowest level global scaling theory is not merely designated the "physical vacuum"; however, the frequency spectrum of the natural oscillations of the vacuum comprises many orders of magnitude and is fractally developed, like a melody. This "melody of creation" is, according to the theory, the cause of the logarithmic-hyperbolic, scale invariant, fractal distribution of frequencies of most varied measure – from the elementary particles to the galaxies.

part contains all other parts. This implies that any part can affect every other part and can be a measure of every other part.

To illustrate this, let's look at an example. It is well known that silver particles in a beaker of water will kill bacteria. What is not so well known is that if the colloidal silver was placed in a nearby gas discharge tube, the electromagnetic emissions from this will also kill the bacteria. If one also closely simulated the silver spectrum using light energy, the electromagnetic radiation from this light source would also kill the bacteria.

We can clearly see that it is not the physical contact of the silver ions with the bacteria that are killing them, but the specific information pattern inherent in the silver atom that is responsible. So, manipulating the information aspect of the silver can alter the information aspect of the bacteria in such a way as to 'kill' the bacteria.

The diagnostic methods described in this book use the human energy field to derive health-related information. For instance, thermography records the thermal properties of the human energy field. The VEGA EXPERT measures electrical energy flow in specific energy channels of the body, known as meridians which are all connected to the Living Matrix. This will be registered after stimulation with a different energy field (a food item, a medical drug, a toxin, a mineral or a vitamin supplement).

Autonomic Response Testing (ART) is a way of measuring energy changes in the autonomic nervous system, which is connected to the Living Matrix - using this method it is possible to understand what stresses the body on an energetic level.

Some people gifted by birth, such as mystics and healers, have been speaking and writing about the energetic nature of the human being and the interconnections with the sea of energy around us for thousands of years. Barbara Ann Brennan, a healer as well as a physicist, bridged her natural gift with the science of physics in her book entitled, *Hands of Light: A guide to Healing through the Human Energy Field.*[153]

Many writers have contributed to this body of knowledge as well, some naturally gifted, others less so. Many were ordinary scientists, relying on indirect observation using special instruments or biochemical tests to infer on the impact of energetic treatments.

---

[153] Brennan, BA. Hands of Light: A guide to Healing through the Human Energy Field. USA: Bantam Books, 1987.

Vibrational Medicine by Dr. Richard Gerber[154], and *Energy Medicine: The Scientific Basis*[155] by James Oschman provide excellent overviews of the scientific basis of energy medicine. The fact remains that many energetic therapeutic interventions work, some of them with exceptional results. The practitioners who employ them do not wait for the blessing of conventional medicine, with all its vices, to be ready to explain the why and the how.

Visual Medicine: Seeing the effects of energy on water

Masaru Emoto[156] is a Japanese author known for his controversial claim that if human speech or thoughts are directed at water droplets before they are frozen, images of the resulting water crystals either take on a beautiful geometric pattern or a disorganized, ugly one, depending upon whether the words or thoughts were positive or negative.

Emoto claims this can be achieved through prayer, music or by attaching written words to a container of water. Dr. Emoto is at the forefront of the study of water. By using high-speed photography under high-power microscopy to photograph water freezing quickly, he has shown that thoughts and feelings affect physical reality. By producing different focused intentions through written and spoken words and music and literally presenting it to the same water samples, the water appears to "change its expression".

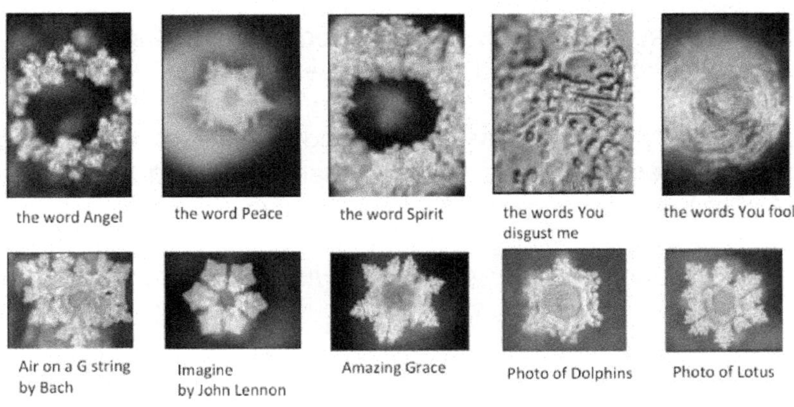

Fig 3. Crystalline patterns of water

He found that water from clear springs and water that has been exposed to loving words shows brilliant, complex, and colourful snowflake patterns (Fig 3). In

154 Gerber, R. Vibrational Medicine (3rd edition). USA: Bear and Company, 2001.
155 Oschman, J.L. Energy Medicine: The Scientific Basis. UK: Harcourt Publishers, 2000.
156 Emoto, M. *The Journal of Alternative and Complementary Medicine*. February 2004, 10(1): 19-21.

contrast, polluted water, or water exposed to negative thoughts, forms incomplete, asymmetrical patterns with dull colours.

The implications of this research create a new awareness of how we can positively impact the earth and our personal health. The success of his books[157] outside Japan has been remarkable. Dr. Emoto has been called to lecture around the world as a result and has conducted live experiments both in Japan and Europe as well as in the US to show how indeed our thoughts, attitudes, and emotions as humans deeply impact the environment.

The Cymascope

The CymaScope is a new type of scientific instrument that makes sound visible. Its development began in 2002 and the inventor is John Reid[158] from the UK. Basically, this scientific instrument allows sound to be imprinted on the surface of ultra-pure water. The surface tension of water has high flexibility and fast response to imposed vibrations, even with transients as short-lived as a few milliseconds.

Therefore, water can translate many of the sinusoidal periodicities - in a given sound sample - into physical sinusoidal structures on the water's surface. Current limits to imprinting sound on water occur in the higher harmonics and are due mainly to there being insufficient energy available in this area of the audio spectrum to cause excursions of the surface tension membrane.

I have recently bought a Cymascope and am beginning to use this fascinating instrument that has you in awe when you see what beautiful geometric patterns are imprinted on water.

Fig. 4 shows a CymaGlyph (image of sound) of a male voice mandala. Most of us do not pay much attention to our voices on a day-to-day basis, as we take for granted our ability to talk, shout, whisper, laugh, and even groan. It is not until we notice a temporary and self-limiting voice change that we begin to listen to our tone of voice. Our voices can say a lot about our health, with tone fluctuations happening frequently with several minor illnesses, but sometimes it can signify a more serious problem.

A croaky voice or the loss of voice entirely, most often derives from an infection in the throat or from overusing the voice. The changes in pitch -the highness or lowness - occur when there are changes in the shape of the gap between the

---

[157] Emoto, M. *Messages from Water, Vol. 1,* Hado Publishing, 1991; Emoto, M. *Messages from Water, Vol. 2*, Sunmark Pub, 2001; Emoto, M. *The Hidden Messages in Water*, Beyond Words Publishing, 2004.
[158] www.cymascope.com

vocal cords. However, it is the shape of our throat, nose and mouth that will determine the quality of our sound, which is why everyone's voice sounds different.

One day we will be able to use the Cymascope to identify health issues from a person's voice. As Cymascopy is such a new science, this work still has not been done, but probably will soon, as I personally intend doing many such experiments on my Cymascope.

There are some other CymaGlyphs illustrated that show the beta brain waves recorded by EEG, and heart ECG and a spinal Electromyelogram (EMG).

We are going to see much more scientific work using the Cymascope that makes sound visible.

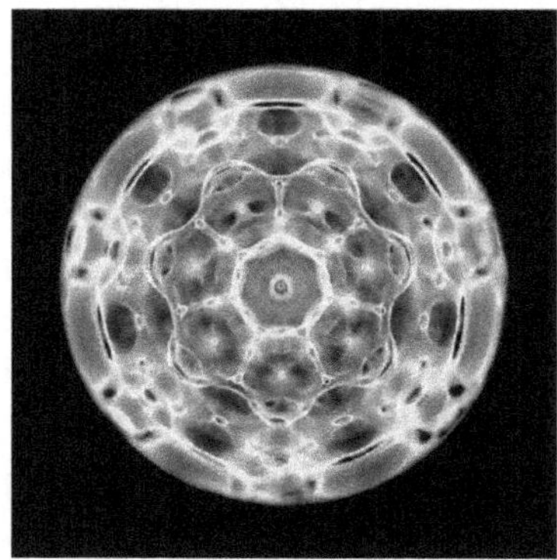

Fig 4. A CymaGlyph of male voice mandala[159]

[159] Printed with permission of John Reid, inventor of the Cymascope

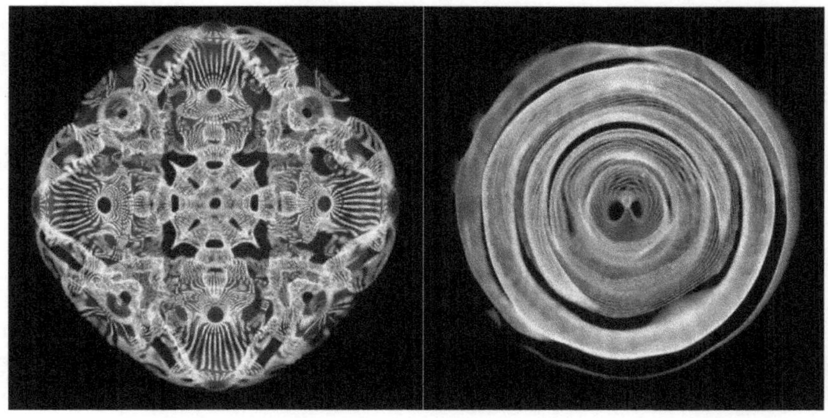

Beta brain wave Heart ECG

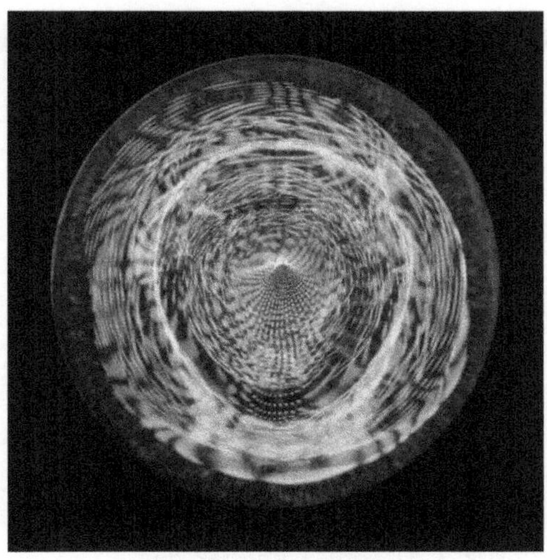

Spinal EMG

The Human Bioenergetic System

Humans consist of more than physical nerves, muscles and bones. We are part of a larger dynamic, multidimensional system of energy and light; we are simply much more than the physical body. Our physiological systems comprising of organs and tissues are not only supported by oxygen, glucose and other nutrients, but also by higher vibrational energies which provide life to the physical body.

These higher energies are regulated by the chakra-nadi system and the physical-etheric interface, which include the acupuncture meridian system. The etheric energies provide ways of organizing cellular structure and function.

The fine network of nadis distributes high-frequency energies coming in through the chakras to all the body's organs and tissues. This high-frequency energy helps to provide balance and order at the molecular level of expression. It's like a higher dimensional homeostatic system. When energetic disturbances occur at these higher frequency levels, these will manifest in the physical body as symptoms and disease.

If we could widen our perspective and see humans in their multidimensional anatomy, consisting of higher vibrational bodies, chakras, nadis, and meridians (Fig 4), then it would be possible to explain much of what allopathic medicine cannot explain about disease processes. Humans are not closed, physiological boxes but open energy systems in a dynamic equilibrium with a multidimensional electromagnetic environment.

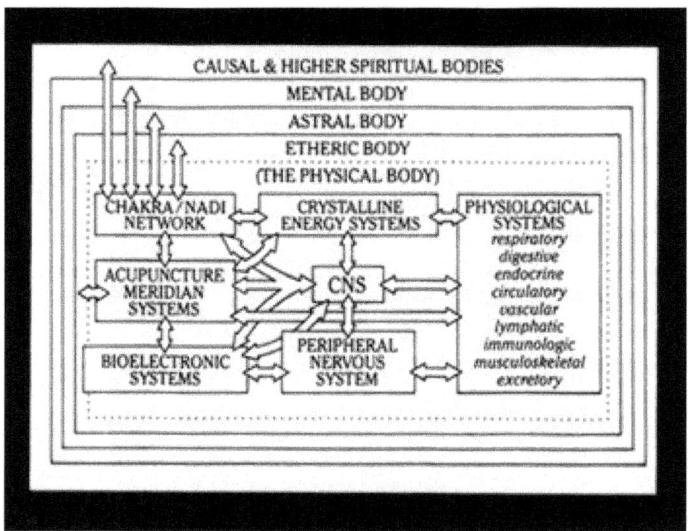

Fig 4. Human Multi-dimensional Bioenergetic System

The real future of Holistic Medicine will depend on the integration of vibrational medical therapies and clinical practice alongside all the other healing modalities. The holistic physician will need to integrate the physical, emotional, mental and spiritual elements of life in order to truly cure the patient on all these levels. The ultimate approach to healing will be to remove the subtle-energy imbalances that led to the manifestation of illness in the first place.

Even though allopathic physicians have acknowledged for some time that stress contributes to diseases such as stomach ulcers, ulcerative colitis, psoriasis, asthma and more, there have been very few attempts to address the underlying pathogenesis of these diseases, other than using anxiolytic drugs such as valium and the like. These drugs may help in the short-term with acutely stressful situations, but only tend to suppress the symptoms and overlook the primary, underlying causes. It is much more constructive for the holistic physician to integrate and rebalance the elements of the mind and body with the element of spirit.

For many years, physicians have looked at and treated the physical body as a separate entity to the mind and the spirit. There has begun a paradigm shift away from this dualistic thinking of old into a new model that accepts the health effects of the mind on the physical body.

Still, it is early days, and most medical doctors are still only trying to direct therapeutic strategies toward organ systems instead of treating the whole person. Humans are greater than the sum of their physical organs and physiological systems. The physical body interacts with complex subtle structures and networks that help the life-force and energies of consciousness to maintain a homeostasis required for the health of the physical body.

Many practitioners will say, "*Well that's all well and good, but how can we measure these 'subtle energies' and help get a better understanding of how they adversely affect our patients?*" This is an excellent. There are many different technologies and techniques that have been developed over the years for doing just this. However, it must be said that all these technologies are still in the process of development and there is not one system that can purport to measure the subtle energies of the body on all their levels and correlate them with the physical body yet.

Subtle Energy Diagnosis

Personally, as a practicing holistic medicine clinician, I have had the opportunity of using many of these 'subtle energy measuring devices.' Even though these are not yet fully developed, it is better to get a broader understanding of at least some of the subtle energies that have been responsible for their health problems, as opposed to ignoring these completely.

Let's look at some of these modalities that I mainly use in the Da Vinci Holistic Health Centre and am very familiar with. This is by no means a comprehensive list of all the measuring devices – it would take another book much thicker than this one to list them all. We will examine the Vegetative Reflex Test (VRT) using the VEGA and the DETA PROFESSIONAL devices; Bioresonance therapy using the BICOM and PROFESSIONAL; as well as Rife frequency generators.

The Vegetative Reflex Test using Bioresonance Devices

One system, which is beginning to grow in popularity among doctors and dentists, are devices known as VRT Bioresonance devices. There are a number of them now on the market, but I personally use the VEGA EXPERT VRT device (Fig 5), and the Deta Elis PROFESSIONAL (www.deta-elis-uk.com) device (Fig 6).

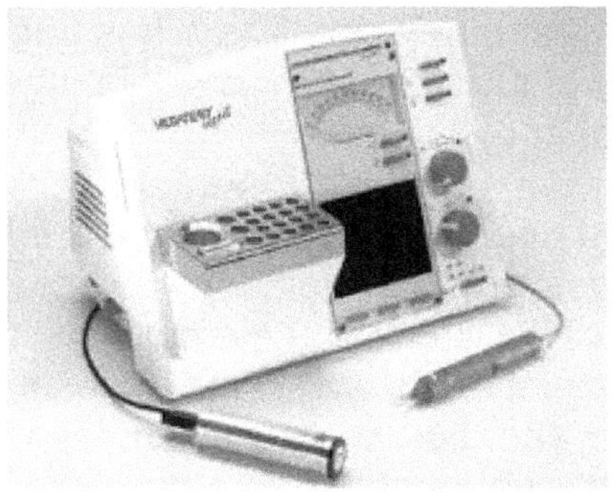

Fig 5. The VEGA VRT device

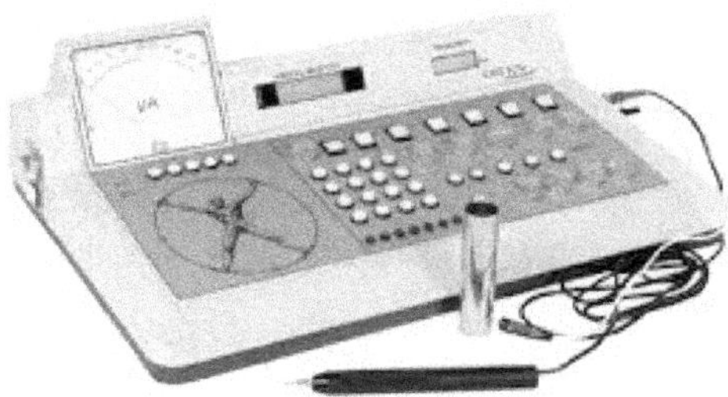

Fig 6. Deta Elis PROFESSIONAL device

Both the VEGA and PROFESSIONAL[160] Vegetative Reflex Test (VRT) represent an advanced development of the "Electroacupuncture according to Voll" (EAV)[161] concept. It features a combination of electronic measurements of skin resistance on specific energy meridian points (acupoints) that disclose vital health information through vegetative (autonomic) reflexes and resonances.

These devices can highlight the underlying causes of illnesses by using homeopathic bionosodes. This is usually a small portion of diseased tissue from a diseased organ that is ground up and made into a homeopathic remedy. When a

---

[161] Voll, R. The phenomenon of medicine testing in electro-acupuncture according to Voll. *American Journal of Acupuncture* 8:97-104, 1980.

particular bionosode is placed on the honeycomb or resonator plate of these devices, it induces a resonance reaction in the acupoint, which infers a relationship between the diseased organ being tested and the related organ of the patient.

If the patient does not have a diseased liver, for example, then they will not resonate with a bionosode of a diseased liver placed on the honeycomb of the device. Even bacteria, viruses, fungi, stealth organisms and more can be tested for resonance with the patient and be identified much quicker than any other type of biological testing.

The Vegetative Reflex Test (VRT) can help the clinician in the following ways:

- Discovery of pathophysiologic processes that escape the standard clinical examination.
- Determination of the existence of focal infections.
- Determination of sub-clinical infections and energetic functional conditions in different quadrants of the body, as well as different organs.
- Show the condition of the immune system and of the immune- related tissues (spleen, thymus and lymph nodes).
- Determination of emotional stress and disturbances.

- Identification of the pathogenesis of disease (the root causes and where they began from with their interrelationships).

- Testing for allergies from environmental factors as well as food intolerances.

Personally, as a clinician, I have found VRT testing very useful in the following cases and circumstances:

- When all conventional diagnostic tests (physical and biochemical) reveal no clues to the cause of a patient's complaints, the disorders are most likely functional in nature rather than morphological. The VEGA reveals about 80% of the otherwise un-diagnosable cases of migraines, backaches, chronic fatigue syndrome, systemic Candidiasis, bowel distention, IBS, Crohn's disease, sleep disturbance and more.

- When conventional examination cannot fully or correctly explain the patient's complaints, the VEGA is highly indicative. It is superbly suited for the diagnosis of functional ailments (about 70% of all patients) and of clinically obscure, sub-clinical disorders. These make up about 20% of all indications.

There are about 40% of patients who have many symptoms, but conventional laboratory tests yield negative results. These patients are often referred to psychologists or psychiatrists resulting in needless suffering and are a waste of time and money.

These Bioresonance devices are capable of going beyond the diagnosis of energetic imbalance levels in particular systems. It is frequently capable of finding the actual causes of the energetic dysfunction, as well as potential cures for the disorders.

Bioresonance Therapy

New methods are evolving all the time which move us closer to the goal of individualized treatment. One such method, BIORESONANCE, also known as BRT (Bioresonance therapy), can be used to treat a wide range of disorders. BRT has been tested and approved throughout Europe and Canada, and it is in use in 85 countries worldwide. In Germany, where it was developed by Regumed,[162] BRT has been in use for over 25 years.

Bio-resonance promises not only to address the unique needs of each patient, but also, as it becomes more widespread, to provide an answer to the nagging question: *"Why do some individuals do well with one type of medication, while others improve only slightly or not at all?"*

At the Da Vinci Natural Health Centre we use a couple of Bioresonance devices: the BICOM, a German-made device (Fig 7) and the DETA PROFESSIONAL made by Deta Elis, a Russian company (Fig 8). The patient's body signals are conducted from the right hand into the input of the device using a brass electrode. These devices can filter out the disharmonious frequencies and invert them. These inverted therapeutic oscillations are now given back to the patient via the left hand using another electrode.

---

[162] http://www.regumed.de

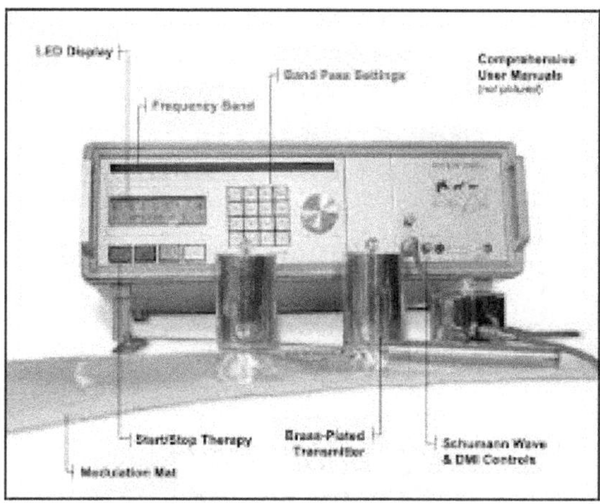

Fig 7. BICOM Bioresonance Device

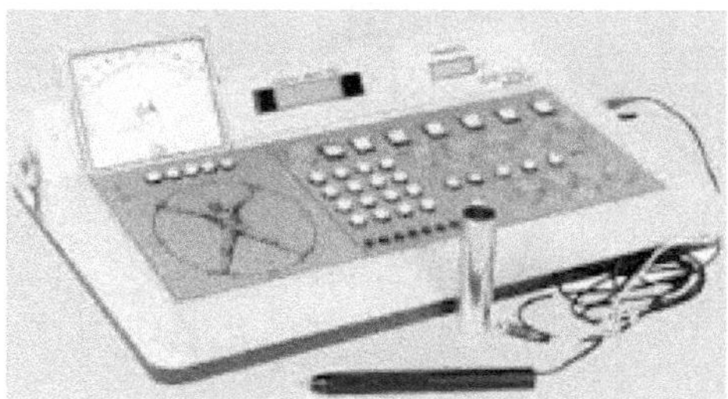

Fig 8. DETA PROFESSIONAL

Central to its application is the idea that all life is made of energy. Although humans tend to think of themselves as relatively solid creatures, we are just a mass of compressed energy. We emit our own electromagnetic fields and, as with all things, we each have our own unique “vibration,” or oscillation. This oscillation can easily be measured with electronic equipment. When we are healthy, our bodies produce a smooth, regular oscillation. When the body is under stress, the pattern becomes jagged and irregular.

The treatment of pathological oscillations involves returning them back to the body in a modified form - in this case, as a mirror image. This action is based on the principle well-known in physics, that oscillations are influenced by their exact mirror image. Returning the oscillation to the patient in this modified form can diminish, or even eliminate, the pathological oscillations of the allergen or toxin, allowing the body’s own healthy oscillations to become dominant. If the practitioner decides that medicine would also be useful in treatment, the oscillation of that specific medicine could also be returned to the patient.

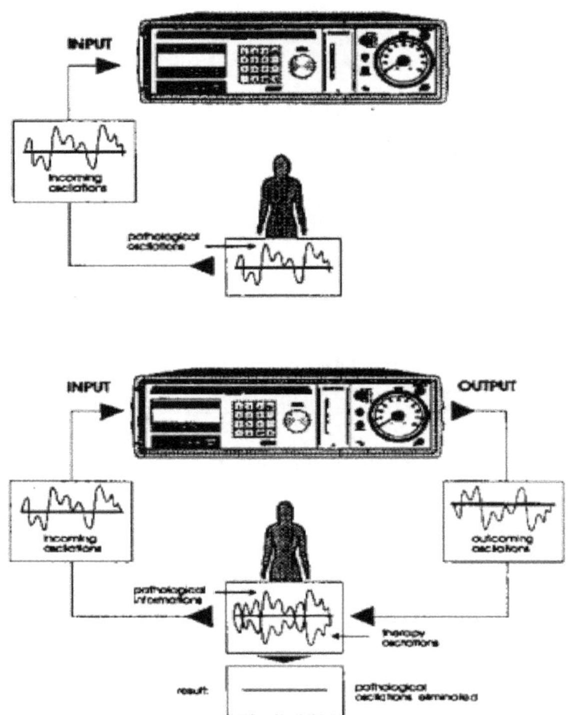

Fig 9 Returning Oscillations of Bioresonance Therapy

These returning oscillations (Fig 9) help to balance the patient electromagnetically and are again fed into the Bioresonance device for further analysis. The process is repeated constantly in fractions of a second. The pathological signals in the body are consequently reduced and finally extinguished and the physiological endogenous regulatory forces can regulate the biological process unhindered.

There has been a lot of recent media coverage on exposure to electromagnetic fields causing illness by altering the body's own electric "chemistry". However, practitioners of bio-resonance believe that the reverse is also true; healthy electrical signals transmitted into the body, in this case via hand-held electrodes, can re-harmonize it. Similar to homoeopathy and acupuncture, bio-resonance aims to relieve the body of stress factors and improve its regulatory systems.

There is considerable ongoing research in the field of Bioresonance, specifically using the BICOM device. One such study was conducted by Machowinski at the Naturopathy Outpatients Clinic of the Carsten's Foundation, University of Heidelberg, under the direction of Dr. Gerhard.

It was a prospective, randomized controlled study with 28 patients suffering with chronic hepatocellular damage, as reflected by elevated laboratory values of hepatic enzymes such as GOT, GPT and gamma-GT. There were 14 patients in the treatment group using the BICOM and 14 in the control group not receiving any treatment.

On completion of the study, the hepatic values of the BICOM-treated group were within normal limits, while the values of the control group were still within the pathological range with no change (Table 1). The following table shows the percentage decrease in the values:

Hepatic values	Decrease towards normal of excess values (BICOM treatment)	Decrease towards normal of excess values (Control group)
GOT	42 %	4 %
GPT	50 %	5 %
Gamma-GT	38 %	7 %

Table 1. Results of BICOM and control group

In the treatment group, the geometric mean values for the degree of improvement were 45% for GOT values (5% for control group), 55% for GPT activity (control group displayed a slight deterioration) and 45% for gamma-GT activity (slight deterioration in the control group).

It is clear from the experimental evidence presented that treating minor hepatocellular damage with BICOM therapy in the frequency range between 10 Hz and 150 kHz can bring about reconstitution of damaged hepatic cells.

The MINI BRT - Bioresonance Device

Recently, Russian companies such as Deta Elis have come up with a true innovation – one of the very first "Mini" portable Bioresonance devices in the world that is truly unique. The device is called the DeVita BRT[163] – BRT stands for Bioresonance Therapy – we briefly mentioned it at the beginning of this chapter.

For many years now, natural health practitioners have used Bioresonance devices in their offices and clinics to successfully treat a myriad of different health conditions. This entailed the patient going to the practitioner's office once or twice

[163] www.deta-elis-uk.com

a week or more and being plugged into large devices such as those in the image on the right.

Now, you can purchase and use your own portable Bioresonance device and use it on yourself and your loved ones, in the comfort of your own home.

The NEW Devita BRT device is easy to use and is designed for a wide range of users. It is basically a hand-held, portable bioresonance therapy (BRT) device that is very user friendly. It contains two brass hand electrodes and two brass foot electrodes.

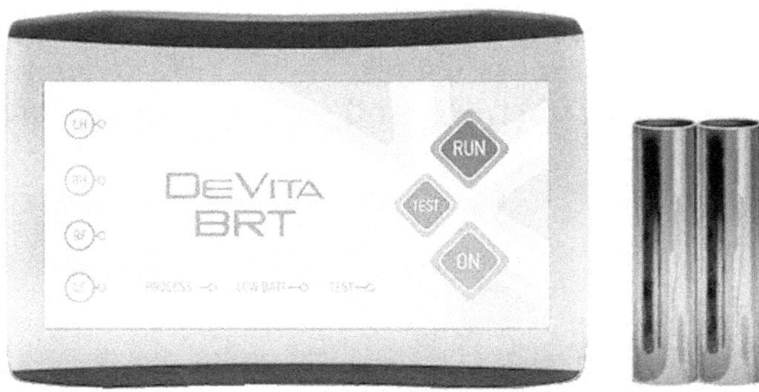

Dr. Rife Technology

Another famous technology that uses the principle of energy medicine is the frequency generator invented by one of the most incredible geniuses of our time, Dr. Royal Raymond Rife, who back in the 1930's had cured 16 terminally-ill cancer patients with this electronic resonance device. This was an incredible feat, not only then, but also by today's standards. He had invented a Universal microscope[164] (Fig 10) with nearly 6,000 parts that could magnify up to 17,000x without killing the specimen. This is how he identified the cancer virus.[165]

164 Siedel, RE., Winter, EM. The New Microscopes, Annual Report, Smithsonian Institute, USA, pp. 193-220, 1944.

165 Annual Report of the Board of Regents of The Smithsonian Institution, 1944, The Rife's Microscope, The Smithsonian Report, 1944.

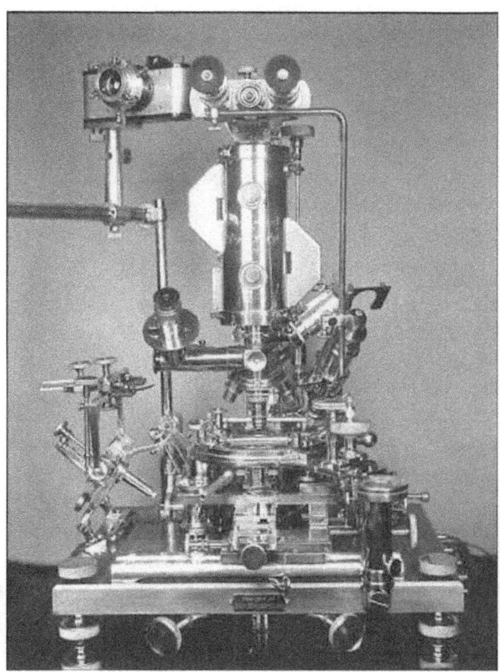

Fig 10 Universal Microscope

Royal R. Rife, born in 1888 (Fig 11), discovered that when a cell was exposed to some form of energy to which it is resonant, this energy would be absorbed by the resonant structure. Should the resonant energy be greater than the cell can effectively dissipate, Dr. Rife found that this cell would fail structurally, often resulting in cell death.

A simple way to understand resonance is to think of an opera singer who can break a wine glass with her voice. The wine glass resonates at a certain frequency. If the opera singer can match that natural frequency with her voice, then the glass will absorb this resonant energy and smash.

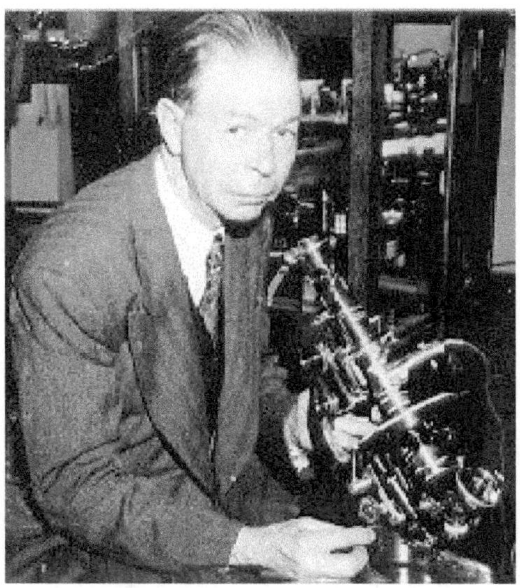

Fig 11. Dr Rife with his Universal Microscope

This simple principle can be applied to living organisms too, such as bacteria and viruses. This is what Dr. Rife managed to do. He discovered a resonant frequency that he called the mortal oscillatory rate (MOR) for over 55 major bacterial diseases. He also found the MOR for cancer after arduous years of experimentation using the sophisticated Universal microscope that enabled him to see micro-organisms live, without killing them by staining. Using this equipment, he isolated the cancer virus that he called the "BX" virus.

In time, Rife was able to prove that the cancer micro-organism has 4 forms:[166]

1. BX (carcinoma)
2. BY (sarcoma - larger than the BX virus)
3. Monococcoid form in the monocytes of the blood of over 90% of cancer patients.
4. Crytomyces pleomorpha fungi

Rife wrote in his 1953 book:

> *"Any of these forms can be changed back to the 'BX' within a period of 36 hours and will produce in the experimental animal a typical tumour with all the pathology of true neoplastic tissue, from which we can again recover the 'BX' micro-organism. This complete procedure has been duplicated over 300 times with identical and positive results."*

---

166 Rife, RR. History of the development of a successful treatment for cancer and other virus, bacteria and fungi. Rife Virus Microscope Institute, San Diego, USA, 1953.

There is no doubt that Rife was a perfectionist to the greatest degree.
What did Rife mean when he said that the other forms could be changed back to the 'BX' form? If we take what Pasteur has taught the world as the absolute truth, then no micro-organisms can change back to other types. Pasteur taught bacteriology based on Monomorphism; there is basically one micro-organism that causes each of the different diseases.

So, for every disease, there is a different bug. However, this is not what Dr. Rife and other researchers such as Beauchamp, Gaessens and Prof. Enderlein saw in their microscopes.[167] Using a darkfield condenser with an iris objective, they could see different forms changing in front of their own eyes. This went directly against Pasteur's theory of Monomorphism, to one of Pleomorphism.

It seems rather remote that all these researchers had reported seeing the same phenomenon of pleomorphism using their microscopes. It is also interesting that monomorphism - one bug for each disease - is still the paradigm that is taught in all medical schools around the world.

By using Live Blood Analysis, it is possible to show that the more toxic the internal milieu of the body, the more these micro-organisms change forms to more and more virulent and pathological types which causes degenerative diseases. The ultimate stage would be the 'BX' virus that Rife had not only isolated but found in over 90% of cancer patients.

As Rife declared in 1953:

> *"These successful tests were conducted over 400 times with experimental animals before any attempt was made to use this frequency on human cases suffering from carcinoma and sarcoma."*

In 1934, Dr. Rife opened a clinic, which successfully cured 16 of 16 cases within 120 days. Working with some of the most respected researchers in America, along with leading doctors from Southern California, he electronically destroyed the cancer virus in patients, allowing their own immune systems to restore health.

A Special Research Committee of the University of Southern California oversaw the laboratory research and the experimental treatments until the end of the 1930s. Follow-up clinics conducted in 1935, 1936 and 1937 by the head of the U.S.C. Medical Committee verified the results of the 1934 clinic. In his 1953 book, Dr. Rife wrote about the cancer clinics on December 3rd, 1953:

---

167 Poehlman, Karl H. Synthesis of the Work of Enderlein, Bechamps and other Pleomorphic Researchers. Explore Vol. 8, No. 2, 1997.

"The first clinical work on cancer was completed under the supervision of Milbank Johnson, M.D. which was set up under a Special Medical Research Committee of the University of Southern California. 16 cases were treated at the clinic for many types of malignancy. After 3 months, 14 of these so-called hopeless cases were signed off as clinically cured by the staff of five medical doctors and Dr. Alvin G. Ford, M.D. Pathologist for the group.

The treatments consisted of 3 minutes' duration using the frequency instrument, which was set on the mortal oscillatory rate for 'BX' or cancer (at 3 day intervals). It was found that the elapsed time between treatments attains better results than the cases treated daily. This gives the lymphatic system an opportunity to absorb and cast off the toxic condition that is produced by the devitalized dead particles of the 'BX' virus. No rise of body temperature was perceptible in any of these cases above normal during or after the frequency instrument treatment. No special diets were used in any of this clinical work, but we sincerely believe that a proper diet compiled for the individual would be of benefit."

Independent physicians utilizing the equipment successfully treated as many as 40 people per day during these years. In addition to curing cancer and other deadly diseases, degenerative conditions such as cataracts were reversed. Rife had been able to determine the precise electrical frequency that destroyed individual micro-organisms responsible for cancer, herpes, tuberculosis, and other illnesses. His work was described in Science magazine, medical journals, and later the Smithsonian Institution's annual report.[168]

Unfortunately, Rife's scientific theories and method of treatment conflicted with orthodox views. His work was stopped, and both the research and the treatments were forced underground. The AMA took him and his associates to court. This trial would start Rife on a long road of deterioration, alcoholism and depression, as the deaths from cancer mounted year after year. While the court case was taking place (and afterwards), the AMA visited all the doctors involved. Those who didn't stop using the Frequency Instrument would lose their medical license.

One of his main co-supporters, Milbank Johnson died under mysterious circumstances (possibly poisoned), and records of Rife's work were destroyed. No medical journal was ever permitted to print Rife's work, except one by the Franklin Institute that slipped by the censors. In 1946, Rife's problems forced him to sell off his laboratory piece by piece.

Doctors secretly continued curing cancer patients for 22 years after the original

168 Lynes, B. 1992. The Cancer Cure that Worked. Marcus Books, Ontario, Canada.

success of the 1934 clinic, but always with opposition from medical and governmental authorities.

However, from 1950 to the mid-1980s, several research scientists, working independently, have slowly been verifying the scientific principles upon which Rife's clinical cures of the 1930s were based. A body of recognized scientific evidence now overwhelmingly supports the original cancer theories articulated and demonstrated by Rife 50 years ago. This includes modern AIDS researchers.

In the next chapter we will look at emotional, psychological and spiritual factors can play a significant role in the cause and maintenance of various diseases – I would say ALL diseases!

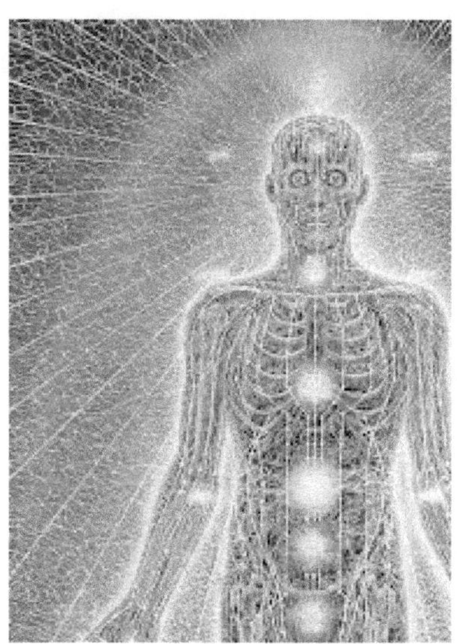

Chapter 8

Emotional, Psychological & Spiritual Roots of Disease

Emotional pain often exacts a greater toll on the quality of your life than physical pain. The stress and negative emotions associated with any trying event can even lead to physical pain and disease.

In fact, emotional stress is linked to health problems including chronic inflammation, lowered immune function, increased blood pressure, gut and stomach problems, altered brain chemistry, increased tumour growth and more.

Of course, emotional pain can be so severe that it interferes with your ability to enjoy life and, in extreme cases, may even make you question whether your life is worth living.

Whether it's a simple spat with your spouse or long-held resentment toward a family member or friend, unresolved conflict can go deeper than you may realize - it may be affecting your physical health.

The good news: Studies have found that the act of forgiveness can reap huge rewards for your health, lowering the risk of heart attack; improving cholesterol levels and sleep; reducing pain, blood pressure, and levels of anxiety, depression and stress. And research points to an increase in the forgiveness-health connection as you age.

"There is an enormous physical burden to being hurt and disappointed," says Karen Swartz, M.D., director of the Mood Disorders Adult Consultation Clinic at The Johns Hopkins Hospital. Chronic anger puts you into a fight-or-flight mode, which results in numerous changes in heart rate, blood pressure and immune response. Those changes, then, increase the risk of depression, heart disease and diabetes, among other conditions. Forgiveness, however, calms stress levels, leading to improved health.

Psychological Inflammation and Physical Illness

A study published in the Proceedings of the National Academy of Sciences suggests that psychological stress directly interferes with your body's ability to regulate inflammation, which leads to the progression of disease.

Stress wreaks havoc on the mind and body. Until now, it has not been clear exactly how stress influences disease and health. Now researchers have found that chronic psychological stress is associated with the body losing its ability to regulate the inflammatory response. The research shows for the first time that the effects of psychological stress on the body's ability to regulate inflammation can promote the development and progression of disease.

"Inflammation is partly regulated by the hormone cortisol and when cortisol is not allowed to serve this function, inflammation can get out of control," said Sheldon Cohen, a Professor of Psychology at Carnegie Mellon University, which sponsored the research.

Cohen states that psychological stress causes immune cells to become insensitive to cortisol's regulatory effect. In turn, runaway inflammation promotes the development and progression of many diseases.

Cohen's earlier work showed that people suffering from psychological stress are more susceptible to developing common colds and used the common cold as the model for testing his theory. He showed the common cold to be a side effect of the inflammatory process that is triggered by the body's attempts to fight infection.

In other words, if your life causes you emotional stress that weighs on you daily, then you are on the path toward chronic inflammation and physical disease.

Stress and the Gastrointestinal Tract

Let us now move on from this important spiritual component of our lives, the power of prayer, back to the biological mechanisms of how stress can affect the GI tract specifically.

The stress response causes several detrimental events in your gut, including:

- Decreased nutrient absorption
- Decreased oxygenation to your gut

- As much as four times less blood flow to your digestive system, which leads to decreased metabolism

- Decreased enzymatic production by as much as 20,000 times.

It is interesting to note that we have the same type of tissue in our gut, as we do in our brain. During foetal development, one part turns into your central nervous system while the other develops into the nervous system of your gut.

These two systems are connected via the vagus nerve - the tenth cranial nerve that runs from your brain stem down to your abdomen.

This "brain-gut axis" is what connects your two brains together and explains why you get butterflies in your stomach when you're nervous, for example.

Likewise, stress results in alterations of your brain-gut connection, which can contribute to, or directly cause, numerous gastrointestinal disorders, including:

- Inflammatory bowel disease (IBD)

- Irritable bowel syndrome (IBS)

- Peptic ulcer

- Gastroesophageal reflux disease (GERD)

- Food antigen-related adverse responses (food allergies)

- Other functional gastrointestinal diseases

Harvard Reviews How Stress Can Cause Stomach Disorders

The wise Father of Medicine, Hippocrates, once said 2,500 years ago, *"All diseases begin in the gut."* It's also widely known that stress is a trigger that causes multiple chronic disease processes to occur.

These two health dogmas are intricately intertwined, as stress is detrimental to your gut health, and together stress and a damaged gut can contribute to multiple inflammatory diseases and conditions, such as:

- Crohn's disease

- Ulcerative colitis

- Multiple sclerosis
- Type 1 diabetes
- Rheumatoid arthritis
- Osteoarthritis
- Lupus
- Chronic skin conditions
- Kidney problems
- Urinary conditions
- Allergic and atopic conditions
- Degenerative conditions
- Chronic fatigue syndrome
- Fibromyalgia
- Myalgic encephalomyelitis (ME)
- Inflammatory bowel diseases

To put it simply, chronic stress (and other negative emotions like anger, anxiety and sadness) can trigger symptoms and full-blown disease in your gut. As Harvard researchers explain:

> *"Psychology combines with physical factors to cause pain and other bowel symptoms. Psychosocial factors influence the actual physiology of the gut, as well as symptoms. In other words, stress (or depression or other psychological factors) can affect movement and contractions of the GI tract, cause inflammation, or make you more susceptible to infection."*

In addition, research suggests that some people with functional GI disorders perceive pain more acutely than other people do because their brains do not properly regulate pain signals from the GI tract. Stress can make the existing pain seem even worse. Interestingly, the connection works both ways, meaning that while stress can cause gut problems, gut problems can also wreak havoc on your emotions. The Harvard researchers continue:

"This connection goes both ways. A troubled intestine can send signals to the brain, just as a troubled brain can send signals to the gut. Therefore, a person's stomach or intestinal distress can be the cause or the product of anxiety, stress, or depression. That's because the brain and the gastrointestinal (GI) system are intimately connected — so intimately that they should be viewed as one system."

Imbalances in Your Gut Can Make You Depressed, Anxious and More

Research using a probiotic containing the friendly bacteria Bifidobacterium longum NCC3001 has been shown to normalize anxiety-like behaviour in mice with infectious colitis.

Research published in 2011 also demonstrated that probiotics have a direct effect on brain chemistry under normal conditions - in such a way that can impact your feelings of anxiety or depression.

In addition, other research found that the probiotic Lactobacillus Rhamnosus had a marked effect on brain chemicals that lowered the stress-induced hormone corticosterone, resulting in reduced anxiety and depression-related behavior.

The authors concluded:

"Together, these findings highlight the important role of bacteria in the bidirectional communication of the gut-brain axis and suggest that certain organisms may prove to be useful therapeutic adjuncts in stress-related disorders such as anxiety and depression."

Interestingly, neurotransmitters like serotonin are also found in your gut. In fact, the greatest concentration of serotonin, which is involved in mood control, depression and suppressing aggression, is found within your intestines, not your brain!

Psychic Masochism

There are probably a number of people that you have encountered who simply don't "let go." Why do we remain in these detrimental psychological states of conflict, anxiety, anger and frustration, even when we know they are not helping anyone and causing us to become ill?

A psychiatrist from the days of Freud by the name of Edmund Bergler answered that very question. So far, the mental health community has shunned Bergler's ugly truth. Here it is in layman terms:

We *like* misery.

Unconsciously, misery and unhappiness are so familiar and self-justifying that we cling to them, regardless of the consequences.

So, we end up subconsciously doing things that give us more of what we hate. When a chance for true happiness and fulfilment appears, we turn away. Bergler called it **psychic masochism**, or the tendency to take unconscious pleasure in *displeasure*. The result is self-sabotage, which may be the one universal mental health concern. In general, we gravitate toward the negative, refusing to let go of the negativity as if our very lives depended on it.

Learn how self-sabotage develops and what to do about it by watching this free video. It's a real eye opener.[169]

We Live in an Insensitive World

We have all watched on television as a family comes out of the courthouse with a guilty verdict for the killer, and unbelievably, they state that they have forgiven the killer! Some would find this concept bizarre. Those who think about it a bit more, however, may realize that harbouring a grudge, anger and hurt against someone who has harmed you only causes damage to you!

In real life, it's not killers that we deal with on a day to day basis, it's the people we have everyday dealings with. The most important are our friends and loved ones.

It is a fact that we live in a world where many people are insensitive to other's feelings and needs – it is quite an egocentric world, and selfish behaviour from others is likely to hurt us in many ways.

Common offences include betrayals of trust, rejection, lies and insults.

Whether you've been cut off in traffic, slighted by your mother-in-law, betrayed by a spouse, or badmouthed by a co-worker, most of us are faced with a variety of situations that can cause us a lot of stress and inflammation that leads to disease.

We have no control over these wrongs committed by others – we can encounter insensitive or angry people at any time of our lives.

---

[169] http://inlpcenter.org/aha-process-self-sabotage

What Happens When You are Hurt

Once hurt, people can rehearse painful memories and harbour grudges. This can perpetuate negative emotions and the physiological responses to these emotions.

When people hold a grudge, they stay in the victim role and perpetuate the negative emotions. Some people hold onto this for reasons of 'saving face' or to give themselves some sense of control. This is because a lack of control causes stress. However, nursing a grudge is a commitment to staying angry and this keeps all the negative health effects going.

Revenge is Disease

Society's main metaphor for revenge is disease. By default, we tend to think of revenge as a sickness that invades a vulnerable host (perhaps one whose resistance to the infection has been weakened by a poor psychological constitution or a bad childhood), consumes the host (morally, physically, and psychologically), and then has destructive effects on the avenger and the object of his or her vengeance.

Sometimes this disease spreads from one avenger-host to another until the outbreak reaches epidemic proportions. When you hear reporters describe "outbreaks of violence" that are fuelled by the lust for vengeance, that's the disease metaphor at work.

This disease model of revenge received modern psychology's seal of approval in 1948, when an influential psychoanalyst named Karen Horney described how the desire for revenge could absorb people for a moment in time, or for lifetime — becoming, effectively, a chronic illness:

"This drive can be the governing passion of a lifetime to which everything is subordinated, including self-interest. All intelligence, all energies, then, are dedicated to the one goal of vindictive triumph."

Horney went on to argue that people prevented from exercising their vengeful impulses may exhibit symptoms such as headaches, stomach aches, fatigue, and insomnia. In short, the desire for revenge produces such a powerful psychological toxin that it literally makes you sick.

So, what do we do in these circumstances where others have hurt and upset us? One of the most powerful healing tools that we all internally possess is to forgive these people and move on. The alternative would be to harbour these feelings and allow them to ruminate inside us, causing inflammation and disease.

One of the definitions of forgiveness involves letting go of the negative feelings you have and adopting a merciful attitude or good will towards the offender.

What is Forgiveness?

Generally, forgiveness is a decision to let go of resentment and thoughts of revenge. The act that hurt or offended you might always remain a part of your life, but forgiveness can lessen its grip on you and help you focus on other, more positive parts of your life. Forgiveness can even lead to feelings of understanding, empathy and compassion for the one who hurt you.

Forgiveness doesn't mean that you deny the other person's responsibility for hurting you, and it doesn't minimize or justify the wrong. You can forgive the person without excusing the act. Forgiveness brings a kind of peace that helps you go on with life.

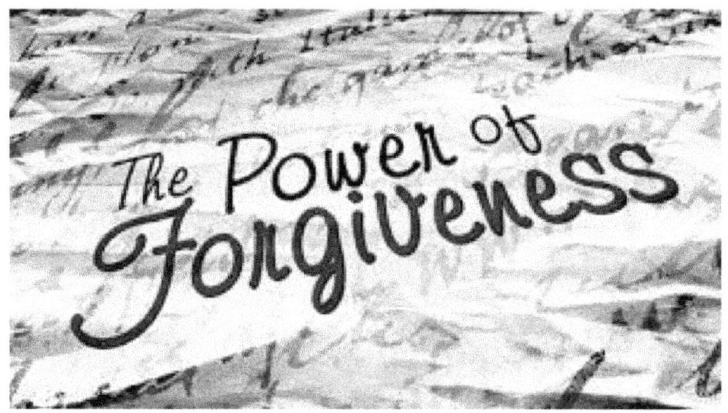

What are the Benefits of Forgiving Someone?

Letting go of grudges and bitterness can make way for happiness, health and peace. Forgiveness can lead to:

- Healthier relationships
- Greater spiritual and psychological well-being
- Less anxiety, stress and hostility
- Lower blood pressure
- Fewer symptoms of depression
- Stronger immune system
- Improved heart health
- Higher self-esteem

Why is it So Easy to Hold a Grudge?

When you're hurt by someone you love and trust, you might become angry, sad or confused. If you dwell on hurtful events or situations, grudges filled with resentment, vengeance and hostility can take root. If you allow negative feelings to crowd out positive feelings, you might find yourself swallowed up by your own bitterness or sense of injustice.

What Are the Effects of Being Unforgiving?

If you're unforgiving, you will:

- Bring anger and bitterness into every relationship and new experience
- Become so wrapped up in the wrong that you can't enjoy the present
- Become depressed or anxious
- Feel that your life lacks meaning or purpose, or that you're at odds with your spiritual beliefs
- Lose valuable and enriching connectedness with others

How Do I Reach a State of Forgiveness?

Forgiveness is a commitment to a process of change. To begin, you should:

- Consider the value of forgiveness and its importance in your life at a given time
- Reflect on the facts of the situation, how you've reacted, and how this combination has affected your life, health and well-being
- Actively choose to forgive the person who's offended you, when you're ready
- Move away from your role as victim and release the control and power that the offending person and situation have had in your life

The Challenges of Forgiveness

Forgiveness can be a challenge for several reasons. Sometimes forgiveness can be confused with condoning what someone has done to us: “That's OK. Why not do it again?” The distinction between accepting someone's bad behaviour as "okay" and accepting that it happened, and you must let go of anger to move forward, can be difficult because these two are easily confused.

Forgiveness can also be difficult when the person who wronged us doesn't seem to deserve our forgiveness. It feels like we are letting them "off the hook" when *they* are the one who wronged *us*. It's hard to remember that forgiveness benefits the forgiver more than the one who is forgiven.

Ultimately, forgiveness is especially challenging because it's hard to let go of what's happened. It can be difficult to accept some things in life, and forgiving someone who has committed unacceptable behaviour can be difficult when we are having trouble letting go of anger about the events and accepting what happened to us.

Can You Learn to Be More Forgiving?

Forgiveness is not just about saying the words. "It is an active process in which you make a conscious decision to let go of negative feelings whether the person deserves it or not," Swartz says. As you release the anger, resentment and hostility, you begin to feel empathy, compassion and sometimes even affection for the person who wronged you.

Studies have found that some people are just naturally more forgiving. Consequently, they tend to be more satisfied with their lives and have less depression, anxiety, stress, anger and hostility. People who hang on to grudges, however, are more likely to experience severe depression and post-traumatic stress disorder, as well as other health conditions.

But that doesn't mean that they can't train themselves to act in healthier ways. In fact, 62% of American adults say they need more forgiveness in their personal lives, according to a survey by the non-profit Fetzer Institute.

Making Forgiveness Part of Your Life

Forgiveness is a choice. You are choosing to offer compassion and empathy to the person who wronged you. The following steps can help you develop a more forgiving attitude - and benefit from better emotional and physical health:

Reflect and remember - that includes the events themselves, and also how you reacted, how you felt, and how the anger and hurt have affected you since.

Empathize with the other person - for instance, if your spouse grew up in an alcoholic family, then anger when you have too many glasses of wine might be more understandable, says Swartz.

Forgive deeply - simply forgiving someone because you think you have no other alternative, or because you think your religion requires it, may be enough to bring some healing. But one study found that people whose forgiveness came from understanding that no one is perfect could resume a normal relationship with that person, even if that person never apologized. Those who only forgave to salvage the relationship wound up with a worse relationship.

Let go of expectations - an apology may not change your relationship with the other person or elicit an apology from them. If you don't expect either, you won't be disappointed.

Decide to forgive - once you make that choice, seal it with an action. If you don't feel you can talk to the person who wronged you, write about your forgiveness in a journal or even talk about it to someone else in your life whom you trust.

Forgive yourself - the act of forgiving includes forgiving yourself. For instance, if your spouse had an affair, recognize that the affair is not a reflection of your worth, says Swartz.

Forgiveness and Health

Lack of forgiveness has been implicated in the following health problems:

1. Stressing the hormonal system that reacts to stress – the part that involves the production of stress hormones such as cortisol and adrenaline. This will also negatively affect other hormones too, as well as the autonomic nervous system which regulates many bodily functions. These reactions place the body under considerable stress.

2. Mental illness; anxiety, depression

3. Heart disease, heart attack, hypertension, premature death

4. Immune suppression. Studies have shown effects on levels of immune protective cells and anti-cancer cells (Natural Killer cells)

5. Gastrointestinal problems

6. Effects on the reproductive system

7. Anything that follows from increased stress responses would also theoretically occur e.g. irritable bowel syndrome, Crohn's disease, ulcerative colitis, pain, muscle tension, fatigue, infectious illnesses and more.

Empathy

Being able to develop feelings of empathy can help move the person towards forgiveness. Empathy is placing yourself in the perpetrators shoes so that you have some sort of understanding of "where they were coming from".

This may help you understand why they did the offending behaviour. Empathy has been found to reduce stress responses in the body as well as cardiac risk.

Please note that forgiveness still allows you to hold the offender responsible for the offence and does not involve denying it happened, nor ignoring, minimizing, tolerating, condoning, excusing or forgetting the offence.

Now, it's not that easy to just decide to forgive. There is usually a process that most people can go through naturally. Some people are more predisposed to forgive – it's in their nature. Some have more difficulty, or there are circumstances that make it difficult.

It's possible to cultivate a more forgiving attitude by developing empathy and understanding that we are all human and not perfect. If you have been hurt and are finding it difficult to move forward to feeling better about it, you may benefit by seeing someone for psychological help.

In the end, its only you that suffers. So, go ahead and forgive, but not necessarily forget for the sake of your health and relationships.

When we do not forgive, we hold on to bad experiences, to the pain, to the trauma. This can cause fear, depression, frustration, anxiety, self-hatred, and loneliness. It's self-destructive. A writer said that non-forgiveness results in emotional, physical and spiritual bondages. He said that 90 percent of all health, marital, family and financial problems come from non-forgiveness.

According to Dr. Steven Standiford, chief of surgery at the Cancer Treatment Centers of America, refusing to forgive makes people sick and keeps them that way. Forgiveness therapy is thus now being used to help patients with cancer and other chronic illnesses.

Of all cancer patients, 61% have forgiveness issues, Dr. Michael Barry, author of *The Forgiveness Project*, said, *"Chronic anxiety and anger produce excess adrenaline and cortisol in the body which depletes the production of natural killer cells or antibodies which are the body's foot soldiers in the fight against cancer, most people do not realize what a burden anger and hatred are until they let them go."*

Spirituality and Well-being

As the director of Duke University's Center for Spirituality, Theology, and Health, Dr. Harold Koenig has been studying the connection between spirituality and well-being since 1985. Koenig's latest project is a $1.5 million study comparing the outcomes of secular and spirituality-based therapies.

How did you come to study the connection between spirituality and health?

"I became interested in the topic as a medical resident. When I asked people with illness how they were coping, they would often talk about their religious faith. I was very moved by their responses and began to look for ways to study it. Many other researchers are exploring this intersection. There's been a tripling of the data in the last 15 years or so."

What are the health benefits of spirituality and religion?

"They run across the board. Religious involvement, particularly if there is a strong spiritual component, is associated with less depression and anxiety, greater well-being, and less drug and alcohol abuse. Research using MRIs suggests that it alters the structure of the brain in people at high risk for depression.

It's also linked to better physical health and health behaviours — less smoking, more exercising, a better diet. Religious people have less cardiac disease and hypertension and better measurable immune function. Many studies show religious and spiritual practices delay the onset of memory loss associated with aging and slow dementia related to actual memory disorders like Alzheimer's. They also confer a longevity benefit - an extra 7 years of life among whites and 14 years for African Americans."

Are these perks a good reason to become more spiritual?

"I'd caution against doing it just for health reasons. The cake is not the health. The health benefits are unintended side benefits of being religious because it gives your life greater meaning."

Spirituality means different things to different people. What aspects of a person's spirituality or religion matter most when it comes to health outcomes?

"It turns out that belief itself doesn't mean much. It's whether the belief is carried out through some sort of action, such as gathering with others in a faith community, spending time in prayer or meditation, reading scripture, or volunteering -generally conforming your life to the teaching of your faith. That's where the biggest benefits are."

What can doctors learn about spirituality to better tend patients' health?

"Most medical schools sensitize students to the importance of spirituality in the lives of patients. But only about 10 percent of doctors address these issues in practice. I'd like to see all physicians assess their patients' spiritual needs and, if need be, refer them to someone who can address those needs. There's enormous healing potential in our spiritual practices and faith traditions."

Prayer is Popular

Prayer has been called the science of sciences and art of arts, and rightly so. Prayer is the most widespread alternative therapy in America today.

A research study conducted by the University of Rochester at 20 sites across America and funded by the National Cancer Institute and the American Cancer Society showed that over 85 percent of people confronting a major illness pray. That is far higher than taking herbs or pursuing other non-traditional healing modalities. And increasingly the evidence is that *prayer works.*

Health Benefits of Prayer

Numerous scientific studies have evaluated the therapeutic effects of prayer. Generally, the research has shown that people who pray regularly are less likely to become ill and that when they do, they tend to recover faster. Interestingly, not only does prayer seem to have healing effects upon the people who pray, it also appears to benefit those who are prayed for by others.

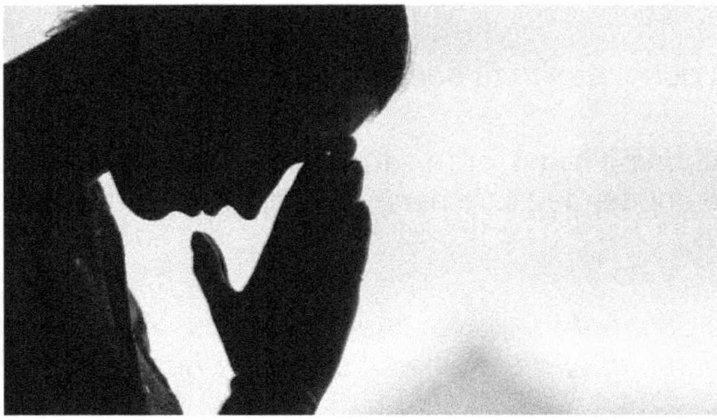

Research reveals that people who pray have lower depression and suicide rates. Prayer even appears to lower blood pressure. In a study funded by the National Institutes of Health, investigators found that individuals who attended religious services at least once a week and prayed at least once a day or studied the Bible frequently, were 40% less likely to have high blood pressure than those who did so infrequently.

In other research, elderly women recovering from hip-fracture surgery who had strong religious beliefs and practices were able to walk greater distances when they left the hospital than those who were not as religious.

A 2011 study of inner-city youth with asthma conducted by researchers at the *University of Cincinnati* indicates that those who practiced prayer and meditation experienced fewer and less severe symptoms than those who had not.

Other studies show that prayer boosts the immune system and helps to lessen the severity and frequency of a wide range of illnesses.

A recent survey reported in the *Journal of Gerontology* of 4,000 senior citizens in Durham, NC, found that people who prayed or meditated coped better with illness and lived longer than those who did not.

But the question remains: *By what physiological mechanisms does prayer impact our health?* Herbert Benson's most recent research suggests that long term daily spiritual practices help to deactivate genes that trigger inflammation and prompt cell death. That the mind can affect the expression of our genes is exciting evidence for how prayer may influence the functioning of the body at the most fundamental level.

Spiritual practice aims to connect the individual with God or a Higher Power, to open one to the Divinity dwelling within the self, and to make one fully present to life in the here and now.

These are not goals that lend themselves to being measured in double blind experiments. The sense of deep peace and radiant well-being that spiritual practitioners in different religious traditions report are also not testable by scientific means.

What science *can tell us* is that people who pray and meditate tend to be statistically healthier and live longer than those who do not. Whether these boons are merely unintended side effects of still deeper spiritual benefits remains a matter of faith.

Prayer as a Healing Tool

"He who is able to pray correctly, even if he is the poorest of all people, is essentially the richest. And he who does not have proper prayer, is the poorest of all, even if he sits on a royal throne"

\- St John Chrysostom

Let me begin by saying that I believe in one-God for all the peoples of the world. Religion and religious denominations are man-made, and we need to transcend these often-fanatical beliefs and focus on the one-God that symbolizes true, unconditional love. This is where our hearts need to be open to becoming more loving and empathic beings, so that we can help all those around us, including ourselves.

Intrinsic Characteristics of Love

In this following Scripture, Apostle Paul has given a clear description regarding the intrinsic characteristics of that love:

Love is patient, love is kind. It does not envy, it does not boast, it is not proud. It does not dishonour others, it is not self-seeking, it is not easily angered, it keeps no record of wrongs. Love does not delight in evil but rejoices with the truth. It always protects, always trusts, always hopes, always perseveres (1 Corinthians 13:4-7).

Love is the personification of the character of God.

LOVE is always patient and kind; it is never jealous.
Love is never boastful or conceited; it is never rude or selfish.
Love does not take offense, and it is never resentful.
Love takes no pleasure in other people's sins, but delights in the truth.
Love is always ready to excuse, to trust, to hope, and to endure whatever comes.
Love does not come to an end.

– Saint Paul the Apostle
1st Letter to the Corinthians: 13

Love is not an abstract. Love is not a feeling. Love is not really an attitude. Love is a deed. Love is an activity. In the original Greek, the word is a verb, not a noun. It describes an *action*.

Apostle Paul in Corinthians lists sixteen characteristics of love. Every time I read this list I feel deeply challenged. I know how far short of all these characteristics I often am – it is humbling:

- ✓ Love never gives up, love is patient
- ✓ Love cares more for others than for self
- ✓ Love doesn't want what it doesn't have
- ✓ Love doesn't strut
- ✓ Doesn't have a swelled head
- ✓ Doesn't force itself on others
- ✓ Isn't always "me first"
- ✓ Doesn't fly off the handle
- ✓ Doesn't keep score of the sins of others
- ✓ Doesn't revel when others grovel

- ✓ Takes pleasure in the flowering of truth
- ✓ Puts up with anything
- ✓ Trusts God always
- ✓ Always looks for the best
- ✓ Never looks back
- ✓ But keeps going to the end.

Praying to the One-God

So, irrelevant of our religious denomination, we can all pray to the one-God that should be in everyone's hearts. Prayer may be a requirement for Christians, but it is not only for Christians – God listens to all of us, no matter our colour, creed, or religion.

Years ago, I never used to pray. I thought nothing really ever came of it. However, in my later years, I began to master the art of prayer and now systematically pray daily - it is an inherent and important part of my life. I pray many times per day; for my children, for my wife, for my patients, for those that are suffering, for the politicians who wish to harm us, as well as all those that do not pray and those who have their focus on materialism and consumerism and other mundane interests.

Prayer is an *experience*. It is not a feeling, even though prayer is from the heart, not the mind. As we learn the art of prayer, we experience things happening in our lives and the lives of others that cannot be explained logically – it is like small miracles happen that are against all probabilities.

There is nothing more important or enriching than having a personal relationship with God. When you take time to walk with God each day through prayer, your relationship will grow with him – this is the goal of prayer.

Prayer is the most powerful way to experience God, but we often fall short. However, when we work at our prayer lives daily, and make it a point to be accountable with God, we begin to enter a space of full vulnerability and openness to receive God's work in our lives. Be open and allow God to guide – you will often be surprised at the positive outcome and usually what you witness is not what you planned personally. God will often nudge us to evolve Spiritually, to open our hearts, to love our family, friends and neighbours. This is what God wants from all of us – just surrender yourself to Him and let him guide.

Prayer is more personal and powerful when we accept prayer not as a daily or daunting task, but as a way of life. When we strive for closeness with Him, we grow in our intimacy with Him and can ultimately deal with the everyday challenges we face. Let go and let God in your life today.

How Should We Pray?

People often ask: how should we pray, in what words, and in what language? Some even say, *"I do not pray because I do not know how; I do not know any prayers."* You do not need any specialized skill for prayer. You can simply talk with God. We can pray to God in the language we use when speaking with people, when thinking.

Prayer should be very simple. St. Isaac the Syrian said: *"The whole fabric of your prayer should be succinct. One word saved the publican, and one word made the thief on the cross heir to the Heavenly Kingdom."*

Let us recall the parable of the Publican and the Pharisee:

Two men went up into the temple to pray; the one a Pharisee, and the other a publican. The Pharisee stood and prayed thus with himself, God, I thank thee, that I am not as other men are, extortioners, unjust, adulterers, or even as this publican. I fast twice in the week, I give tithes of all that I possess. And the publican, standing afar off, would not lift so much as his eyes unto heaven, but smote upon his breast, saying, God be merciful to me a sinner (Luke 18:10-13).

And this short prayer saved him. Let us also remember the thief who was crucified with Jesus and who said to Him: *Lord, remember me when Thou comest into Thy kingdom* (Luke 23:42). This alone was enough for him to enter Paradise.

Prayer can be extremely brief. If you are just starting out on your path of prayer, begin with very short prayers, to allow you to focus. God does not need words; He needs hearts. Words are secondary; of paramount importance are the feeling and disposition with which we approach God.

To approach God without a feeling of reverence or with distraction is much more dangerous than saying the wrong words in prayer.

Distracted prayer has neither meaning nor value. A simple law is at work: if the words of prayer do not reach our heart, they will not reach God. Therefore, it is very important that each word of prayer should be felt deeply by us.

We do not need to say long prayers or read from a prayer book. Perhaps the most famous and often-used prayer amongst Christians is the Jesus Prayer, it is simple and short, but very powerful and can make profound changes in our hearts when repeated many times each day.

One ascetic struggler said that if we could, with the full force of our feelings, with all our heart and soul, just say the prayer *"Lord, have mercy,"* then that would be enough for salvation. But the problem is that, as a rule, we cannot say this with all our heart; we cannot say this with our whole life. Therefore, in order to be heard by God, we tend to use many words.

The Jesus Prayer is very simple:

"Lord Jesus Christ, have mercy on me"

If you are including others in your prayers, then it is often enough to say: *"Lord Jesus Christ, have mercy on us"* while thinking of your children or patients or whoever – God knows who you are praying for, without even mentioning their name.

The words are really quite simple, but we need them to reverberate from the heart, and this requires us to quieten the mind, believe in the importance of prayer and make time during our day; have empathy and let the words touch your heart – after much practice this will begin happening automatically, and the changes in your life and those of others that you pray for will change for the better.

The Secrets to Maximum Prayer Power

Perhaps the most interesting and important detail of all this research is that certain factors do affect how powerful the benefits of prayer will be. Those factors are basically qualities of human consciousness, like:

- Caring
- Compassion
- Empathy
- Love

The stronger these qualities are, the greater the benefits of prayer. One thing holds true for all the studies on prayer — and that is that **it's not important** *what specifically you* **believe in. What matters is whether you believe in something, and** *how you* **put that belief into practice.**

Mind-Heart Connection

Research has also shown that the heart is a key component of the emotional system. Scientists now understand that the heart not only *responds* to emotion, but that the signals generated by its rhythmic activity play a major part in *determining the quality of our emotional experience* from moment to moment.

All thought or form is neutral - neither positive nor negative - in its pure form. All feeling has either a positive (Love-based) or negative (fear-based) charge or vibration. There is no such thing as a "neutral" feeling. If you are "feeling" neutral, it means there is an absence of emotion, or substance, to your thought.

When the Heart field is coherent, the energy and information sent to the Body results in improved health and wellbeing, better performance at work, improvement in relationships, increased problem-solving abilities, intuition, and much more. In other words, when images in the Mind (thought + feeling) are Love-based, the Body benefits in many ways.

At the Da Vinci Centre, patients going through the Da Vinci Universal Treatment protocols[170] will also learn about the importance of the mind-heart connection through a series of videos. In addition, they will have the opportunity to practice achieving this beautiful state of being by practicing using the emWave® educational self-regulation technology and the tools and techniques of the HeartMath System, incorporating over 23 years of scientific research on the psychophysiology of stress, emotions and heart-brain interactions.

References

Journal of Physiology and Pharmacology December 2011; 62(6):591-9.

Neurogastroenterology and Motility 2011 Dec;23(12):1132-9.

Proc Natl Acad Sci U S A. 2011 Sep 20;108(38):16050-5.

[170] https://www.naturaltherapycenter.com/da-vinci-universal-treatment-protocols/

Disclaimer

The information contained within this book is offered for you to make educated health decisions so that you can optimize your health. If there are serious health conditions, then you should always consult your primary care physician before beginning any other treatment regime.

The health information in this book is not advice and should not be treated as such – it is provided without any representations or warranties, express or implied. We do not warrant or represent that the medical information in this book is true, accurate, complete, current or non-misleading.

You must not rely on the information in this book as an alternative to medical advice from your doctor or other professional healthcare provider. If you have any specific questions about any medical matter, you should consult your doctor or other professional healthcare provider. If you think you may be suffering from any medical condition, you should seek immediate medical attention. You should never delay seeking medical advice, disregard medical advice or discontinue medical treatment because of information in this book.

While every attempt has been made to provide information that is both accurate and cutting-edge, the author cannot be held responsible for any decision that the reader may take while reading the guide, nor can a guarantee be provided that this guide and the remedies that it recommends will help everyone.

Summary and Concluding Remarks

Modern medicine has become a dictatorial, monopolistic endeavour that attempts to eradicate disease without understanding the body's attempts to self-heal. It appears that disease is something we have no control of and that new drugs are the answer to all of man's ailments. This is the biomedical model of disease that has completely missed what the Father of Medicine, Hippocrates taught over 2,500 years ago. Ironically all doctors take the Hippocratic oath when they qualify.

The social control of the population by the medical industry reinforces a morbid society, with its principal economic and profit-making activities. These economic motivating factors are what prevent people from mobilising their self-healing powers as turning the patient into a drug-dependent customer is far more important. It's as if the disease can be controlled by the routine prescription. This fostering of a drug-dependent culture with its principles of "symptom-suppression" leads to moral degeneration and prevents disease from being cured.

Medical treatments have become the suppression of the natural survival mechanisms that are so vital for protecting the body against all types of disease. The holistic model of health does not want to suppress symptoms, to the contrary, the symptoms are an important part of unravelling and understanding where the body has lost its balance and why.

Listening to the body was an art that was admired many years ago before technological medicine came in and doctors were taught to pay more attention to the blood tests and scans, while literally ignoring the important information that is being shared by the patient.

When the blood tests and other scans come back "within normal parameters," even though the patient is feeling very sick, the doctor will simply conclude that "it's all in your head, or it could be genetic". This is a very soul destroying for the patient, and very demoralising.

It is my hope that this book will help these patients to understand some of the underlying causes of their symptoms that are not always looked for by the medical profession. It is a stimulus to think outside the box and begin looking at a more holistic way of approaching your health and disease.

From my experience as a clinician for many decades, I know that the holistic model works well – identify the underlying causative factors, whether they be somatic, energetic, social, psychological, emotional, Spiritual, toxicity, nutritional deficiencies and so much more. Once these are identified and eliminated using the correct treatment protocols, then the innate intelligence of the body takes over and true healing takes place.

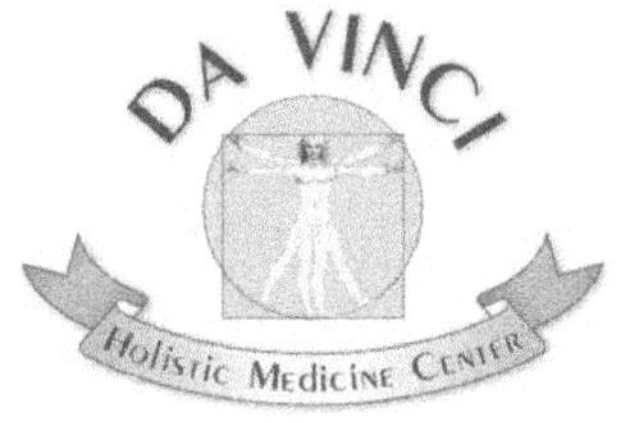

Clinical Consultations
To book appointments to see Dr Georgiou at the Da Vinci Holistic Health Center in Larnaca, Cyprus simply call the Center or email.

Tel: +357 24 – 82 33 22
Email: admin@naturaltherapycenter.com
Web: www.naturaltherapycenter.com

Da Vinci Institute of Holistic Medicine

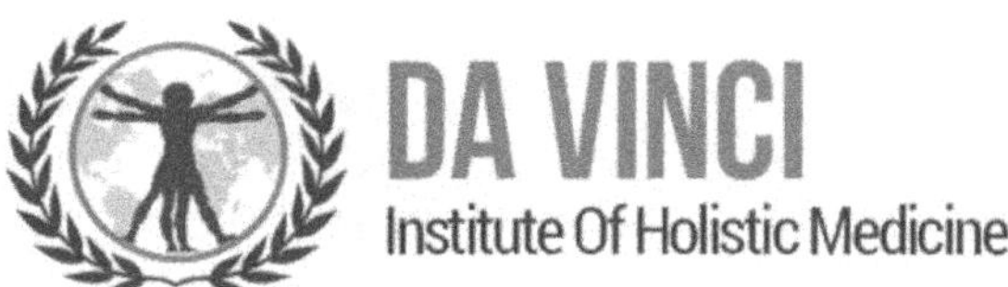

Holistic Medicine Education
Anyone interested in completing studies in Holistic Medicine can apply directly to the Da Vinci Institute of Holistic Medicine.

Tel: +357 24 – 82 33 22
Email: admin@collegenaturalmedicine.com
Web: www.collegenaturalmedicine.com

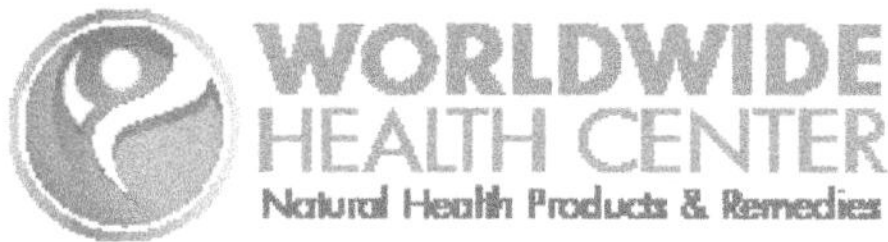

Natural Supplements
Most of the supplements mentioned in this book can be obtained from this website.

Tel: +357 24 82 33 22
Email: admin@worldwidehealthcenter.net
Web: www.worldwidehealthcenter.net

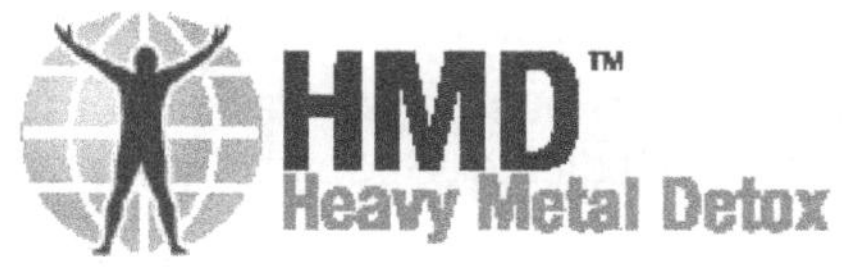

Heavy Metal Detox
Products related to the natural detox of toxic metals can be purchased here - sent globally.

Tel: + 357 24 82 33 22
Email: admin@detoxmetals.com
Web: www.detoxmetals.com

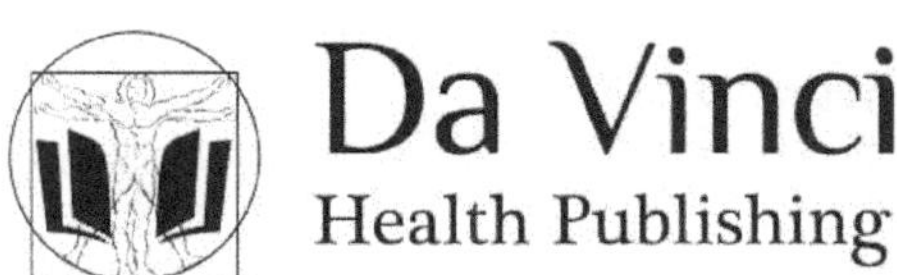

Ethical Publishing
Health practitioners that want to publish their books, but do not want to lose their copyright, while gaining most of the royalties, can apply to Da Vinci Health Publishing – the ethical publishers!

Tel: + 357 24 82 33 22
Email:
admin@davincipublishers.com

ABOUT THE AUTHOR

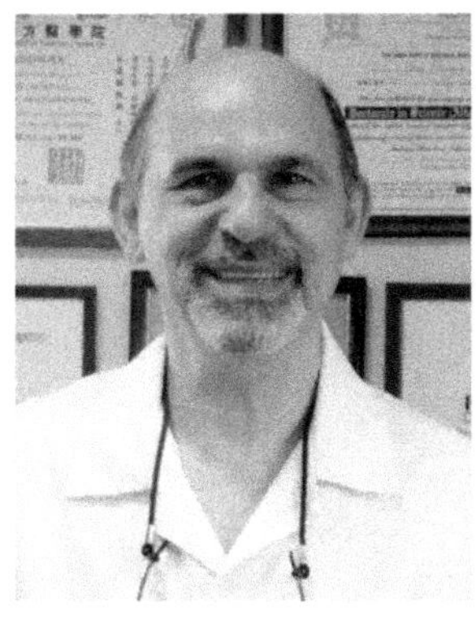

Dr. George John Georgiou, 62 years old, has 11 degrees and Diplomas spanning 25 years in various topics ranging from Biology, Psychology and Natural Medicine. Specifically:

1. Bachelor of Science (B.Sc) honours degree in Biology/Psychology from Oxford Brook's University, Oxford, England
2. Master's of Science degree (M.Sc) in Clinical Psychology from the University of Surrey, Guildford, England
3. Doctor of Philosophy degree (Ph.D). in Clinical Sexology from The Institute for Advanced Study of Human Sexuality, San Francisco, USA.
4. Doctor of Science (D.Sc (AM)) degree in Alternative Medicine from the International Open University of Alternative Medicine
5. Clinical Nutrition (Dip.ION - Distinction) from the Institute of Optimum Nutrition (ION), London, England
6. Diploma in Electronic Impulse Therapy (Dip.E.I.Th) from the Euro College of Complementary Medicine, UK
7. Diploma in Naturopathic Iridology from the Holistic Health College, UK and Diploma in Iridology from the Society of Iridologists, UK
8. Diploma as a Master Herbalist (MH) from the Holistic Health College, UK
9. Diploma in Homeopathic Medicine (DIHom) from the British Institute of Homeopathy, UK
10. Diploma in Su Jok Acupuncture from Onnuri College, Almaty, Kazakhstan
11. Doctor of Naturopathic Medicine (Pastoral) – N.D. (P) from the Sacred Medical Order of the Knights of Hope, US – Licence number: L1016988.

He is the Director Founder of the Da Vinci Holistic Health Centre in Larnaca, Cyprus – see www.naturaltherapycenter.com This is a multimodality centre specializing in treating chronic diseases of all kinds. This model of healthcare using a holistic approach has been illustrated in his 23 books that he has written to date.
Research is also one of his passions and he is considered an expert in natural heavy metals detoxification, having been awarded a Doctor of Science in this topic. He has spent over three years formulating and testing using double-blind, placebo-controlled trials with over 350 people a natural toxic metal chelator called HMD™ (Heavy Metal Detox). He is presently the worldwide patent-pending holder on this product which is sold worldwide at www.detoxmetals.com

There are many papers that Dr Georgiou has published in peer-reviewed journals that are available on his websites at www.naturaltherapycenter.com and www.detoxmetals.com
Dr Georgiou has also been Knighted as a Knight Hospitaller by the Sovereign Medical Order of the Knights Hospitaller (www.smokh.org), one of the oldest Christian charitable organizations in the world with over 200 medical knights all practicing holistic medicine using natural medicine formulated by the monks of old practicing monastic medicine. They have built 5 hospitals and clinics worldwide all running on charitable donations to help the poor. As the Diplomatic Cultural Attache for Cyprus he is presently in the process of setting up the St. Luke's Health Care Charity to help people in need through Holistic Medicine.

His research interests have made him the Principle Investigator for the World Health Organization (WHO) in studies on AIDS and Drug Use, as well as other research involving alcoholism, drug abuse and sexual dysfunctions. He has lectured to Master's students in Psychology at an external campus for Indiana University, USA, and has been a prolific writer of health articles for the general public, having written literally thousands in both English and Greek languages.

Regarding his career in Clinical Sexology, he was the first professional sexologist to ever work in Cyprus, making history in this respect. This was back in 1983 when sexology was unheard of in this sexually repressed country.

His doctoral dissertation in Clinical Sexology was entitled *The Sexual Attitudes of Greek Orthodox Priests* – a unique study never before studied in the Orthodox religion. There was considerable antagonism from certain spheres of the Orthodox Greek church regarding the results of the study.

In 1990 he had his own live radio programme on Saturday lunchtime entitled *Human Sexuality.* This was far ahead of its time and in a two-year period Dr Georgiou managed to cover 96 topics of human sexuality with the audience asking questions reflecting the ignorance, taboos and prejudices of the time. This was the first such programme in the history of Cyprus.

In 1999 he published the first book ever written in the Greek language on the treatment of Premature Ejaculation, published in Greece. He is also the Editor for the chapter on Cyprus in the International Encyclopedia of Sexuality, Volume 4.

As Dr Georgiou has two doctorates, one in Clinical Sexology and one in Alternative Medicine, he has formulated protocols for the treatment of sexual dysfunctions that involve the integration of both these disciplines. He has coined this *Naturopathic Sexology* which is a unique term pertinent to himself – if you Google this term it will bring you back to his websites.

He is presently the Director Founder of the Da Vinci Holistic Health Center[171] in Larnaca, Cyprus, as well as the Academic Director of the Da Vinci Institute of Holistic Medicine,[172] a distance-learning educational institution, and the Director/founder of the Da Vinci BioSciences Research Center.

He is a Member of the following Associations/Institutes:

- The Society of Biology, UK (MSBiol.)
- Chartered Biologist, UK (C. Biol)
- Member of the Royal Microscopy Society, UK
- The General Council and Register of Naturopaths, UK (GCRN)
- Full Member, The British Naturopathic Association, UK
- Member of Oncology Group, British Naturopathic Association

---

171 www.naturaltherapycenter.com

172 www.collegenaturalmedicine.com

- The Register of Naturopathic Iridologists, UK (M.R.N.I.)
- The British Association of Nutritional Therapists, UK (BANT)
- The Association of Master Herbalists, UK. (AMH)
- Fellow of the British Institute of Homeopathy, UK (FBIH)
- The American College of Clinical Thermology, USA
- The International Su Jok Therapy Association, Russia
- The British Holistic Medical Association, UK (BHMA)
- Member of the Institute of Complementary Medicine, UK (ICM)
- National Iridology Research Association, USA (NIRA)
- Associate Fellow of the British Psychological Society, UK (AFBPsS)
- Chartered Psychologist, UK, BPS (C.Psychol)
- Member, Health Professions Council, UK – registered as Clinical Psychologist (PYL15128)
- Member of Cyprus Psychologists' Association, Cyprus.
- Diplomate of the American Board of Sexology, USA (ABS)
- Registered Sex Therapist with ABS, USA
- Member, The American College of Sexologists, USA (ACS)
- Fellow of the American Academy of Clinical Sexologists, USA (FAACS)
- Member, World Association for Sexology (WAS), USA
- Member of the Cyprus Association of Alternative Therapists (N.D.).

Dr. Georgiou is married to Maria, a Psychotherapist/Lecturer and has 4 children aged between 18 and 31 years. His hobbies and interests include flying a private plane, classic antique motorbike and car restoration, antique furniture restoration, playing the Bouzouki, horology (repairing antique pocket watches), web master, travelling, writing, running his private lab researching energy medicine and bioresonance, microbiology and cellular biology, bee keeping and running an organic farm.

More Books written by Dr Georgiou:

1. Surviving a Nuclear War: Save Your Family and Loved Ones
2. Candida Cure: Healing Naturally in 90-Days – 5,000 Successful Cases!
3. Gallstones: Ridding Stones Naturally in 24 Hours
4. Diabetes: Natural Treatments that Really Work!
5. Curing the "Incurable" with Holistic Medicine: The Da Vinci Secrets Revealed
6. Acid Reflux: Natural Healing for GERD in 90 Days
7. Lupus: Natural Treatment Protocols for Complete Recovery
8. Haemorrhoids: Natural Healing That Really Works!
9. Cholesterol Cure: Heal Naturally Without Medication
10. Diverticulosis: Natural Healing That Really Works
11. Why Am I Sick? Eliminate the Causes and Be Well Forever!
12. Eczema: Heal Naturally, Without Medication
13. Celiac Disease: Natural Approaches for Optimal Living
14. Fibromyalgia: The Natural Approach to Pain-Free Living
15. Gout Cure: Natural Treatments that Really Work!
16. Osteoarthritis: Natural Treatments Without Medication
17. Psoriasis: Natural Treatments That Really Work!
18. IBS: Heal Your Gut Naturally in 90 Days
19. Hypothyroidism: Natural Healing That Really Works!
20. Weight Loss Secrets Revealed: No More Dieting!

CPSIA information can be obtained
at www.ICGtesting.com
Printed in the USA
BVHW060827211221
624586BV00004B/101

9 789925 569366